Wessel — <u>Natural Childbirth & the
Christian Family</u>

LLL of Olympia, PM.

NATURAL CHILDBIRTH
AND THE CHRISTIAN FAMILY

Natural Childbirth

AND THE

Christian Family

FOURTH REVISED EDITION

HELEN WESSEL

1817

Harper & Row, Publishers, San Francisco

Cambridge, Hagerstown, New York, Philadelphia
London, Mexico City, São Paulo, Sydney

This book is lovingly dedicated to
my sons and daughters
and their sons and daughters

References to Scripture translations are as follows: New American Bible (NAB); New English Bible (NEB); New International Version (NIV); King James Version (KJV); Living Bible (LB); Phillips' New Testament (Phillips); Revised Standard Version (RSV).

This book has also been published under the titles *Natural Childbirth and the Family* and *The Joy of Natural Childbirth*.

Designer: Jim Mennick

Library of Congress Cataloging in Publication Data

Wessel, Helen, 1924–
    NATURAL CHILDBIRTH AND THE CHRISTIAN FAMILY.

    Rev. ed. of: Natural childbirth and the family. Rev. ed. 1974, c1973.
    Bibliography: p.
    Includes index.
    1. Natural childbirth.   2. Christian life—1960–
I. Title.
RG661.W45 1983   618.4'5   82-48943
ISBN 0-06-069314-2

Contents

Acknowledgments

Many people have contributed in many ways to this book. It is not possible to thank them all by name, but I would like to express my appreciation to the following persons:

To my husband, *Walter W. Wessel*, Ph.D., for his constant praise, encouragement, and helpful criticisms. He has never discouraged my searching for answers in the areas in which, as a biblical and linguistic scholar, he is the expert and I am the novice. He has patiently corrected my mistakes and placed all his resources for biblical research freely at my disposal.

To my father, *John Albert Strain,* for the use of his poems "The Sculptor" and "The Rock." Most of all, I am grateful to him for having taught me, by the example of his life, the lesson of implicit faith in a loving God.

To the late *Dr. Grantly Dick-Read,* whom I was never privileged to meet but whose teachings confirmed my intuitive belief from childhood that the goodness of God is not limited in its expression in any area of our lives—not even in the experience of giving birth.

To *Carol Nelson,* for her beautiful line drawings illustrating the book.

To *Sister Mary Meyer,* for her dedication to family-centered birthing, and for the inspiration of her continuing efforts for community-wide childbirth education.

To *Ilene Rice,* breastfeeding consultant at St. Joseph's Hospital, St. Paul, Minnesota, and mother of three children, for contributing helpful material included in the chapter "Breastfeeding."

To *Donald Singerman,* librarian of the Mount Zion Temple library, St. Paul, for his patient, friendly assistance in locating necessary Jewish source material.

In addition to my appreciation to those mentioned above, I want to express my special thanks for help in this fourth edition to *Kathy Nesper,* Director of Apple Tree Family Ministries, which I founded thanks to her inspiration so that natural childbirth can be taught in our churches.

I also am most grateful to my editors at Harper & Row for their continued encouragement and support: *George W. Jones,* now retired, my editor for the first edition; *Harold E. Grove,* now retired, my editor for fourteen years and a warm personal friend; and *Clayton E. Carlson* and *Roy M. Carlisle,* my current editors. Thank you, each one!

Foreword

I first met Helen Wessel at the Fourth International Childbirth Education Association (ICEA) Convention held in 1968 in Los Angeles. As a past president of the Association (1964–1966), she spoke out with authority, courage, and clarity against many of the inhuman practices some childbearing women must face. The sparks of admiration I felt for Helen at that time have since ignited into a deep friendship as we have striven for common goals—the dignity of woman, the strengthening of the couple, and reverence for the child.

"One of the main tenets of natural childbirth is that every pregnant and parturient woman must be cared for on an individual basis, according to her own physical and emotional needs and desires. A woman longs to remain a *person* throughout her childbearing experience," Helen Wessel writes. It is our observation that a positive experience of childbirth is of great value in increasing a woman's feeling of self-worth. "It should be her hour of greatest dignity," says Dr. Pierre Vellay of Paris, "a real step forward, not only in the liberation of the woman, but also in the liberation of the couple." My husband and I have found this to be true, not only among the Zulus of South Africa, the people of Papua, New Guinea, but also among couples in the United States and Europe.

In teaching Family Life Seminars throughout the world, we have placed a strong emphasis on natural childbirth with the active participation of the husband as an avenue of emotional and spiritual enrichment of the marriage. The attitude of a husband intelligently supporting his wife during the hours of labor and then present at the moment of birth of their child is different from the attitude of one who is barred admission to the delivery room. "I shall never forget the joy of that moment, even if I live to be a thousand years old!" one husband writes.

If the whole experience of childbirth can be remembered with joy, then it is carried over in the attitude toward the child. Käthe Kollwitz, well-known German artist and mother of two sons, wrote the following in her diary at the age of forty-three: "I repeatedly dream that I again have a little baby, and I feel all the old tenderness again—or rather more than that, for all the feelings in a dream are intensified. What I have in these dreams is an inexpressibly sweet, lovely physical feeling. First it was Peter who lay asleep and when I uncovered him it was a very small baby exuding the warm bodily fragrance of babies" (*Diaries of Women*).

Mastering labor and childbirth is a skill to be learned—one that affects the future of the child as well as the parents.

I am especially thankful that Helen Wessel does away with the misinterpretation of Genesis 3:16, which has led many to think of childbirth as a curse. Instead she opens the door to make childbirth an experience of redeeming joy and favor. The fact that the author speaks not only about the physical and psychological, but also about the spiritual aspects of childbirth, makes this book unique.

INGRID TROBISCH
Family Life Mission

Preface to the
Fourth Revised Edition

It has been a joy to work on this latest edition, for I still feel—perhaps now more than ever—the necessity and importance of promoting the kind of natural childbirth I believe in and have experienced myself in the births of our last three children. Increasing numbers of young women are now having their babies without medication or intervention, in any position comfortable for them, with their husbands assisting, and often in their own homes.

But this does not mean that wisdom prevails in obstetrics as it is practiced today. Instead, obstetrics has moved in two directions. One trend, to be sure, is toward more wholesome, safer, physiological birth. The other major trend is toward increasing obstetric intervention in childbirth for every woman who enters the hospital in labor. Routine procedures include tranquilizers, artificial rupture of the membranes, intravenous glucose and/or oxytocin, fetal monitors, analgesics in labor, and local infiltration or general anesthesia for the birth. Women are still often confined to bed for labor and transferred to the delivery room for birth, where they are pinned flat on the delivery table with their legs in the air. In some hospitals, even manual removal of the placenta is routinely being done!

Accompanying all this intervention is the shocking increase in the number of cesarean births. Fifteen to thirty percent of women in labor in some hospitals have a cesarean delivery with its accompanying risks, especially for the mother. (Maternal morbidity and mortality, while still low, are much higher in percentage for cesarean than for vaginal births.)

I had thought that by this time my work in promoting natural childbirth would no longer be needed. My own children are all grown and my husband and I have an ever increasing number of grandchildren. Far from being over, the need for the truths of these principles is still so great that I have founded Apple Tree Family Ministries, with Kathy Nesper as Director, so that these things can be taught in Christian circles, with this book as one of the texts. Many of you through the years have asked me to prepare such teaching material, and I have finally done so. (Please see Appendix A for more details.)

More information on sexuality is included in this new edition, because of the intertwining of a couple's sexual relationship with good childbearing. Their sexual adjustment has a profound effect on the proper functioning of the woman's body during birth, just as the kind of birth she experiences in turn affects their sexual harmony. There is also more information on the importance of good nutrition. In addition, several chapters have been completely rewritten to reflect childbearing practices in this latter portion of the twentieth century.

In this edition, for convenience, a baby is usually referred to as "he" to distinguish the baby from the mother, "she."

May our loving Lord Jesus grant to each of you a wonderful "birth" day for your little girl or boy.

And please, let's keep on working for a safe, comfortable birth experience for every woman and for the healthy, undrugged child she will bear, who will be received into the daddy's loving hands at the moment of birth.

HELEN WESSEL

Preface to Previous Editions

Giving birth is one of the most beautiful spiritual and physical experiences woven into the tapestry of a woman's life. This has been proven in the lives of many thousands of women like myself, who have had the privilege of giving birth to babies naturally. By following the teachings of the late Dr. Grantly Dick-Read, the great pioneer of the natural childbirth philosophy, we have found it true that childbirth is a normal physiological function of the human body and is not meant to be painful.

Dr. Dick-Read's kind heart was touched in his early days of medical practice when he observed the pain of women in labor—women who were suffering in spite of all the medication and relief that science had to offer. He dedicated his life to research for ways to prevent this pain by natural means, rather than by attempting to blot it out with ineffective, dangerous drugs. He searched for normal, commonsense ways it could be prevented, because he had faith that God did not intend women to suffer in childbirth. He followed this leading of his heart to success. Our society owes grateful tribute to the memory of his dedicated life.

Giving birth to a child is a "natural" event, but one must learn how to work in harmony with the processes of "nature," just as it is necessary to learn the basic principles of good health. Adequate education and training for natural childbirth are necessary for both husband and wife. Relaxation and proper breathing habits for good health need to be applied during pregnancy for their use to be easy and natural during labor and birth. The mother should have the loving support of her husband as well as of the birth attendants she has chosen, so that she may give birth actively and happily, rather than being passively "delivered."

Because of the importance of maintaining a warm and understanding relationship between husband and wife during labor and birth, as well as during courtship, marriage, pregnancy, and parenthood, this book emphasizes birthing as a family experience. After all, God did not create human life to exist in a vacuum but invented the first "family" concept.

The material presented is given in two parts. The first is the "story" of John and Mary, who demonstrate by example wholesome attitudes toward sex, marriage, and the birth of a child. The story form is used to make the material more easily understood. It should be noted, however, that the labor and birth experiences of the young wife and her friend are not "idealistic fiction," but are based on the actual experiences of women bearing their first child, women I have known personally.

The second part of this book consists of more detailed discussion than is possible in the story, and it will be helpful not only to young couples, but also to the doctors, nurses, nurse-midwives, birth attendants, pastors, educators, and others who have the responsibility of counseling them.

Many have asked how I became interested in natural childbirth and if all our children were born in this way. My own deep concern over current childbirth practices occurred as the result of my suffering at the birth of our third child. I had not been happy about the births of our first two children, but I did nothing about it.

When our first child was born, I was completely anesthetized for the birth, without any warning that this would take place. I awakened from the anesthetic angry and disappointed that I had been denied the right to be present at the birth of my own child, an experience I had looked forward to with keen anticipation. I expected to breastfeed my baby, but she was never brought to me. Finally, I asked a nurse, "Why don't they bring me my baby to breastfeed?"

She gave me a startled look, and then said, "You can't breastfeed your baby," and left. When the doctor came in, I asked the same question and received a similar answer, with no explanation. This surprising disappointment was so upsetting that I cried all night.

Labor for our second daughter began with gentle, regular contractions. The doctor examined me on my arrival at the hospital, and I was suddenly startled by a rush of water. "I just ruptured the membranes," he explained, "to speed things up." I was deeply annoyed, but it was too late to object. Heavy medication kept me asleep during labor, but I awakened to find myself bearing down hard, was taken to the delivery room, and given a spinal anesthetic.

What a joy to be awake to see my daughter's little body lifted up before my own eyes! But my lower body was as void of sensation as if it were dead. The paralysis lasted for long hours, until I began to wonder if I could ever move my legs again. "Does it sometimes happen," I asked the nurse, "that one can become permanently paralyzed by a spinal anesthetic?"

"Hush," she whispered. "We don't talk about such things here!"

For days following the birth my head ached whenever I raised it from the pillow. I was informed that this was a common aftereffect of spinal anesthesia.

No women in this hospital were allowed to breastfeed their babies, for an epidemic had occurred earlier in the year in a nearby hospital in which twenty-five babies died in a week. Thus all babies were kept in the nurseries continually until discharge. The first time I held this little daughter was the day we left the hospital.

Three years later I was back in the hospital—for extensive repair of damage to the cervix caused by the birth—and was discharged three days later. The cervical damage may have been partly due to the premature rupture of the membranes and to the fact that I was bearing down under sedation, no doubt before the cervix was fully dilated. Whatever the cause, it was left unrepaired at the time of the birth. The physician who repaired it said I would never be able to carry a fetus longer than three months without the repair.

The third pregnancy was complicated by threatened premature labor from the fifth month on, so that every few days I had to go to bed under strong medication to quiet the restless uterus. My physician was highly qualified and kind, insisting that I call him any time of the day or night when contractions began and that I not take any medication to stop them without his express permission. Under his conscientious care I kept the baby until full term, although I was physically and emotionally exhausted from the long months of anxiety. It was a great relief when labor began, and I walked confidently into the most excruciatingly painful and shocking experience of my life.

The labor was brief, with powerful, almost continuous contractions that seemed to accomplish nothing. Suddenly, while still alone in the room, the cervical scar tissue violently ruptured. Nurses came running, dashed me down the hall on a gurney and onto the delivery table. A saddle block anesthetic was given, my hands and legs strapped down, and a blindfold and oxygen mask clamped over my face. But the saddle block had no time to take effect, and as the birth began I experienced the most blinding pain I have ever known. My screams were totally ignored, and as the intensity of pain increased I lost consciousness. When I came to shortly after, those around me were talking nonchalantly as if nothing had happened!

The mask was removed, I was shown the baby, the doctor prepared to repair the episiotomy, and then said softly under his breath, "My gosh! We're going to be here all night!." But after forty-five minutes of patient stitching he finished the repair and I was taken to my room, still stunned and in a state of shock. My husband came into the room beaming, leaned over, and said, "The doctor tells me you had a *very easy delivery*. I'm so glad!" I stared at him in astonishment, and then closed my eyes without answering until he went away. It was as if a curtain had fallen between me and every other human being, even the one I loved best.

For days I was too weak to lift my head, turn myself in bed without assistance, or even eat, for a fork was too heavy to hold. There was no question of breastfeeding this baby, for I didn't even want to see her bruised and swollen face. One day when the nurse brought her to the room for me to see, I said, "Please, not today," and turned away.

"You don't want your *baby?*" she asked indignantly.

"No," I whispered. She marched away, her footsteps echoing down the long hallway. Then, for the first time, I cried. Tears of shame and guilt rolled down my cheeks, into my ears, and splashed onto the pillow. I didn't even want my own baby! I felt too wicked even to pray.

A little Mexican grandmother came softly into the room, pushing a dustmop. Noticing my tears, she came near the bed and laid her hand tenderly on my leg. Tears of sympathy rolled down her own brown, wrinkled cheeks as she stood there several moments without a word. She may have known no English, but love has a language of its own, and I was comforted, drawn back into the world of human beings who understood. As my tears ceased, she slipped away as quietly as she had come. I never saw her again, but I have thanked God for her ever since.

Not until years later did I learn that the terrible pain had been caused by forceps the doctor was using to control the birth—my flesh crushed painfully between steel and bone, while he assumed the area was anesthetized and ignored my cries because he believed I was "asleep." No one had meant to be unkind.

The following weeks and months were frightening because my strength returned so slowly and I was losing weight continually. I was too ill to give the baby more than minimal care for a long time, and she spent a large part of every day propped up on her daddy's shoulder. If I passed a store window with a man inside wearing a white coat—even a barber—I would break into a sweat and begin trembling all over. Even God seemed changed—he was not the loving God I had always known but an angry God who had damned half the world to such suffering. It just couldn't be. God was not like that. Questions flooded my mind, demanding answers. If mine had been an "easy" birth, what indeed must a "hard" one be? If I was fortunate, as the doctor had said, to have had such excellent medical attention, what indeed must be the plight of the unaided woman?

Then, one day, stepping into the yard, I noticed for the first time that the trees were still green, the sky was still blue. How strange. It seemed that everything should be different, for God was not the loving Savior I had known so intimately before. On returning indoors, I picked up a hymnal at random and flipped it open. "O God, our help in ages past, Our hope for years to come,"—the words leaped out before my startled eyes:

> Before the hills in order stood
> Or earth received her frame,
> From everlasting Thou art God,
> From age to age the same.

God had not changed. Why then—blasphemous thought—had he deserted me and not helped me in my desperate need? One day I picked up my Bible, and God spoke to me unexpectedly in the words of Isaiah 54:8:

For a small moment have I forsaken thee; but with great mercies will I gather thee. In a little wrath I hid my face from thee for a moment; but with everlasting kindness will I have mercy on thee, saith the Lord my Redeemer.

God had permitted this to happen and had a purpose in it for me. It was not "meaningless" suffering. My responsibility now was to find his purpose, so that the experience could be used to honor him and prevent such terrible suffering for others. Prayerfully I began searching the Scriptures day after day to find the answers. At first fearful of what I might find, I was delightfully surprised again and again. God is indeed the loving Savior, the Creator who does all things well. The wonderful biblical truths I discovered are all recorded in this book.

One day, while I was learning these things, God brought into my hands *Childbirth Without Fear* by Grantly Dick-Read. I wept all the way through the book. Here at last was a doctor who understood how a woman feels. Here was a person whose teaching was in harmony with what God was showing me in the Bible. Though still badly frightened, I was determined to have another baby as soon as possible, to discover for myself if these truths were really so. My sanity and my faith depended upon their validity.

My pregnancy had just begun when a letter came, saying that my young cousin Ruth had died at the birth of her first child. It seemed incredible. Ruth, so radiantly healthy and happy—who of all persons would have wanted a natural birth if she had known it was possible— was gone. Just before the birth she had been routinely put under anesthesia, although she had not made one sound of complaint during her entire labor, nor had she asked for an anesthetic. Under anesthesia she vomited, her jaws locked, her throat constricted, the fluid went into her lungs and shut off the air. She never regained consciousness or ever saw her baby, though the doctor tried valiantly for four hours to restore a normal heartbeat. The doctor said she had had "an easy delivery." Easy for whom? Ruth was dead.

It was at this time that I first wrote Dr. Dick-Read, for reassurance, and sent him a treatise I had written called "The Biblical Teaching Concerning Labor and Childbirth." I received a long, beautiful letter in reply. This was the beginning of a cherished correspondence. In one letter he said:

. . . I am making a big effort to have the prayer book of the English Church changed. Their service for the Churching of Women, which is ostensibly to give thanks for the birth of the child, is one of the most heretical misinterpretations of truth I have ever read, and it offends me when women come to me and say, "Yes, I went to Church, but I didn't repeat the service because it wasn't true." I have heard that many times in my life. . . .

Our fourth daughter was born one beautiful Sunday in December, 1954, six weeks prematurely. I had noticed contractions during the morning at church and called the doctor about noon, after having gone right to bed and relaxing completely for a while to see if the contractions would go away. He asked, "Do the contractions hurt?" When I told him I could tell I was having a contraction only by placing my hand on my abdomen, because I was so relaxed, he said, "It's probably only false labor. Call me later if it doesn't stop."

Contractions were already only three and a half minutes apart, but I lay down again, becoming as limp as possible to *stop* labor if possible and keep the baby until full term. But each time I touched my abdomen to see if I was having a contraction, it was hard beneath my fingers. Suddenly, at four o'clock, I realized that not only was I really in labor—the baby would soon be born! We got to the hospital, and I was quickly taken to the delivery room. My husband had been promised he could be with me, but since our doctor was not there, he was shut out by the nurse. The baby was born at 4:20 P.M., so gently that the water sac had not even broken and had to be punctured by the attendant. More remarkable still was that the badly scarred, irregular cervix had received no further injury. My doctor, red-faced, came flying into the room a couple of moments after the baby had arrived.

I felt so marvelous, so elated, I could have picked up my baby and walked back home! But one look at my husband's long face a few minutes later, and I said to myself, "I will *never* have another baby in the hospital. This is one disappointment too many." We named our beautiful little daughter Dorothy, which means "the gift of God," for indeed she was. I wanted another baby as soon as possible.

Fourteen months later our first son was born at home—the most beautiful experience of my life. I planned the circumstances carefully in advance and made a backrest for myself. Only the doctor and my husband were present, while the other children were sent to the neighbors for a short time. There was no pain, or hurry, and the baby arrived in an atmosphere of dignity and peace. Afterward, I felt so refreshed and exuberant that I got up, took care of the baby myself, combed my hair, and put the room back in order. And then, because it seemed to be the thing to do, I lay down again, although I felt absolutely marvelous. I feasted my eyes on this precious baby all day long.

For the birth of our sixth child, another son, five years later, I returned to the hospital for the birth, on one condition—that my husband be with me the entire time. The attendants were most cooperative and it was a beautiful birth, marred only by the discomfort of not having a backrest on the delivery table and breast engorgement from not being able to breastfeed on demand. A few weeks later a breast infection and kidney infection developed from the hospital stay, and though my recovery was uneventful the baby refused to breastfeed on the side that had been affected. I had successfully breastfed the first two "natural babies," so I continued feeding this one for several months on the breast he would accept, and he thrived.

To every couple who read this book, looking forward to sharing one of the most precious of life's experiences—the birth of a little son or daughter—I would say:

Faith is the secret of success: faith in the rightness and beauty of conception and birth; faith in a loving God who made our bodies as they are. Rest on this faith when labor begins, relax all tensions and cares and wait patiently for love's reward.

HELEN WESSEL

PART I

1. God's Design

He who finds a wife finds happiness;
it is a favor he receives from the Lord.
—Proverbs 18:22, NAB

Twilight slowly wrapped the world with silent fingers as the long shadows of the cedars and pines crept stealthily up the hillside, thrown into silhouettes by the setting sun. John and Mary Thomas paused a moment in their walk to watch its final burst of glory before it slipped out of sight behind the blue Pacific. The only sound to be heard was the distant rhythmic rumble of the surf, and Mary gave a little start when John broke the silence suddenly.

"We'd better be getting back. It'll be dark soon, and there are no paths near us here."

"Just a minute, honey. It's so beautiful now. See that little cloud just above the horizon? It reminds me of the poem I wrote in high school, 'The Maiden.' "

" 'The Maiden'? Hey, that sounds interesting. I like maidens, especially this one! Remember what Solomon said? 'There be three things which are too wonderful for me, yea, four of which I know not: The way of . . .' "

"John! Be serious a moment! I'm not talking about *that* kind of maiden. I'm talking about, well—nature—you know, that sort of thing."

"That's right, I married a poet, didn't I? Okay, let's hear this nature thing, or whatever it is."

"John!"

"I'm only teasing, honey. C'mon, let's hear it."

John listened quietly as Mary shared her creation. He loved the way her voice rose and fell in rhythmic cadences and was as fascinated by the soft curves of her cheek and chin in the growing dusk as he was in the lovely phrases she had so carefully woven together—

In the solemn stillness of an early dawn is heard
The crystal-throated reveille of a waking bird.

Donning golden slippers arises then the Day
   And flings across the morning sky her crimson negligee.

Enchanting now, she saunters forth to spread abroad her charm
   And shakes perfume from every flower to smooth upon her arm.
She paints the children's bodies brown, their faces rosy fair,
   And with soft fluting of the wind breathes kisses through their hair.

Shrill piccolo of the cricket warns that night at last has come!
   She gathers up her flowing skirts and hastens quickly home.
But looking up into the sky, a wary child might find—
   She left her veil of mauve chiffon trailing far behind.

"Mary, that's beautiful! You know what? You can write all the poetry you like—as long as you don't get so lost in your reveries that you forget all about your little ol' husband and go wandering off after some pipe dream."

Mary turned away, pretending to be cross. "That just shows what *you* are. You may think I'm an unrealistic, dreaming poet, but I think you're a preacher!"

Laughingly they turned and started arm in arm down the hillside toward their little cottage, delighted not so much with their own joking as with the fun of knowing that they were going to be together for ever and ever.

The day of the wedding had been sunny and warm. There had been a good many misgivings in Mrs. Johnson's mind about the feasibility of an outdoor wedding, knowing the fickleness of the weather, even in early June. She had been anxious to please her daughter, but all the same she had planned how she would manage indoors in case of rain. The tears came to her eyes as she pictured what a lovely bride her Mary had been, moving gracefully over the lawn on her father's arm to the little bower that had been arranged for the altar.

"It seems so right, Mother," Mary had told her earlier, "that we should be married out of doors. God's world is so beautiful. I don't see how we could ever decorate a church to look half so nice. Remember the time I wrote that poem about the world being like a cathedral?"

Mrs. Johnson remembered all right. She had saved every scrap of her daughter's poetic scribblings—had them tucked away in a special box. She gazed out of the window a moment and smiled to herself as she thought of one of Mary's birthday poems for her, carefully decorated with a drawing of a very lopsided blue cake—

I love you Mother More and more
Even though Your thirty four.

How old was Mary then. Eight? Nine? Well, it didn't matter, only it seemed such a short time ago.

And it seemed such a short while since the starlit night when they had been driving home from a day at the seashore. Jo Lynn was asleep in the back seat, and Mary was snuggled in the front seat with them. Suddenly she had whispered, "Look, Mama 'n' Daddy—the sky has on its polka-dot pajamas!"

Jo Lynn had been a pretty bridesmaid too. I'm fortunate to have such beautiful daughters, Mrs. Johnson thought. Unless I'm prejudiced. But they really *are* pretty, even though Jo Lynn is so different—athletic and jolly, like her Dad. It's a good thing she saw where the ring rolled when Paulie dropped it! We never would have found it in the grass otherwise.

Absently Mrs. Johnson turned away from the window and sank into the nearest chair, engrossed now in the scene of the wedding. It was just like Mary, she thought, to turn a little farther toward us when she recited her verse to John, so Grandma could hear her clearly too—

John, "Where you go, I will go, and where you stay I will stay. Your people will be my people and your God my God. May the Lord deal with me, if anything but death separates you and me."

There had been no danger of Grandma's not hearing John's reply, spoken with such profound sincerity!

Mary, I promise to love you and cherish you, even as Christ also loved the church, and gave himself for it!

Mrs. Johnson's thoughts turned to the short wedding sermon on the founding of a godly home that Pastor Dirkson had given the young couple during the ceremony. She gratefully reviewed all that he had said and prayed in her heart that his words might become reality in John and Mary's lives.

"It was not the Creator's plan," the pastor had said, "for the people of the world to live alone, even though he created each one of us as a distinct individual. The Bible tells us that he brings joy to lonely hearts by setting 'the solitary in families.' When he created Adam, he said, 'It is not good that the man should be alone. . . .'

"God did not give Adam a family at once—just one person with whom he could share. It is God who has put within our hearts the need to share with someone special our deepest thoughts and feelings and emotions. This 'someone special' is a person of the opposite sex, for 'he created them male and female.' Man and woman each have unique gifts with which to complement the other, climaxed by the unity of the marital embrace. Thus it was that Adam felt his loneliness, and Eve was taken from his own flesh by the Creator to be given back to him as his wife.

"Notice God's order in the establishing of the home: man was created first, then the woman. Now some have seemed to think that because of this order man is more important than woman and that she is an inferior creation. But if one is arguing of the importance of the *order* of creation, it is well to remember that God created the angels and *every living creature as well* before he created man! Since we are clearly told in Corinthians that man is higher than the angels, if we are to use order as a sign of intrinsic worth, it will be necessary to conclude that in creating a lovely wife for Adam, God had saved the best for the last!

"The order of creation does not indicate the superiority or inferiority of man or woman but, rather, God's pattern for the harmonious functioning of a godly home. There is to be no competition between husband and wife but only a sense of completion and fulfillment. The husband lovingly serves his wife, and she in turn serves him. Both share in the responsibility of rearing children, for it says in Proverbs: 'Listen, my son, to your father's instruction, and do not forsake your mother's teaching.'

"Much unhappiness has arisen over a misunderstanding of God's plan. He did not intend that a man should 'lord it over' his wife or that she should be strictly limited to responsibilities within the home. Because of their intrinsic worth as individuals, each was to be free to develop his or her potential abilities to full capacity, secure and confident in their marriage relationship. It is sometimes overlooked that the description of the perfect wife in Proverbs 31 shows her to be a woman of many talents. Here she is not only industrious in the home, feeding and clothing her family, but we find her also in the marketplace selling her merchandise, in the countryside purchasing land, and among the poor 'reaching forth' her hands to the needy. She was free to use the talents God had given her. Because she really loved her husband, in renunciation of herself, continually putting his needs and those of her children before her own, his heart safely trusted in her: 'Her children rise up and call her blessed; her husband also, and he praises her.'

According to the Bible, women desire to please their husbands. This is brought out in Genesis 3:16 where it says of Eve, 'her *desire* shall be to her husband.' The Hebrew word for 'desire' can also be translated as 'longing.' In a Greek translation of the Old Testament (the Septuagint) this phrase reads: *kai pros ton andra sou hē apostrophē sou* (your *turning* will be to your husband).

"How true to life that in the times of her deepest need a wife longs to turn to her husband for his love and understanding. In the Song of Solomon there is a picture of this relationship between man and wife. 'I sat down under his shadow with great delight,' says the young bride, 'and his banner over me was love.'

"So do not be afraid, Mary, to yield to John's loving concern for you, confident that his greatest desire is to see all your own God-given talents find opportunity for expression. May your attitude be, 'I am his willing partner. He has captured my devotion!'

"But what if you disagree with John on some important matter, even after an honest discussion? The God-given principle is that you are to yield to his decision, even though you feel it is wrong. If instead you resist, either by silent resentment or by open anger and rebellion, your attitude will be destructive both to you as a person and to the marriage. Remember that you always have resource to a higher authority than John, so take your complaints freely to the Father in heaven, and let him work out the problem.

"And, John, although in God's plan the husband is the head of the wife, remember that Paul goes on to say that this is to be 'even as Christ is the head of the church.' The 'headship' of Christ is not one of tyranny, or of domineering, but one of tenderness and concern. His example is that of a renunciation of himself—a sacrificial and a giving love, *even to the point of death* for the sake of his bride, the church. Surely no higher standard than this could be given for a husband's behavior toward his wife.

"Nor is this all. God has included in his plan for married love a sharing with himself in the making of little children. Thus it is that when a child is born into the atmosphere of harmony and self-giving love of a godly home, we can see the beauty of the unfolding pattern of God's design: husband, wife, child.''

2. Bear and Forbear

Live together in harmony, live together in love, as though you
had only one mind and one spirit between you. Never act from
motives of rivalry or personal vanity, but in humility think more
of each other than you do of yourselves—

Philippians 2:2–3, PHILLIPS

John and Mary gathered up the breakfast dishes and carried them to the
sink. They hoped to leave their honeymoon cabin while it was still
early, as it might get quite hot on the road before they reached Uncle
George and Aunt Emma's.

"I'll be back in a few minutes, Mary," John called over his shoulder as he strode out to the car, letting the screen door bang behind him.

Now where is he going? Mary wondered, annoyed. She hurried to
call after John, but he was already driving away. I suppose he wants to
get something done to the car for the trip, or maybe get gasoline, she
thought. At least he could have told me where he was going and not
just go whamming out the door like that! We could just as well have
stopped along the way somewhere.

Mary didn't fret long, however, since there was much to be done.
She finished putting away the dishes, and packed her suitcase. John
was still not back, so she stepped out the door onto the soft carpet of
grass, inhaling deeply the delightfully refreshing fragrance of the evergreens, the trees she most loved. She stood quietly a few moments
watching their stately branches featherdusting the sky under the touch
of a gentle breeze, enjoying a bird's song from somewhere in the
branches. Her sensitive ear caught the gurgling of a little stream nearby. What a lovely place this was! She wished she had a piece of paper
so she could jot down some of the phrases forming in her mind for a
new poem.

My toothbrush! she thought suddenly and rushed back into the cabin. Sure enough, it lay on the window ledge of the cramped bathroom.
She had thought of it just in time, for the car was already turning into
the lane.

"Ready?" John asked.

"Yes. Everything's all packed. Where have you been? You might at least have told me where you were going!" Mary didn't mean to sound cross, but she certainly did.

"Why, honey, I just went to get some gasoline while you got your things gathered up. I thought it would save us some time. I'm sorry if I worried you."

"It's all right," Mary shrugged. "Let's put the suitcases in the car and be on our way."

Soon they were out on the highway. "You look so fresh and pretty this morning," John volunteered, hoping to make amends for offending her.

"Thanks," she smiled and leaned her head against his shoulder.

"You sure you got everything, sweetheart?"

"Oh yes, I'm quite sure. I . . . " Suddenly she remembered that her hiking boots were probably still by the door of the front room. "I might have left my shoes," she said hesitantly.

"Your shoes!" John exploded. "How in the world could you forget something like that!" John was an orderly person who seldom had anything out of place.

"I don't quite remember," Mary stammered.

"You don't remember! We'd better stop and be sure." John pulled over to the side of the road. Several minutes of shuffling through the trunk were of no avail.

"But, honey, I was *sure*—"

"You may have been sure, but they're not here. We'll have to go back. Now it'll get really hot and we'll be late!" Angrily he spun the car around and headed back.

Mary's eyes filled with tears, and she sat quietly the twenty minutes back. If only she had checked through the cabin more carefully, rather than wasting so much time outdoors!

"I'm sorry, John. I really am."

"It's all right, honey. I didn't mean to be cross." John pulled her over near him, ignoring the hazards of one-arm driving. "We'll just enjoy the extra traveling time together. I should have helped you check through the cabin myself, instead of rushing off to fill the tank."

They drove in silence for a few minutes, when a thought suddenly occurred to John. He glanced over at Mary with a sly grin and asked impishly, "By the way, write any poems this morning?"

"No!" Mary said, half truthfully. She turned away to look out the car window so he could not see the guilty color rising in her cheeks.

"This was sure a good idea, Mary." John reached into the grocery bag for the apple juice. "Would you hand me the bottle opener?"

Mary was spreading the plastic picnic cloth on the grass just off the highway. "It's a good thing you spotted that store back there. I was beginning to think we weren't going to find anything open. I like this so much better than eating indoors—we can be by ourselves, and we can walk around a bit. What are you smiling about?" she asked, as she happened to notice his amused expression.

"H'm? Oh, I was thinking of the lady who played the organ in that little outdoor chapel we visited last month."

"She was a riot, all right," Mary agreed. "She was so short I don't see how she could manage the pedals at all. It didn't seem to matter to her how many notes she missed, just so she impressed everyone by playing as loudly and as fast as she could. It almost spoiled the service for me." Mary handed John a sandwich on a napkin, and they both sat down.

"Thanks, honey," John munched on his sandwich a while as he studied the landscape around them. "I don't know what made me think of the organist," he said between mouthfuls, "unless it's the way this spot reminds me of the chapel. Notice the hill sloping down toward the water fountain"—he gestured, with a sweep of his arm—"the way the hill sloped down toward the pulpit in the chapel. And the logs set around here for benches are the same kind, only here they're put every which way, not in neat rows."

"I loved the service," Mary reminisced with him, "except for the organist. I liked what the minister said about the God of Creation also being a God of love."

"I appreciated the sermon too. To think that God is interested in every little detail of our lives! I don't think I ever heard anyone preach on the 145th Psalm before, but the contrast is there all right!—the mighty God where it says 'Great is the Lord, . . . and his greatness is unsearchable'; and then the gentle and loving God where it says 'The Lord is good to all: and his tender mercies are over all his works.' "

"I liked what he said about God's perfect love casting out fear of a terrible God," Mary added.

"So did I—especially the way he compared this to the Israelites at

Sinai who thought that the God of Creation was so powerful and so dreadful that they were afraid to come near him, with the fact that Jesus came to show us God is Love, and to take away all our fear.''

"Hadn't we better be on our way?'' Mary asked, nudging him back to the present moment. Together they gathered up their things and were on their way.

Uncle George and Aunt Emma kept going to the door and looking down the road in anticipation of their young guests. But the tranquil silence of the late summer afternoon was interrupted only by the lowing of a cow in the pasture. And if it had not been for the occasional ambling of a heifer in search of a more choice morsel of grass, the scene just beyond their doorway would have been as motionless as a watercolor in a frame.

"They're coming, George!'' Aunt Emma called suddenly, as the car came into view down the road. Uncle George eased himself out of his rocking chair and came to wait beside her.

"Hello, Uncle George 'n' Aunt Em,'' John called as he stepped out of the car. "Look who I've brought. He helped Mary from the car and drew her toward them. "This is my wife, Mary. Mary, this is Uncle George and Aunt Em.''

"We're *so* glad to meet you, Mary,'' Aunt Emma said warmly, putting out her hand to draw Mary's arm through hers.

"Uncle George, I can see by the twinkle in your eye that you're going to ask to kiss the bride,'' John noted amiably. "You may.''

"Thanks, John. How'd you know?'' Uncle George gave Mary a kiss on the cheek. "I must say I admire your taste. Prettiest bride I ever saw! Except one,'' he added quickly, with a sly glance at Aunt Emma.

"Come on in,'' Aunt Emma told them, ignoring his banter as she led them into the house. "You must be tired, and supper's ready and waiting. This will be your room, if you'd like to freshen up a bit.'' She opened the door to the guest room—really their own bedroom, but she and George were going to sleep on the porch that night so their young guests could have the only bedroom.

"You shouldn't do this,'' John chided her. "Mary and I can just as well sleep on the porch.''

"Now, John, you just do as we say and don't argue,'' Uncle George advised. "Aunt Em and I decided on that before you came, and that settles it!''

"Okay, Uncle George," laughed John. "C'mon, honey," he called to Mary, "we can bring our bags in here."

Supper was a simple one. Aunt Emma had fixed cold chicken and fruit, not knowing when the young folks would arrive. But she popped biscuits into the oven as soon as they came so there would be something hot.

"Are you still working in the lumberyard during summers?" Uncle George asked, absently stirring the third spoonful of sugar into his coffee.

"Yes," John replied. "I enjoy the outdoor work. It's a refreshing change from the classroom all winter, although I like teaching more than I thought I would. The best thing about my teaching is that it's in Pinedale. If I'd gone to some other school I might never have met Mary!" He smiled at her across the table. "By the way, Mary's quite a poet. You ought to hear some of the things she's written."

"May we, Mary?" asked Aunt Emma politely.

Mary blushed. "I'd—rather not, now. John is always bragging about me."

"Writing poems is nothing to be ashamed of, Mary," Uncle George told her gently. "I rather like to try my hand at it sometimes too. Em, where is that piece I wrote about the creation of the craggy cliff?"

"I think it's in the desk, George, in the lower lefthand drawer. Or maybe in that box of photos and clippings in the bedroom. Just a minute, I'll go see." Aunt Emma excused herself, returning a few minutes later with a yellowed paper. "Now wait a minute before you read it till I can bring out the pie."

After everyone had been served dessert, Uncle George held his poem up to the lamp, cleared his throat, and read, in a voice almost as craggy as the cliff—

> Thou relic of an ancient glory
> Tell me, O rock! What is your story?
> What sculptor formed your stately ridge
> And chiseled it an arching bridge?
>
> Whose fingers moved to form thy face
> That time and tide cannot erase?
> Which ancient worker knew just how
> To hold his tools to shape your brow?

Who molded thy protruding chin
That stands so firm against the wind,
And planted trees upon thy shoulder?
O tell me this, thou time-worn boulder!

Who rounded out your stubby nose
And gave you rippling waves for clothes;
Who chiseled place for deep-set eye?
What was his name? Come! Make reply!

Then, as the breeze sighed through the pines,
I thought I heard him say these lines—
"The God who made earth, sky, and sea
Is He who also molded me."

"George reads his poems to people every chance he gets," commented Aunt Emma, "but I don't mind. Fact is, I enjoy them more each time I hear them."

"This one fits right in with the sermon we heard last month about God being such a wonderful Creator," John remarked. "You want to tell them about it, Mary?"

Mary declined. "You make a much better preacher than I do, honey. You tell them."

"Now that's a good combination!" chuckled Uncle George. "We have a poet and a preacher in our family too. I'm the poet," he added, with a wink at Aunt Em.

Aunt Emma didn't mind his joking. Mary helped her clear the table and do up the few dishes while John helped Uncle George carry some chairs out onto the porch.

The steady creaking of the porch swing attested its great age as John and Mary sat in it together later, in the warm, gray-dark of the summer evening.

"Your father always loved that swing when he was a little boy," Aunt Emma remarked to John. "Many's the night I sat there with him in my arms after Mother died and talked and sang to him until he fell asleep."

"I know. Dad's told me, Aunt Em. I loved this swing when I was little too. It's amazing that it still holds together. Maybe one of these days it'll just fall apart all at once!"

They all laughed. Uncle George hitched his rocker forward a little so he could see the stars. "I courted your Aunt Em in that swing," he said, "and if it could talk, what stories it could tell!"

"I'd like to hear them," said Mary, and they all laughed again.

"The swing can't talk—good thing," he winked at Aunt Em, "but I can tell you a story someone told us when we were first married. It's about the two bears that should be in every marriage. Ever hear it?"

"I've heard about the three bears," Mary volunteered, "but not about two."

"Now it's this way," Uncle George explained. "When two people fall in love, they can't see any fault at all in the loved one. Either their lover seems perfect to them, or else what little faults they notice don't matter at all. But after they're married, they find they're both human, after all. Each of them does things a little differently from the other, since they weren't brought up in the same home environment, and little habits of the other person begin to annoy. Sometimes unhappiness and cross words creep in even before the honeymoon's over."

John and Mary had stopped swinging. Each was thinking sheepishly of the cross words that had passed between them that very morning.

"Now if the two bears become a part of the marriage, everything will be all right," Uncle George went on. "The first bear is this: 'Bear one another's burdens, and so fulfill the law of Christ.' You'll find that one in Galatians if you look," he added with a twinkle in his eyes. "This sharing of burdens should be done not only with big problems, but with little ones as well," he continued. "If the husband always tries to see things from his wife's point of view, and the wife from her husband's, it will help them share each other's burdens and will keep them from offending each other even in little things.

"The second bear is this—the one in Colossians—'Forbearing one another, and forgiving one another, . . . even as Christ forgave you.' Married love is to be a forgiving love—putting up with the little things in the other person that annoy, in a spirit of love, not of martyrdom."

John reached for Mary's hand and pressed it tightly within his own in the dark. "Bear and forbear. Thank you, Uncle George. We'll try to keep the two bears a real part of our marriage."

"Who did George say was the preacher in our family?" smiled Aunt Emma. "We should let these children go to bed, George. They've had a long day traveling."

"Good night, Aunt Em," said Mary softly, as she and John walked toward the door. "Good night, Uncle George."

3. Let Me Count the Ways

Let your fountain, the wife of your youth,
be blessed, rejoice in her,
a lovely doe, a graceful hind, let her be your companion;
you will at all times be bathed in her love,
and her love will continually wrap you around.
　　　　　　　　　　　　　—Proverbs 5:18, 19, NEB

Mary was humming to herself as she dusted the last few pieces of furniture in their little home. The doorbell rang just as she entered the bedroom to pick up the curtains she was making to brighten up the kitchen. She hurried to the door.

"Why, Mother! I wasn't expecting you this morning. Come on in." She gave her mother a quick embrace.

"I hadn't expected to stop by, Mary." Mrs. Johnson set her hand-bag on the counter as she spoke. "I just thought that since I was out shopping, I might as well drop by for a minute. We still miss you so much at home."

"I'm glad you came, Mother. I've been having so much trouble with these curtains. Isn't this pretty material?" Mary held up the color-ful print. "I picked the brown and yellow because John likes these colors best. But they won't hang straight, no matter what I do!"

Mrs. Johnson picked up one of the basted curtains and looked it over with an experienced eye. "Mary, you haven't drawn the threads. These will have to be done over. Don't you remember how I've shown you how to draw a thread at each end so the curtain will hang by the straight of the goods?"

Mary let out a discouraged sigh. How many times had her mother had her rip things out and sew them over!

"Don't be discouraged." Mrs. Johnson picked up one of the cur-tains and carried it over to the table. "Hand me the scissors, and I'll stay and help you pull the threads and hem these up again."

They both sat down and worked on the curtains for several minutes, while Mrs. Johnson gave the latest news of Jo Lynn's many activities.

"By the way, Mary," she asked, attempting to sound offhand, "how are you and John getting along?"

"Just fine, Mother. I'm so glad now for all the things you taught me about how important it was to respect myself and keep my body pure for the man I would one day marry. I wouldn't have thought of wearing my wedding dress before the day of the wedding! Now I'm glad I kept myself for John too."

Mary absently let her curtain fall into her lap. "So many of my friends have the idea that as long as they 'love' somebody, they can do what they like with each other! But now," she sighed and picked up the curtain again, "they don't seem as happy as I am. And some of them have such problems."

"I'm glad for you, Mary," her mother said quietly, reaching for a thread and needle. "I believe that God has planned one special person for each of us, if it is his will for us to be married." She hemmed with neat, firm stitches as she spoke. "Marriage is more than a piece of paper. It is a commitment to each other before God and the community. Sexual indulgence for 'love alone' doesn't hold people together when trouble comes. It becomes harder to trust someone else. And although there is forgiveness in Jesus for every sin—including sexual sin—there is still the pain of repentance and the need for inner healing. Married love has an especially deep meaning to those who have kept themselves true to just that one special person."

Mrs. Johnson hesitated. She wanted to say more but did not like to pry into her daughter's privacy. "Mary, this hem is fixed, and I really must go now." She laid down the finished curtain. "Just one more thing I'd like to say—if you have any problems at all with the physical adjustments of marriage, don't hesitate to go back to Dr. Gordon for advice."

"We won't, Mother, although we really don't need to now. He gave us such helpful advice when we went to him before our marriage. Thanks so much for sending us to him." She gave her mother a kiss and a wave as she went out the door.

After her mother had gone, Mary picked up the curtain and bent over her work again. Her cheeks flushed a little as she thought back to the conversation she and John had had with Dr. Gordon, and of how much it had helped them to find pleasure in their physical relationship.

"I assume that you young people are familiar with the physiology of the male and female," Dr. Gordon had said. "This information is now taught in the biology and family courses in most schools. You know how the male glands secrete a solution called *semen,* in which are contained the tiny *sperm* that fertilize the *ovum,* or egg, of the female? When intercourse, or *coitus,* takes place, the male's *penis*—which becomes hard and erect when excited—*ejaculates* semen into the *vagina* of the female. When the *ovum,* or egg, of the woman is present at this time, the sperm fertilizes it and a new life begins to grow. You are familiar with this information?"

Both John and Mary nodded, so Dr. Gordon went on. "Now it has been assumed by some people that when God created us 'male and female' it was only for one purpose—the procreation of children—and that the pleasure and excitement of mating had no other justification. But if this is true, why is it that we're made so that the sexual urge doesn't disappear when childbearing age is past? We know, and the Bible teaches, that the act of mating is one that God planned in every detail and one he meant to be a beautiful experience for the two people involved. The New Testament has some sound ideas on this. Remember the passage in Hebrews?" He reached for the Bible on the bottom shelf of his bookcase. "Here it is—Hebrews 13:4—'Marriage should be honored by all, and the marriage bed kept pure.' Corinthians is even more specific." The doctor turned the pages back to the passage. "Listen to this—'Do not deprive each other except by mutual consent and for a time, so that you may devote yourselves to prayer. Then come together again.' What Paul is saying is that neither the husband nor the wife has the right to avoid having intercourse with the other, unless they mutually agree to do so for a specific purpose, such as prayer. The abstinence is to be temporary—for a reason they have talked about and agreed on. The wife is not to withhold her body from her husband, nor does he have the right to withhold his body from her. Each belongs to the other.

"In Ephesians 5 we even read that the sexual relationship between a man and his wife is a symbol of the relationship between Christ and the church. 'This is a great mystery!' Paul says. The sexual relationship, of course, is itself a symbol of the 'oneness' of the marriage. Marriage is an institution created by God in which each partner is 'one' with the other all the time as well as during the sexual act, hurting or helping the other in everything each one does.

"In the Old Testament, too, we read of the beauty of the marriage relationship, especially in the Song of Solomon, which describes in allegorical form the physical pleasures of marriage. And in the Talmud it says that a Jewish wife even had the right to demand that her husband perform his sexual obligations to her!

"So we know that as an ideal the intercourse of marriage is holy and right in God's sight and that it's intended to be a delight for both husband and wife. The question in your minds just now, and in that of most young couples about to be or just recently married, is how to make this ideal a reality in your own experience.

"Lovemaking can be satisfactorily fulfilled only where there is complete trust in each other, which is possible only in marriage. Yet it is such a revelation of the 'self' that even in marriage either partner can be deeply hurt by being casually 'used' by the other only for 'self'-satisfaction. Only where there is complete trust can lovemaking become such a delightful abandon of two persons to each other that they are 'one,' body, soul, and spirit.

"When this trust and abandon is present, the mechanics of intercourse and its climax for both the man and the woman become the marvel that God's creative genius intended. For each of the pair, the *climax,* or *orgasm,* consists of involuntary, rhythmical contractions. It is imperative that the man be able to reach this climax so that he can send his fertilizing semen into the woman, or the human race would not survive. But because a woman can become pregnant without reaching this climax, it has often been assumed that the pleasure of sex was meant only for the male."

"I know that isn't true, doctor," John interrupted, "but the guys I know—" he paused, blushing slightly, "these guys say some girls never do reach a climax. I want Mary to be able to."

"Are these guys married, John?" the doctor asked.

"Well, no, but I know some married guys who make the same complaint."

Doctor Gordon smiled. "Remember what I said about the ability to 'abandon' oneself in absolute trust to the other? This is seldom possible outside marriage. Both partners are cheated, and the man's mechanical orgasm is a poor substitute for the rich experience God intended it to be in marriage. This is true even when the young woman has learned— from the free flow of sexual information today—how to achieve orgasm. For each partner, outside of marriage, coital orgasm is attained more for self-satisfaction sexually, than out of concern for the total needs of the other person.

"Another inhibiting factor for a virginal bride and groom is the natural modesty of revealing oneself to another more fully than ever before. It takes time to learn to communicate verbally about these things, learning the little details of how best to please each other. The sexual relationship between husband and wife should grow ever richer and more pleasurable as the years pass, as communication deepens.

"Further, the couple may find that their sexual union is immeasurably sweeter after they have shared in the birth of their first baby. Intercourse is only an early step in a woman's sexual cycle. A healthy pregnancy, a happy birth experience, and pleasurable breastfeeding often give her more self-confidence, poise, and inner satisfaction with being a *woman* than she has ever known before. She may be able to abandon herself more freely to her husband and achieve a climax more easily. She may be less inhibited about skin-to-skin contact with her husband, just as she has learned to enjoy the skin-to-skin contact of her nursing baby fondling her breasts as he or she sucks contentedly. The husband too, who shares in the birthing of his own baby and bonds with him or her skin to skin, both at birth and in the weeks that follow, may be healed of some of his own inhibitions. Husband and wife must learn to *give* themselves to each other freely, in this love-bonding.

"But let me go back now to the mechanics of sexual orgasm, which for both consists of a series of involuntary rhythmical contractions of a ring of muscular tissue. Much of life is rhythmical in similar ways. Our lungs expand and contract rhythmically as we breathe. Our heart and blood vessels rhythmically expand and contract. At the height of the male orgasm the ring of muscular tissue at the base of the erect penis contracts involuntarily and rhythmically to propel the semen as far as possible into the vagina of the woman. And at the height of female orgasm, the ring of muscular tissue a third of the way inside the vagina involuntarily contracts rhythmically around the penis of her husband, sending waves of pleasure diffusing through her entire body.

"The basic difference in the sexual responses of the man and the woman is that the husband's desire is aroused more quickly and fades more quickly once orgasm is reached. The woman's desire is not only more slowly aroused, but once she reaches orgasm these involuntary vaginal contractions may recede, and then recur again and again several times over a period of twenty minutes or more. The involuntary contraction of the vaginal muscle stimulates contractions of the uterus as well until her whole being is caught up in the pleasure of this rhythm. Even her breathing rhythm may add to the total pleasure.

"This is the mature female orgasm, and it recedes slowly. The husband must continue to give her his attention and affection until it begins to fade, revealing how much he is interested in *her*, and not just in his own pleasure."

"But, doctor," Mary observed soberly, "are you saying that I won't be able to enjoy a climax until we've been married for years?"

"Not at all," the doctor laughed. "But you can reach this goal much more quickly by observing and practicing a few simple rules. The first one is to learn to contract your vaginal muscles *voluntarily*."

Mary frowned. "What do you mean? I thought you said the climax consisted of *in*voluntary vaginal contractions."

"It does. But if you learn to contract and relax these muscles alternately at will, this helps to trigger the involuntary contractions that bring such pleasure in intercourse."

"How do I do that? I don't even know where these muscles are!"

Patiently the doctor explained. "The vaginal wall is capable of the tremendous expansion necessary in the birth of a child. It is composed of layers of tissues drawn up tightly into folds by muscle fibers. The *sphincter muscle* that keeps the vagina closed is directly attached to the muscles that close the *anus* and the *urethra*. When one contracts, all three outlets contract. When one relaxes, all three relax. These muscles help form the 'floor' between the legs that give added support to the internal organs. If you cannot feel where these muscles are, cough.

"When you cough sharply, you will feel these muscles push out. Now reverse this pushing out and tighten these muscles, drawing them up toward the inside of the body. Hold them tightly for a count of three, then relax them slowly. If you are not sure you have relaxed them enough, cough again.

"Do this until you have learned to 'feel' exactly where these muscles are and can tighten them or relax them at will. To practice, tighten, relax, tighten, relax, in a slow, even rhythm, up to twenty times.

"In preparation for intercourse, John, you should realize that in a woman the areas of sexual response are widely diffused. It is important to enjoy a period of caresses before attempting insertion. Notice, for example in the Song of Solomon in the Bible, the emphasis upon fondling the hair, neck, lips, breasts, navel, and the references to the mount (pubic mound) and the hills. Genital caresses are spoken of as entering the wife's garden and uncovering her fountain, the vagina.

"The genital caresses should include the *vulva* and *clitoris* as well as the vagina itself. The vulva includes the *pubic mound* and the *outer lips* and extends on down around the anus. (During orgasm, the anal sphincter muscle also tenses up and contracts rhythmically.) Medical literature has described the clitoris as 'a miniature penis' but it is far more than that. New definitions of the clitoris include not only the *shaft* and the *glans,* but also the skin over the hood which joins underneath (called the frenulum) and then divides into the *inner lips* which thin out and surround the vagina. The clitoral opening to the vagina is the skin at its base, called the fourchette, which can be stretched and thinned to allow for insertion of the penis. An understanding of this interrelated tissue as all part of the clitoral mechanism helps one know how to achieve early arousal.

"Genital stimulation causes the glands at the base of the vagina to release a secretion to moisten the entrance, making insertion easier. It also causes the clitoral skin of the fourchette, inner lips, frenulum, and hood to fill with blood and become rigid, increasing erotic pleasure. This in turn presses down on the shaft of the clitoris, causing it to become erect in excitement. Ordinarily it is pulled back up under the pubic bone where it is protected from injury.

"When both husband and wife are ready, there are still two things that may cause difficulty with the first attempts at penetration by the husband. Just inside the vagina is found the *hymen,* often called the 'maidenhead.' It is a small membrane composed primarily of connective tissue. It has no glandular or muscular elements and few nerve fibers. The hymen usually tears during the first intercourse. In some brides, the hymen may be so thick or resistant to penetration that this causes pain. For this reason it should be gently dilated with the fingers first, and if it doesn't respond after five or six attempts at intercourse, it should be treated by a physician. In other women, however, the hymen may be quite fragile and easily broken. It may already have been broken during some childhood accident.

"The second thing that may cause difficulty is a spasm of the vaginal muscles. One young wife said to me, 'But, doctor, I'm just too small for my husband!' Of course this wasn't true. What happened was that this young bride was so fearful and anxious that she was not able to relax the sphincter muscle that closes the vagina. This resistance of the vaginal muscles is also an important cause of pain during childbirth. A woman *must* learn to relax these muscles at will.

"If she has not learned to do so before, it will help to open her mouth and inhale deeply, trying at the same time to 'let go' of the tension in the vaginal walls, and cough a time or two to help relax the outlet. The husband should then guide the penis carefully and gently so that it follows the slope of his wife's vagina and doesn't cause her discomfort. Often she can direct it herself so that it's comfortable for her.

"The insertion of the penis into the vagina is not the climax of intercourse, although this may cause such excitement to the young husband that it precipitates the climax for him. This may be disappointing to them both unless they realize that this is an experience to learn together, and that a sense of humor and a deep affection for each other will overcome all obstacles as time passes. One does not become a concert musician the first time he or she touches an instrument, nor can two beginning musicians play in absolute harmony. Time and experience, patience and humor will make the lovemaking more harmonious, more fulfilling, as time goes on. And even at the start, it can be fun!

"Once the penis is inserted about halfway, the husband should let it lie perfectly quiet. The walls of the vagina have few nerve endings, so that a rapid back and forth movement will only bring on a rapid climax for him, and not give pleasure to the wife. Immediately in back of the vaginal walls, however, are tissues with many nerve endings which respond pleasurably to *pressure* on the sides of the vagina. As the husband lies quietly, the wife should begin to consciously contract and relax the vaginal muscle rhythmically around her husband's penis. This adds to the pleasurable pressure in the vagina without overstimulating the husband. As she consciously contracts and relaxes this muscle and pleasure increases, before long the muscle of its own accord will involuntarily begin to do so, and she will have reached the threshold of orgasm. At this time the husband may begin to move the penis *slowly*, back and forth, pressing firmly against the vaginal walls as he does so, until his climax occurs. And when it does, he must be careful to continue showing his wife affection until her own excitement begins receding.

"A young husband can learn to control the timing of his ejaculation by not thrusting rapidly back and forth after insertion, and also by a better understanding of his own sexual anatomy. For example, *erection* results from the trapping of blood in the tissues of the penis which causes it to increase in size and makes insertion into the vagina possible. A husband can learn to maintain an erection for fifteen to thirty minutes, *even in the vagina,* and it is important for him to learn to do so. By allowing the penis to lie quietly in the vagina for some time, his wife is better able to reach the threshold of orgasm with him.

"Maintaining an erection in the vagina is possible because the process of erection is controlled by nerve centers other than those controlling ejaculation. The male sex glands, the testes or *testicles,* lie in the sac-like structure called the *scrotum.* The testicles produce male sex hormones and *spermatozoa,* the male reproductive cells. Each testicle is capped by an *epididymis,* a very thin, convoluted tubelike organ that stores the sperm. But sperm cells do not go directly from the epididymes into the penis. Rather, they are carried up into the abdomen through tubes known as *vas deferens,* which make a loop up past the bladder, down past the *seminal vesicles* and on into the *prostate gland,* where they join the *urethra* which goes on down through the penis. Fluid is secreted by the seminal vesicles and the prostate and mixes with the sperm in the seminal vesicles at the time of ejaculation. A system of valves within the prostate make it impossible for urine and semen to enter the urethra at the same time.

"When a husband realizes intellectually that erection and ejaculation are two *separate* phenomena, he is better able to control the timing of each. If after several months of marriage he still is ejaculating before he wants to, there are some techniques he and his wife can try to help him learn control.

"It may be helpful for the wife to be in the above position, in which she very gently and slowly inserts the penis into the vagina as she leans forward at about a 45-degree angle. Once it is inserted, she should remain motionless until the husband has a chance to achieve control. The lateral position may also be tried, in which the wife lies on her right side and extends her right leg behind her while she leans on the husband's chest. He bends his left knee, keeping it under her leg and flat against the bed. These positions allow both partners greater freedom and control than with the husband above the wife.

"In addition, the wife may apply the 'squeeze technique' if necessary. When the husband fears ejaculation is near before desired, she grasps the penis between her thumb and forefingers, with the thumb just below the head of the penis on the underside where the shaft ends, and squeezes *hard.* (This causes no pain on the erected penis.) This pressure will immediately make him lose the desire to ejaculate. Each time the husband approaches unwanted ejaculation during a lovemaking session, he can give his wife a signal, and she can move away from him and apply the squeeze technique. This can be done several times in one session, until they agree to allow the climax to occur. By doing this during each lovemaking over a period of weeks or perhaps months, the husband will gradually learn control so that he will ejaculate only when he desires to do so.

"Keep in mind that the real goal is not just to come together to reach a climax, for this is only one small though important part of the total experience. The real goal is to enjoy each other throughout the entire lovemaking and give each other pleasure. To focus on the climax only is to inhibit its occurring properly and to miss much of the other joy that rightfully accompanies this whole experience."

The doctor paused, as if weighing over what he had said, and then added, "One other thing. John, there are some men who only show affection and caress their wives when they want coitus. If this is true of you, Mary may soon become resentful and sex will lose its true meaning for you both. The subtle meaning behind every hug and kiss then becomes for her a signal that you want your sex hunger satisfied, rather than a sign that you really love her. The ability to show affection, hugging and kissing one's wife and children, makes a man a better husband and a better father, so that his children learn from the time they are small how to convey affection through cuddling and touch, and his wife feels secure in his love. Do you two want children?"

"Oh yes!" Mary said quickly. "John and I have already talked about having children. We are ready to start our family now. But what do you think about birth control, doctor?"

"There are times, Mary, when it is wise to prevent a baby from being conceived in order to give a young couple time to adjust to each other after marriage before assuming family responsibilities, when used to conserve a young mother's energy, or in order to make sure the family can support the children they bring into the world. However, I believe that any means used for birth control is wrong when it's employed for purely selfish reasons—to avoid the trouble and expense of raising children."

"What about overpopulation?" John asked. "From all one hears about it, sometimes I wonder if it's right to have children at all."

"The world wouldn't last long if that were true," the doctor smiled. "My personal belief is that this is a matter between a married couple and their God. Only he knows what children he wants born into their home, which particular children are to be born into which home. I do not believe this is a matter to be dictated by a government or even by a social code that says a couple may have so many and no more. Since we know how to prevent conception, we already are able to prevent having an unlimited number of children who cannot either be fed or clothed. But God may guide some parents to have five or six children and others to have only one. This is an intensely personal matter, and God's guidance will not be the same for each couple."

"What form of birth control do you recommend, doctor," John queried, "if we ever decide not to have any more children?"

"First, let me describe briefly several methods, and then I'll suggest what I think might be best for you, although it is really up to you.

"The first and oldest form of contraception (birth control is really 'conception' control) is simply *abstinence*—not having intercourse at all. Although certain religious elements in our society have objected to coitus except for the purpose of having children, abstinence is neither scriptural nor advisable, except for short periods of time under special circumstances, as we discussed earlier.

"The second simple and old form is *coitus interruptus*—withdrawal of the penis before ejaculation. This is most unsatisfactory for both husband and wife, and she may become pregnant anyway, if a few sperm had escaped before withdrawal.

"The *condom*—a thin rubber sheath that is pulled over the husband's erect penis—is simple and inexpensive, but it does detract a little from the pleasurable sensations involved, for there is not the sensitivity of skin-to-skin contact.

"The wife can be fitted by a doctor with a *diaphragm,* a rubber cup-shaped protection that she inserts into the vagina over the *cervix,* or mouth of the womb, prior to intercourse. The diaphragm must be used in combination with a *spermicide* (sperm-killing) cream, to be completely effective. The diaphragm is a bit of a nuisance to have to stop and insert before lovemaking, but it is highly effective, and does not in any way prevent the pleasure of the act.

"However, neither the condom nor the diaphragm is effective without the use of spermicide creams. And there is some concern that birth defects are occurring in some infants conceived in spite of these attempts to prevent it. The birth defects may have been caused by sperm damaged by the spermicide cream.

"A permanent form of preventing conception is surgical *sterilization* of the husband or wife, in which the *fallopian tubes* (in the wife) or the *vas deferens* (in the husband) are severed. Unfortunately, it is not always as 'permanent' as has been thought. Six out of every thousand women who undergo tubal sterilization will later become pregnant. The operation also increases the risk of *ectopic pregnancy* (in which the fertilized ovum begins growing in the tube because it cannot move on down into the *uterus*, or womb), which can become a life-threatening situation for the mother. In males, sterilization has been found to interfere with the autoimmune system, making them more vulnerable to certain health risks.

"So far we have been talking about ways to prevent conception," the doctor went on. "But you should be alert to the fact that much of what is called 'birth control' actually aborts the infant that has already been conceived. For example, *intrauterine devices* (IUD), which can be implanted in the uterus by the physician, work by irritating the lining of the uterus so that a fertilized ovum cannot attach itself to the uterine wall and is expelled from the body.

"Thus the IUD is an *abortifacient;* that is, it causes very early abortion if conception has taken place. It can create problems for the woman too. It sometimes causes inflammation of the fallopian tubes. Occasionally it becomes imbedded in the uterine wall. The irritation within the uterus due to the presence of a foreign object makes it more vulnerable to infection. It has been known to cause toxic shock syndrome (TSS) and even death, because the string of the IUD acts as a wick to draw germs up into the uterus. I learned just last week of a young woman who died because of this."

"Why couldn't I just take *birth control pills?*" Mary wanted to know. "I have lots of friends who take them and they say it's really easy. They don't have to worry about fooling with any of these other things."

"Mary, there are other things you will want to consider beside how 'easy' it is. You see, the pill works in two ways: it is supposed to inhibit ovulation so that no egg escapes from the ovaries each month, but it also changes the lining of the uterus so that if a baby is conceived, it will be aborted. Thus the so-called birth control pill is also an abortifacient if a child has been conceived. There is even a new contraceptive under research that need be taken only once a month, but whose purpose is also to prevent a fertilized egg from taking hold in the uterus and beginning to grow. It works by altering the hormones in the woman's body. Many Christians who would never think of aborting a baby have been using the IUD or some form of birth control pill because they have been ignorant of the fact that they are abortifacients.''

"That's a sobering thought," John said. "Can you explain a little more about abortion?''

"I'd be glad to, John. It is important to distinguish between preventing conception from taking place and taking a life after it has been conceived. We have been talking about abortifacients, which cause the conceived baby to be aborted early, usually without a woman even knowing she has conceived. *Therapeutic abortion* is performed after a woman knows she is pregnant, most often in the first few weeks of pregnancy. In this procedure the baby is killed by injecting a saline solution or other solutions into the uterus, by trying to induce contractions to expel the baby, by surgically scraping the lining of the uterus, or by having the baby drawn out in fragments by suction. A woman often suffers psychological consequences later on at any reminder that she has destroyed her own child, and her future childbearing is also affected to a greater or lesser degree.

"Many today support 'abortion on demand'; they believe abortion should be available when a woman and her doctor agree to destroy the living fetus. But the Bible says that this is a matter in which someone else is involved—the living God who formed that child in the womb and who alone knows for what purposes that child was meant to live.

"But let me finish my explanation about the birth control pill. In addition to its role as a possible abortifacient, it also creates health problems for some women. Some are predisposed to the risk of blood clots and the greater likelihood of earlier heart attacks or strokes. It upsets the natural hormone balance of the body so that a few women suffer from depression or other mental disorders. It should only be prescribed for a woman by a doctor well acquainted with her medical history. And there is an additional problem: when she stops taking the pill in order to become pregnant, it may be a long time before ovulation and her menses return, so that she is infertile and unable to have a child during that time. In a few women, fertility never returns.

"For all these reasons, I cannot recommend any of the above methods of birth control, though many couples choose to use them even with full knowledge of their risks and effects. My suggestion is that you learn and practice *natural family planning*, the method that allows you to prevent conception by recognizing the short period of fertility in the woman each month and avoiding genital contact during that time. It will be helpful for you to begin learning all you can now, Mary, before you become pregnant, as it will help you to become more familiar with your own body. And it will help you both to recognize the symptoms of fertility after your baby is born. It will make it easier for you to apply the method during breastfeeding, when symptoms can seem confusing if you have not learned them in advance.

"Natural family planning not only makes any artificial means of preventing conception unnecessary, it also can be of great benefit in helping a couple work out their sexual relationship, increasing communication and intimacy. A woman is fertile for only a few days each month. The difficulty is that no two women have exactly the same fertile days. Even for the same woman it may vary a few days from month to month, but there are ways in which she can learn to recognize her fertility. She and her husband agree to abstain from genital contact during those fertile days, if they wish to postpone or prevent a pregnancy. Would you like to know more about this method?"

"Yes, please," John and Mary exclaimed, almost simultaneously.

"All right," Dr. Gordon agreed. "I'll give you a brief summary and then suggest some material you can study more carefully. You already understand that there are two ovaries, one on each side of the uterus, suspended just below the fallopian tubes which branch out on each side of the uterus. Once each month an ovum is released from the ovary (*ovulation*), usually from the fifth to the fourteenth day after the first day of the menstrual period. Once the ovum is released, it is drawn up into the fallopian tube and propelled slowly along it toward the uterus, where it passes on through and is expelled from the body. From the time the ovum is first released, it is capable of being fertilized by a sperm from the male, if genital contact takes place (even though the penis is not actually inserted into the vagina). Furthermore, since sperm can live up to five days in the woman's body, genital contact *before* the ovum is released can result in pregnancy. But once the ovum has passed out of the body, conception is no longer possible until the next menstrual and ovulatory phases.

"There are several ways in which a woman can recognize by her body's signs that she is in the ovulatory cycle. One of these is by the white loss, a small discharge of stringy, stretchy whitish mucus from the vagina, which means that the unfertilized egg is about to leave the ovary. This mucus helps the sperm to survive longer as it waits for the ovum to be released. Once the peak of this moist, lubricative, egg-white type of mucus is over, it is still possible to conceive for another three or four days. Intercourse should not be resumed until the evening of the fourth dry day.

"A second sign of fertility/infertility is the change in a woman's *basal temperature,* the temperature of her body at rest. It is helpful to keep a chart on which the basal temperature is recorded day by day. There is a temperature rise as the fertile phase is ending. When the basal temperature has been elevated 4/10 to 6/10 of one degree above the pre-ovulation base for at least three consecutive days (after the final day of the fertile mucus), it is certain that ovulation has passed. If there was intercourse *prior* to this rise, pregnancy could result. Pregnancy would be confirmed by a temperature elevation for eighteen days or more.

"Contrary to popular opinion, a woman can be quite fertile during menstruation (if her cycle is short) and afterward, while her basal body temperature is low. Therefore, accurate temperature recording is extremely important. The husband can help by bringing a basal thermometer to his wife each morning before she gets up, helping her take her temperature, and then writing the record down on the chart. His participation in temperature recording enchances his cooperation and understanding.

"There is a *relatively* infertile period for some women between the last few days of menstruation and the onset of ovulation, but very careful observation of the signs is important. After ovulation has passed fertility is no longer possible until the next cycle begins.

"A third sign of fertility/infertility can be recognized by cervical changes. The woman can learn to examine her cervix each day, at the same time and in the same position, by inserting a finger into the vagina. She will note that it is lower, firmer, and drier to the touch during the infertile part of the month. The slight dimple she feels at the center of the cervix is the mouth, or *os.* During the dry phase, the dimple will feel small and tightly closed. As ovulation approaches, the cervix raises, becomes slightly softer to the touch, more moist, and the os can be felt opening up.

"These three signs more or less coincide. By recording them on a chart, a couple can learn to be very efficient at recognizing the wife's period of fertility and infertility. Here," the doctor paused, spun around in his chair and pulled a book off the shelf, "take this home and look it over. If you find it helpful, you'll want to buy your own copy to keep, so you can learn the method.

"Oh, one more thing," he added. "Occasionally a woman may have all the symptoms of fertility without actually ovulating. In this case, she still will not ovulate until the next cycle. This is why a very few women who are observing the signs faithfully in order to *become* pregnant may not conceive; they may not actually be ovulating, even with all the symptoms. Even so, observing the signs in order to have intercourse *during* the fertile signs is the most certain way to achieve a pregnancy.

"Often an inability to conceive may be related to the faulty nutrition of either husband or wife, or both," the doctor continued. "This brings up the subject of good nutrition, which is of utmost importance. Not only is good nutrition important during pregnancy, it is of vital importance *before* conceiving a child. If the wife has been properly nourished before conceiving, she will feel much better all during pregnancy and may experience little or no nausea or other pregnancy-related problems. Her baby is more likely to be normal and healthy.

"But good nutrition is just as important for the husband before conception is attempted, for *either* parent may contribute to abnormalities in the germ plasm—the sperm of the male and ova of the female. Abnormal sperm or ova can result in nonconception, miscarriage, prematurity, stillbirth, mental retardation, and birth defects. Deficiencies in vitamins A and E are known to cause sperm abnormalities. Animal studies have confirmed that abnormal sperm produce gross defects. One researcher has demonstrated that the male is the more important of the two parents in causing genetic deformities. You see, the formation of healthy sperm requires a full assortment of nutrients and a complete set of enzymes, just as is required by any other healthy cell. This is why good nutrition is so important for the husband."

Mary interrupted, "My folks always said nutrition was important, but I thought it was just so *we* could be healthy. I never realized it would affect the children we might have."

"Neither did I," John admitted. "Would you explain what you mean by good nutrition?"

"I'll summarize my view briefly," the doctor said, "but I also encourage you to read all you can on the subject. There is a wealth of information being published today on nutrition. You perhaps already know that it is wise to avoid the use of alcohol, caffeine (found in coffee, chocolate, some teas, colas), and nicotine (found in cigarettes, cigars, and pipe tobacco), and all over-the-counter medications like aspirin. In addition, avoid refined sugars and flours, food additives, and artificial coloring, as well as nonnutritive substances—food substitutes sold as 'food.' It is wise to read all labels.

"Eat fruits and vegetables and grains as close to the natural state as possible, rather than processed or canned. Use fresh or dried fruits, raw vegetables as well as cooked, and include roots and herbs, seeds and sprouted seeds, and legumes (such as peas, lentils, beans) in your diet. Make liberal use of whole grains, soy flour, wheat germ, and nuts of all kinds.

"Eggs, milk, and cheese are valuable. Skimmed milk powder can be added to your cooking for added nutrients. Brewer's yeast is a rich source of balanced vitamins and trace minerals. Choose lean meats rather than the fatty ones, and use poultry, fish, and organ meats more often than the muscle meats. A spoonful of salad oil is needed in the diet each day; it can be used in cooking or salad dressings. Safflower oil is a good choice.

"You will both find yourselves feeling better, looking better, and enjoying life more if you eat in this way. And before conceiving a child, make sure that for some time your bodies have been receiving all the known vitamins and minerals through good nutrition and perhaps some supplements (for each person's needs are unique). Adequate zinc, folic acid, and vitamins A, C, and E are particularly important at this time."

The doctor was silent, waiting for further questions, and leaned back in his chair. When there were none, he reached across his desk for his Bible and opened it to Psalm 139. "The conceived child is extremely precious in the eyes of God," he said soberly, "whether it is a few moments after conception or a few weeks in the womb. This is why natural family planning is so important, for it in no way endangers a child who might be conceived. Let me read you this Psalm from the New International Version:

> If I say, Surely the darkness will hide me
> and the light become night around me,

even the darkness will not be dark to you;
the night will shine like the day,
for darkness is as light to you.

For you created my inmost being;
you knit me together in my mother's womb.
I praise you because I am fearfully and wonderfully made;
your works are wonderful,
I know that full well.
My frame was not hidden from you
when I was made in the secret place.
When I was woven together in the depths of the earth,
your eyes saw my unformed body.
All the days ordained for me
were written in your book
before one of them came to be.

Since John and Mary had no more questions, the doctor stood up, ending the interview. "Thank you, Dr. Gordon, so much," John said. "You have been most helpful."

"The best of happiness to you both," the doctor smiled in response. "Don't hesitate to come in again if you have any problems."

"We certainly won't. Goodbye now."

The bright new curtains were swinging merrily back and forth in the warm summer breeze swishing its way through the open window as Mary hurried to finish the sauce to pour over the baked chicken. This was one of John's favorite dishes and she hoped to have it ready when he came home from the lumberyard where he was working for the summer. As she heard the car door slam, she took the chicken out of the oven, to pour the topping over it and pop it back into the oven for fifteen minutes—just long enough for John to get washed up for supper. A moment later he opened the door.

"Hi, honey! M-m-m-m! That chicken smells good!" He swept her into one arm, but kept the other behind him while he gave her a long kiss.

"John, what's that in your hand?"

"Guess."

"I can't. Tell me."

"It's a present for you, honey. Here. Open it." He handed her a small, flat package.

It had obviously been gift wrapped in a store. Mary was sure John couldn't tie a bow like that! She carefully untied the gold ribbon. She could feel the shape of a book beneath the flowered paper, and as she lifted it out John explained, "I stopped by the bookstore on the way home. I know how much you like the poems of Elizabeth Barrett Browning, so I got a copy of them for you. I've picked one out to read you. Listen."

He opened the book to a place he had marked and slipped his arm around her waist. Mary laid her head on his shoulder as he read—not minding at all that he smelled of sawdust and the sweat of honest labor—

> How do I love thee? Let me count the ways.
> I love thee to the depth and breadth and height
> My soul can reach, when feeling out of sight
> For the ends of Being and Ideal Grace.
> I love thee to the level of every day's
> Most quiet need, by sun and candlelight,
> I love thee freely, as men strive for Right;
> I love thee purely, as they turn from Praise;
> I love thee with the passion put to use
> In my old griefs, and with my childhood's faith.
> I love thee with a love I seemed to lose
> With my lost saints,—I love thee with the breadth,
> Smiles, tears of all my life!—and, if God choose,
> I shall but love thee better after death.

NOTE

Recommended books for further study on marriage, natural family planning, and nutrition may be found in Appendix B.

4. My Father's World

The earth is the Lord's, and everything in it,
the world, and all who live in it.
—*Psalm 24:1, NIV*

The golden warmth of the September sun flooding the landscape was reflected in the brilliant gold, orange, and scarlet foliage of the woodland trees, framed as they were against the dark green shades of the evergreens. The Johnsons and the Thomases were taking advantage of the sunny Saturday for a late drive along the river.

"We must be almost to the bridge," Jo Lynn remarked, leaning forward and tipping her head a little to see out of the windshield past her mother in the front seat.

"It won't be long now, Jo Lynn," her father answered. "The scenery along here is so colorful that it would be a shame to hurry by."

"How much farther is it to the falls after we reach the bridge?" John asked.

"Not very far. I've forgotten exactly," Mr. Johnson replied. "Here's the bridge now." He slowed the car and turned it toward the bridge approach.

"Wow! This is some bridge!" John exclaimed. "We seem to be a mile above the river!"

The teal-blue splendor of the magnificent river far below them stretched in both directions as far as they could see. On their left, its broad expanse plunged toward them through the channel it was forging in the mountains; on their right, its turbulent water churned onward in its restless quest for oblivion within the bosom of the ocean.

As they turned west onto the river highway, they could see, back on the other side, the scenic road that they had just left, drawn like a curved white chalk line through the green and orange foliage along the north bank of the river. After only a few moments on the highway they arrived at the falls.

"Here we are!" cried Jo Lynn, preparing to hop out of the car the minute her father parked it in the lot near the falls.

"Let's take our lunch to those tables up near the little bridge over the falls," Mrs. Johnson suggested, as they all piled out of the car. "Jo Lynn! Come back here and help carry some of these things." Jo Lynn came back reluctantly and took a box to carry. With everyone helping, they soon had the lunch deposited on the picnic table.

"I'll stay at the table," Mrs. Johnson offered, "so you youngsters and Dad can hike the rest of the way to the top of the falls."

Mrs. Johnson opened one of the boxes and began spreading out the picnic cloth. Jo Lynn was already bounding up the mountainside, her dad right behind her, John and Mary close on his heels. The falls loomed above them, a spectacular drop to the river far below.

"John!" Mary gasped. "Please stop."

"Why, honey, what's the matter? Here, sit on this rock a minute." He drew her to the side of the path and had her sit on a small boulder.

"I—don't know." Mary felt very faint and leaned against him until she could focus her eyes more clearly. "I guess—we were going up too fast. I never felt this way before!—I'm better now. Let's go on." She stood up, but John eased her gently back onto the rock.

"What's the matter, Mary?" her dad asked. He and Jo Lynn came back toward them. "Were we setting too fast a pace? You look pale."

"I'm all right now. Let's go on up." Mary got up, but Mr. Johnson took her arm and turned her toward the descent.

"Look, Mary. Let's you and I go back and help Mother set out the lunch. John and Jo Lynn can go on up to the top of the falls. I've been there many times before, but John ought to see it."

Mary consented reluctantly. Jo Lynn gaily took John's arm, swung around flippantly, and looked back at Mary with a broad, teasing wink. Mary made a face at her behind John's back. Usually she didn't mind Jo Lynn's joking, but this time she felt unaccountably irritated.

"Don't mind her, Mary." Her father patted her arm. "John wouldn't look at her twice if they were marooned on a desert island."

"I know that, Dad. It's just that . . . " Mary's sentence trailed off unfinished, as they walked leisurely back down the trail. Mary loved her dad and the way he understood so many things about her without her having to explain.

Mrs. Johnson looked up in surprise when she saw them coming. After observing her daughter's behavior unobtrusively for a moment, she quietly drew her own conclusions.

"There's something that has always bothered me," John remarked thoughtfully. They had parked in one of the places provided along the highway on their way home and were walking over to sit on the stone ledge overlooking the river. "I've been thinking about it all day. I've been so conscious today of God's presence in the world as I've seen the splendor of this area. But, since he is present in our world, *why* is there so much suffering?"

"That's a hard question," Mr. Johnson answered. He paused a moment, looking around him, and then said to his wife, "Honey, come sit over by me. You can see better here, and the wall's a little smoother to sit on." After seeing that she was comfortable, he returned to John's question. "Ever since the time of Job people have pondered over the problem of pain, and there are no easy answers."

"Some people say that all suffering is the result of sin," Jo Lynn interrupted, "but I don't see how that could be. When that little girl in the next block was hit by a car, was it because she was so evil? And is old Mrs. Arkwright all crippled up with arthritis because she didn't live right? It doesn't make sense to me."

"Some suffering is certainly the result of sin, Jo Lynn," her father answered. "Sin has marred the perfect artistry of God, and countless numbers have died beneath bombs we've made with the knowledge God has given us, knowledge we've corrupted. You see, God has given us a free will, and with this freedom of choice comes the peril of our not going the right way, God's way. This leaves a trail of suffering in our path of evil doing. For example, perhaps the fellow who ran over little Laurie was exceeding a safe speed limit or had been drinking. Ignoring the welfare of other people is certainly sin. But this makes the problem harder—often people suffer not because of their own sin, but because of the sins of other people."

"To say that all suffering is the result of sin is too simple an answer then, isn't it?" Mary asked. "But the Jews of Jesus' day seemed to believe this. Remember, Dad, when they asked him about the blind man, 'Who sinned, this man or his parents, so that he was born blind?' and Jesus answered, 'Neither this man nor his parents.' "

"That's right, Mary," her father agreed. "So there must be additional causes for suffering. There are also what we call the 'accidents of nature.' God has set up certain unchanging physical laws that govern the universe, and these laws operate without discrimination. Jesus said of the Heavenly Father, 'He makes his sun rise on the evil and on the good, and sends rain on the just and on the unjust.'

"The small child who falls into a river and drowns is an illustration of this. It wouldn't make any difference if the child was good or bad, a boy or a girl, English or Chinese, Hindu or Christian. The unchanging chemical formula of the water would cause its death. But what would happen if this formula for water was constantly changing? Human life couldn't survive if the balance of hydrogen and oxygen in water wasn't a stable one."

"But then, Dad," Mary said, "wouldn't it be all right to say that suffering either from sin or from an accident of nature is caused by an interference with the harmony of God's natural law?"

"I'm inclined to agree with you, Mary," John spoke up. "So much suffering is caused by ignorance, as in places where nutrition and sanitation aren't understood. This destroys the harmony of God's laws too—but surely he didn't intend for people to be ignorant of the simple laws of the natural world he created, did he?"

"I'm sure he didn't," Mr. Johnson replied. "Some have called this breakdown in the harmony of his laws the theory of a disordered universe, due to the presence of evil forces in the world. The Bible teaches that there is a source of evil that existed even before humankind, and that if it weren't for God's staying hand, the whole universe would be in chaos.

"Jesus identifies this source of evil as 'Satan,' and says that Satan is responsible for much of the ignorance, sickness, and tragedy present in the world. For example, when Jesus saw the woman who had been crippled for eighteen years, he said, 'Should not this woman . . . whom Satan has kept bound for eighteen long years, be set free?' And he healed her."

"But the comforting thing to remember," Mrs. Johnson added as they walked slowly back to the car, "is that no matter what may have caused the suffering, God can bring peace of mind, and restoration of health, or strength to bear the trial graciously." After they had settled into their places and driven back out onto the highway, she went on, "I've been so impressed, in reading Mark again, with Jesus' concern for the sick. Everywhere he went he not only taught the people, but he also healed them. He didn't heal everyone in Palestine, but he did heal all those who came to him."

"Yes," Mr. Johnson agreed. "Jesus is revealed in the Gospels as being concerned for the whole person—body, mind, and spirit. Remember, too, that he taught that God is our Heavenly Father, concerned with every need of ours. The New Testament says over a hundred and fifty times that God is our Father.''

"That reminds me of the song we used to sing when I was a boy,'' John reminisced, "called 'This Is My Father's World'. I haven't thought of it in a long time. I like the part that says that

> Though the wrong seems oft so strong,
> God is the Ruler yet!''

They had recrossed the bridge and were winding quickly along the twisting road on the other side of the river.

"Dad, aren't you going awfully fast?'' Mary finally asked. She had tried to endure the lurching in the back seat as long as she could but was getting sicker by the minute. "I think you'd better stop,'' she warned.

Mr. Johnson pulled off to the side of the road and helped her from the car. "You and Mother trade places, Mary,'' he told her, "and you can sit up in front with me where the riding's smoother.''

"On second thought,'' he added, after glancing into the back seat and noticing the mischievous look on Jo Lynn's face, "why don't you drive, John? Mother and I haven't had a chance to sit in the back and hold hands for a good many years!''

5. Tinier Than a Raindrop

Just as you know not how the breath of life
fashions the human frame in the mother's womb,
So you know not the work of God
which he is accomplishing in the universe. . . .
—*Ecclesiastes 11:5, NAB*

Lift up your eyes on high
and see who has created these. . . .
—*Isaiah 40:26, NAB*

Mary gazed out the window of the doctor's waiting room at the gentle balm of rain. I can't understand why some people feel that the rain is depressing, she thought to herself. So many times as a little girl I lifted my face to feel the raindrops and thought how good God was to me. And now I'm so happy! To think that there's a new life growing in my body seems like a dream—a new life that was tinier than a raindrop at first! I know God's love is within me, all around me, enveloping the whole world as the rain refreshes the thirsty earth. Oh, how I love him! And everybody!

Mary glanced around the room. What a pretty outfit, she thought, a bit covetously, noticing the woman sitting just opposite her. I wonder how far along she is. She looks pretty big—maybe her baby is about due. I can hardly wait to go shopping for my outfits. Won't Joanie be jealous! They've been married two years now. Of course, it would be fun to keep it a secret as long as we could—she glanced over at John, buried in a magazine—but it's so exciting I just *have* to tell somebody. What a darling little girl that is walking by outside with the pink umbrella! I wonder if we'll have a girl, or a boy. We'll have to think about names—

"Mr. and Mrs. Thomas, will you step in now, please?" The nurse's voice broke into Mary's reverie. John laid down his magazine, and he and Mary followed the nurse down the hall to Dr. Gordon's office.

"Hello! Come on in," Dr. Gordon greeted them warmly. "How's the teaching this year, John? I've noticed the team's doing very well this fall." He motioned to the chairs near his desk, and John and Mary sat down.

"It's going pretty well," John replied. "I don't have as many problem youngsters in my history classes, and, of course, we're all happy about the performance of the team. The boys are taking their training rules seriously this year, and it sure makes a big difference in their game."

"I'm hoping to get to tomorrow night's game, but don't count on it." Dr. Gordon had seated himself behind his desk. "What can I do for you young people today? You're not having any problems, I trust?"

"No, it's just that—" Mary blushed slightly, "I think we're going to have a baby."

"That's good news. Can you tell me what makes you think so?"

"Well," Mary answered, "I've missed my last two periods, and this has never happened to me before. Also, I've noticed that my breasts are a bit larger, and more tender when bumped or touched."

Dr. Gordon nodded. "These are good indications of pregnancy. Other signs may include more frequent urinating, as the growing uterus presses against the bladder, or slight skin changes. Sometimes fatigue and nausea occur. Have you had any problem with either, Mary?"

"No," she said, thinking back, "except for one time when we went to the falls with my folks. I was rather miserable part of the time, but then we did quite a little hiking, and Dad drove home pretty fast."

"Nature puts out little warning signs when we're doing too much," Dr. Gordon smiled. "A woman who's carrying a child soon learns that she'll have to make a few adjustments and take things at a more leisurely pace. Real fatigue in pregnancy, though, if one is not overactive, may be a sign of poor nutrition, or it may indicate that inwardly the mother is a little unhappy over being pregnant. We're learning more all the time about the important relationship between the state of a person's mind and the functioning of his or her body.

"The same thing is true of nausea. Occasionally, the glandular changes that take place when pregnancy begins cause disturbances of other functions, but many women have no difficulty with this at all. Frequently, when nausea persists, I suspect that there are other problems creating tensions that show up in this way as well as in fatigue. Sometimes there are financial or marital difficulties that the mother is worried about, or she may be anxious because this is a new and untried experience for her. Nausea may also be a sign of a nutritional or vitamin deficiency, particularly a lack of the B-complex vitamins.

"Learning to relax helps to relieve nausea if it has been caused by tension or worry. Eating small meals frequently rather than three large ones or munching crackers between meals helps. Sometimes a light breakfast in bed before getting up will prevent discomfort in the morning."

"I get the hint!" John grinned. "Now don't start pretending to have nausea, Mary, so you can have breakfast in bed!"

"Not a bad idea," Mary laughed, "and how could you tell if I was pretending?"

"I don't want to get involved in a family controversy!" Dr. Gordon laughed, "but let's stay on the subject a bit longer. Not only is it absolutely essential, Mary, that you follow the outline of good nutrition I gave you last time; it is now even more important that you avoid certain common items. We have learned that birth defects, prematurity, low birth weight, and lowered intelligence may be the result of substances taken in early pregnancy—even during the first few days and weeks of pregnancy. This is why it is so important to learn to live without these substances even *before* pregnancy begins, as one may not be aware that pregnancy has started until after the most crucial period in which all the major organs and basic body structure of the embryo are being formed. These common items include both prescription and nonprescription medications (aspirin, cold tablets, sleeping pills, etc.) and stimulants such as caffeine (found in many medications as well as in coffee, tea, colas, and chocolate). The rule is, *no* drugs—either prescription or over-the-counter remedies—*none at all.* I do not even prescribe antinausea medications for my patients, for these have also been implicated as a possible contributing factor in birth defects. Nausea can usually be prevented or controlled by nutritional therapy. If I feel it is necessary to prescribe any medication for you, I will discuss the need with you thoroughly, so that we can come to a consensus as to the need. I expect you to take responsibility for your own health, and I will take your opinions seriously.

"Of course you know that alcohol and tobacco are detrimental to the unborn, as we discussed earlier. Marijuana is particularly dangerous. Some do not realize that even the husband's smoking before and during his wife's pregnancy is harmful. Not only may his sperm have been damaged by tobacco, resulting in a defective embryo, but the smoke his wife inhales also has a detrimental effect on the unborn child.''

''I'm glad you've made that clear,'' John interjected. ''Although I don't smoke, it hasn't been easy for me to impress on the athletes at school how harmful smoking is. Some think it's such a 'macho' thing to do! They need to know it can be harmful to their own offspring someday.''

''Yes, not to mention their own health,'' Dr. Gordon agreed. ''But to change the subject, let me explain, Mary, that next month we'll give you a complete physical examination to be sure everything is progressing normally. As a rule, I like to use the first prenatal visit to get acquainted and go over some of these basic items that are so important. Of course, if you had come in later in your pregnancy, or if there were any indications of a problem, we would have given you a complete physical examination right away. But today the nurse will only check your blood pressure, weight, and test a urine sample; these three things will be done each time you come in. We already have your medical history on file. From time to time we'll test your blood to be sure you're not anemic.

''I want you to call me at once if you notice any persistent headache, swelling or puffiness of your legs or other parts of your body, or any sudden weight gain. I'm not talking about how much you gain, but any *sudden* increase in weight, as these things are danger signals and should be treated at once. Call me right away, too, if you have any vaginal bleeding.

''Normal intercourse is all right, if it is gentle. Of course, if miscarriage threatens it will be necessary to avoid intercourse until we are certain the danger is past. During the later weeks of pregnancy it may be helpful for the two of you to explore positions in which John's weight is not on your abdomen. This is for Mary's comfort only, as it would not hurt the baby.

''Now, it is very important, Mary, that you master the art of relaxation. Learning to relax during pregnancy will make it possible for your baby to be born without your needing sedation, or with very little. Not only will you have a happier, more comfortable labor this way, but it will be safer, too.''

''That's something I've wanted to ask you about, doctor,'' Mary said soberly. ''I've heard so many awful things about women suffering whenever a baby is born, but I just can't believe that it was meant to be that way. It doesn't fit with what I've always been taught about the Creator being a God of love. It seems to me that when he gives us a little baby it ought to be a really happy time—but even Mother won't talk about when Jo Lynn and I were born!''

"I'm glad you asked this, Mary," he answered her, in the same sober vein, "if it's troubled you. You see, we doctors have learned that babies can be born not only without a mother's suffering, but with great happiness for her, in the majority of cases. Even for the small percentage of mothers whose deliveries present difficulties, the ability to relax will make the needed medication more effective. I've changed from my former approach to obstetrics—and it takes a real struggle with our pride for us doctors to admit we've been wrong about anything or to change our minds! But I feel so differently about obstetrics now that sometimes, Mary, when I remember how I delivered babies like you, I feel that I should apologize to your mothers!

"When the labor of childbirth begins, the muscles of the uterus, or womb, contract periodically, gradually and gently pushing the baby's head out of the uterus down into the birth canal. This is the first stage of labor. As the uterine muscles contract, they also shorten, drawing up the cervical muscles of the uterine outlet so that the baby can slip through easily.

"The uterine muscles are 'smooth' muscles, similar in structure and function to muscles of other internal organs that rhythmically contract and relax, such as the stomach, with few nerve endings. A normal uterine contraction causes no more pain than a normal stomach contraction. But during labor the tightening of these uterine muscles causes it to tilt forward against the muscles of the abdominal wall, and the baby begins to move downward against the muscles and tissues of the pelvic floor. When a woman feels the slight pressures from these changes of position, she becomes aware that labor has begun. Her reaction to this awareness determines whether or not she will begin to have pain.

The skeletal muscular tissues of the abdomen, back, and pelvic floor are liberally supplied with sensory and pain receptors. If these muscles are contracted, in fear of the contracting uterus, pain is caused, not in the uterus itself, but in all these surrounding tissues. This is the so-called pain of labor, and it really hurts! But if the surrounding muscular tissues remain relaxed and do not resist the uterus in its work, the cause for pain is absent. Thus a woman creates her own pain by inadvertently tightening her abdominal muscles and thus interfering with the normal work of the uterus.

"So you can see how important it is for a person to be able to 'let go' of muscle tension throughout the body for a comfortable birth. But muscular relaxation is also tremendously important for basic good health in all of life, so you should both learn it well.

"We hear a great deal these days about the stress diseases: nervous indigestion, colitis, ulcers, headaches, backaches, high blood pressure, chronic fatigue, heart trouble. All of these things, in addition to pain in childbirth, are among the adverse effects of stress on the human body. We cannot get rid of stress in our environment, but we can learn to respond without an excess of muscular tension. Some people are so 'up tight' that they never relax their skeletal muscles properly, even in sleep!

"Relaxation is a condition in which muscle tone throughout the body is reduced to a minimum, and all the skeletal muscles are 'limp,' 'loose,' with as little tension as a cooked string of spaghetti or a wet noodle. Why waste muscle energy when we don't need it? We need to give serious thought to the advice of the wise aged black man who was asked how he'd managed to live so long. He said, 'Well, when ah works, ah works hard, but when ah sits, ah sits loose!' "

"This makes sense to me," John spoke up. "I think we live in an awfully tense, fidgety, restless way most of the time today. I try to explain to my athletes that if their muscles are tense all the time their coordination will be poor, and they're bound to fumble the ball a lot more. They have to learn when muscle tension is needed, and how to 'let go' the tension in those same muscles when the tension is not needed in order to play a good game."

"Exactly," the doctor said. "Now, Mary, I'm going to lift your hand to see how well you can relax. You are to let it drop onto the table. No, you're putting it down with your muscles, not letting it drop. Here," he took hold of her forearm again, "let me shake your arm so the hand flops like a leaf in the wind."

Patiently he worked with her until she was able to relax the muscles of her hand enough to let it drop limply. "Now," he said, laying her forearm on the table, her hand down, placing his finger across the back of her wrist, "lift one of your fingers, and tell me when you can feel which muscles are working."

"My finger muscles," Mary said.

"Do it very, very slowly this time and tell me what muscles you feel working *before* you begin to lift your finger, as soon as you feel any tension at all."

"Why, I can feel the muscles pull on the back of my hand and up the forearm, even before I lift my finger!" Mary exclaimed.

"Exactly. Now let's do it again, and this time 'let go' this muscle tension just as soon as you begin to feel it, when you just *think* about raising your finger." Mary did so.

"I see what you're driving at, doctor," John said. "You want her to learn what tension feels like in every muscle, so she'll know when she's *not* relaxed."

"Right," the doctor agreed. Turning to Mary, he said, "I'm giving you these instructions on how to relax, Mary." He handed her a small folder. "The next time you come in I'll test you to see how well you've learned to do it. You can help her with this, John.

"In fact," he added, "it's my conviction that the husband has a most important role to perform throughout his wife's experience. You can help Mary in many ways, John, by encouraging her to learn proper relaxation, to follow my instructions about nutrition and exercises. You should also master the relaxation techniques, John, for your own benefit. And I'm sure the nutritional guidance will be helpful to your own health, not only encouraging Mary to eat properly, but doing so yourself. Junk food never made anyone healthy!

"But most of all, John, you can help Mary by your patient understanding. We have learned in recent years that the psychological and emotional well-being of the unborn child is greatly affected by the mother's emotional health—whether or not she feels loved and protected by her husband. Then when it is time for the baby to be born you will want to be with her and help her throughout the labor and birth. You will be learning in these coming weeks what your role as husband can be to help make it a wonderful experience for you both."

"Thanks, Doctor, for the good advice. And I intend to be with Mary," John added emphatically. "There are so many stories of the useless husband pacing the floor or reading a paper upside down, while his wife's in another room giving birth. It annoys me. I want to help Mary in every way I can."

"But how can we know when our baby's supposed to be born?" Mary asked. "Can you tell exactly when it will be?"

"Not exactly, Mary, but within a few days, either way. When was your last menstrual period?"

"Let's see." Mary thought a moment. "It was about July twentieth. I can check for sure when we get home."

"To arrive at the approximate date, figure back three months and add seven days. That would be April twenty-seventh, wouldn't it?" He marked it down on her chart. "Do you have any other questions? If not, you may go into the laboratory now, Mary, so the nurse can check the things I've indicated.

"By the way," he called them back as they turned to go out the door, "why don't you ask Carolyn Thebes about how her babies were born? She's had three beautiful natural births, and she can spend more time explaining how it should be than I can."

"I'll do that," Mary said. "Thank you for all the time you've given us already." Before following the nurse down the hall, she said to John, "You know who Carolyn is, don't you, dear? She's Paulie's mother."

"You're not really relaxed, Mary," John said to her that evening as she was trying it for the first time. "Your lips are twitching, and you keep shifting your left foot a little."

Mary was lying on her back on the floor, one pillow under her head and shoulders, and another large pillow under her knees. Her feet were about twelve inches apart with each foot falling outward. She was trying to lie as limply and loosely as a rag doll. When John spoke to her, she concentrated on her left foot a moment, tightened its muscles just a little, and then let it fall more limply outward than before. To relax her lips, she tightened them, and then let them fall slightly apart. She squeezed her eyes tighter, before letting the muscles of her eyelids and forehead become limp, too.

"Much better," John told her. "Now lie perfectly still—the folder says you shouldn't shift or move a muscle for thirty minutes. You've got twenty minutes to go. I'll tell you when time's up." He set his watch on the arm of the couch where he could see it and picked up the newspaper. Pulling the footstool toward him, he placed his feet on it, letting them fall limply outward in a relaxed manner, as Mary's were. He took a slow deep breath and then let the muscles of his abdomen and back relax, so that he slumped down comfortably against the back of the couch.

After lying down, Mary had begun relaxing by taking a deep breath, holding it for a count of five, and then letting it out slowly, slowly,

slowly, letting her abdomen and chest wall collapse of its own weight limply as she exhaled. She had paused a second or two, then taken another deep breath, this time concentrating on letting her abdomen rise, rather than her chest, and again she had let her abdominal muscles become limper and limper as she let her breath out slowly. She continued breathing in this way several times after John spoke to her, each time letting all the joints and muscles of her entire body become more limp with each outgoing breath. Soon she was breathing deeply and evenly without needing to give it any more thought. Her arms and legs were beginning to prickle and seemed almost numb, as if they were becoming detached from her body, and she felt as if she were about to float off into space.

"Time's up," John said, when the thirty minutes had passed. "Get up slowly, so you won't get dizzy."

"There's nothing very hard about that!" Mary exclaimed, as she sat up. "I don't think I've ever been so completely relaxed in my whole life!"

"Remember that Dr. Gordon said you must do this *faithfully,*" John warned her. "I'm going to check up on you. You're supposed to learn to become completely limp within a minute or two after lying down."

"I wasn't very relaxed until a few minutes before you called time, but I don't think it'll take so long next time, now that I know how to do it. And I *intend* to practice faithfully, for my baby's sake especially."

"I'm all for you, honey," John encouraged her, as he drew her down onto the couch beside him. "Why don't we read through these instructions once more," he suggested, as he flipped the folder open again, "just to be sure we're doing this right."

RELAXATION

Learning to Recognize Tension and Its Release

There is no such thing as a relaxation "exercise," as the two are direct opposites. But follow the procedure below until you are sure you can recognize the difference between tension and relaxation in your own body.

• Make your hand slowly into a fist, noticing what the muscles feel like as they tighten. Slowly, slowly, "let go" of the tension in the muscles of your hand, noticing at each step how it feels. When the hand seems completely limp, let it relax still more, and more, noticing carefully how it feels as it becomes completely relaxed. Repeat with the other hand, slowly making a fist, slowly relaxing the hand muscles, paying careful attention to how it feels at all stages.

• Tighten the muscles of the right arm slowly, observing the "pull" of the muscles throughout the arm. Very slowly release the muscular tension. When the arm seems completely limp, relax it some more. Relax it still further.

• Repeat this with the left arm, then with each foot, and then with each leg. Lift each leg slowly, noticing how it feels, then let it fall limply. Relax the muscles further. When it seems completely limp, "let go" the muscles still more. You will be surprised at how much tension is still there to "let go"!

• Now tighten the muscles of your chest and shoulders, slowly, slowly, so you can feel each muscle pulling. Now slowly relax them, letting the shoulders droop and the chest collapse, continually noticing how different the muscles feel as they relax.

• Tighten the muscles of your face and neck slowly, and frown. Slowly relax these muscles, thinking all the time of how it feels. When your face seems completely relaxed, relax your forehead and eyelids still more. Relax your neck slowly, until it droops forward on your chest, too limp to support your head.

• Tighten the muscles of the pelvic floor (the area between the legs, including the anus, vagina, and urethra). Hold for a count of three, and then relax slowly, slowly, more and more, and more. Still more.

Procedure for Daily Relaxation

• Empty the bladder before beginning, and remove all tight clothing —shoes, belts, collars, etc.

• Lie on your back on a firm bed, or on a folded blanket on the floor, with one or more pillows under your head and shoulders, whatever is comfortable for you, and place another pillow under your knees. (In later pregnancy it will be more comfortable for you to lie on one side, as will be explained later on.) It may be more comfortable to use one pillow under each knee. Roll the pillows so that the knees are supported four or five inches off the floor and are several inches apart. Rest the arms on the floor, with the elbows bent slightly outward. No part of the body should rest on any other, and every joint should be slightly bent.

• Take a slow, relaxed breath deep into the chest and abdomen, and let it out slowly, relaxing the chest and abdominal wall as the air is released. Pause a moment before taking another breath, then breathe in slowly, breathe out slowly, in slowly, out slowly, relaxing the muscles more and more with each outgoing breath. This is called *sleep breathing,* the abdominal wall gently rising and falling as if you were asleep, and the breathing becoming slower and slower until it is barely noticeable.

• Go limp all over as quickly as possible, letting all joints and limbs be as loose as if you were "falling through the floor."

• Do not shift or move for thirty minutes, even to look at the time. Set an alarm or have someone call when time is up.

• Arms and legs will soon seem detached, as if "floating." They may have transient "pins and needles" as relaxation deepens.

• When the time is up, get up slowly to avoid dizziness.

• Relax all muscles in this manner near the middle of each day. Do it again on going to bed. You will go to sleep quickly and "sleep like a baby."

6. The Joyful Mother of Children

Blessed are all who fear the Lord,
who walk in his ways. . . .
Blessings and prosperity will be yours.
Your wife will be like a fruitful vine
within your house;
your sons will be like olive shoots
around your table.
—*Psalm 128:2,3,* NIV

"Why Mary! Come on in!" Carolyn greeted her warmly as she held the door open. "I haven't seen you since the day of the wedding. You look marvelous! And what a lovely outfit! This *is* a surprise."

"It does seem like a long time since I was here," Mary said, when Carolyn stopped talking long enough for her to answer. "Just think!" she said dreamily, "I was still Mary Johnson then. It seems like years ago."

Carolyn drew up a chair for Mary near the table where she had been working on a pile of mending. "You don't mind if I keep sewing while we visit, do you?" she asked, picking up the button jar and a small pair of overalls.

"Not at all," Mary answered. "Carolyn," she asked, after glancing around the room and noticing the sewing machine placed in the middle of the playpen, "what in the world have you done *that* for?"

Carolyn chuckled as she explained. "Baby Greg is always unhappy when I put him in there, but if I let him out, he and Julie keep trying to climb onto my lap while I'm sewing, or stepping on the machine pedal by mistake, so—I decided to put the machine where they couldn't reach it. Now they can play happily in the room, and I get into the playpen and sew in peace."

"It'd take a genius to think of a solution like that!" Mary teased her, "or a nut," she added slyly. "It seems so quiet here today. Is

Paulie in school? It must be a help to have him out of the house part of the time.''

"Paulie really enjoys kindergarten,'' Carolyn replied, ''but Julie is so lonesome with just the baby, that I often wish he were still here to play with her. By the way, I'm terribly sorry about his dropping the ring at your wedding. I'd stitched it to the pillow with only one loop so it could be pulled off easily, but he must have picked at it beforehand so it fell off.''

"Don't worry about that the least bit,'' Mary reassured her. ''Thinking back on it now, it's even funny—he'd tried so hard to do everything just right, bless his heart.''

"Let's hear the news about you, Mary,'' Carolyn suggested, reaching for another small pair of overalls to mend. ''I didn't expect to see you in a maternity dress already.''

Mary smiled. ''Mother tried hard to convince me to wait longer before buying one, especially since we've been married such a short time—but I've been so happy and excited I've wanted everybody to know about our baby.''

"That's an awfully pretty dress,'' Carolyn observed, ''but you'll sure get tired of it before nine months are over. I've several smocks you can borrow—it's more fun to have several changes. Of course, everyone in Pinedale will know where you got them!''

"I don't mind if they do. That's kind of you, Carolyn.'' Mary hesitated a moment, and then said, ''You know, this is one of the things I came to talk to you about today—I mean about having my baby. Dr. Gordon said I ought to come see you as you'd had three natural births and would have more time to explain things to me than he had.''

"I'll be glad to help you. Ralph and I want to do all we can to help other couples have happy times when their babies are born, as we have. And this is a good time to talk while Julie and Greg are taking their naps.'' She glanced toward the bedroom door to reassure herself that they were still asleep, and then began telling Mary her own experiences.

"We waited eight years, Ralph and I, for our first baby. We both had tests of all kinds that showed that there was nothing wrong, but still we didn't have any success. We prayed about our problem, too, until finally I decided to stop fretting and just relax and trust God. I thought of the verse in the Bible that says, 'He gives the barren woman a home, making her the joyous mother of children,' and I felt that if it was God's will for me, I would really be a mother someday—either to my own, or to someone else's homeless child.

"We had begun to apply to adoption agencies when, one day, we found that our dreams had come true. I began to experience what I had always felt in my heart—that carrying and giving birth to a baby is one of the most wonderful things that can happen to a woman. I wouldn't trade one moment of my experiences for anything in the world!"

"You certainly sound different from others I've heard," Mary commented wryly.

"That's because a lot of women don't understand a natural birth," Carolyn explained, "and they confuse it with stoicism—but it's really so exciting that after Paulie was born, I would have liked to have had a baby every year! The only trouble with *that* is it's too wearing running after too many little tots, when they're so close together.

"When I first became pregnant with Paulie, I went to an obstetrician of good reputation where Ralph was stationed. He did a routine examination but explained nothing to me. As I was going out, he patted my arm kindly and said, 'Cheer up, Mrs. Thebes. This is a sickness that only lasts for nine months!' Believe me, I never went back to him again! A *sickness*, of all things! To me it was a privilege to be pregnant, and I was very happy.

"Before long we moved to Pinedale, and I went to Dr. Gordon. I'll never forget his response when I told him I wanted to have a natural birth. He said, 'Carolyn, I'll do everything I know to help you have the kind of birth experience you want.'

"I asked if I could have my baby at home, and he said yes, since I was in good health and very careful about my nutrition. Of course, if any indication of a problem arose during the pregnancy or labor, he said I would be better off in the hospital.

"He told me that it is important for birth to take place in as relaxing a setting as possible, and there is no place more relaxing for most well-prepared women than at home. He said that Ralph was welcome to be with me during the labor and birth—that he *ought* to be there—and that Ralph could even 'catch the baby' in his own hands. He would show Ralph what to do and would stand by ready to help if there was any problem. I could hardly believe my ears!

"Dr. Gordon explained that another safety factor in the home is that a woman is free to move about, as moderate activity helps stimulate labor. A woman need only lie down when she is tired, or if she is unable to relax sufficiently unless lying down. 'At home,' he added, 'she can assume any position for the actual birth most comfortable for her—squatting, kneeling, standing (leaning over a chair for support), propped up in bed, or lying on her side. The freedom to assume any position without inhibition,' he explained, 'helps her press out her baby more comfortably. The mother can then put her baby to breast at once, while waiting for the afterbirth to be expelled.'

"He did say that I would have to prepare for a natural birth ahead of time in order to have the best possible experience, since women in our culture are often tense and unprepared for the sensations of such a completely physiological event. Just wishing won't help! Mary, you're really blessed to have such an understanding and well-informed doctor. Be sure to do everything he tells you, and learn all you can."

"I certainly will," Mary assured her soberly, "though I don't know if I should have my baby at home or not. I'd need to learn more about it. But, Carolyn, I want a happy experience like yours. Can you tell me what happens when a baby is born? I mean, what does it actually *feel* like to have a baby?"

"It's this way," Carolyn explained patiently. "When labor first begins, the uterus, or womb, contracts rhythmically in order to push the baby gradually out through the cervix, the mouth of the womb, into the birth canal. This is called the *first stage of labor,* when the uterine muscles tighten, relax, tighten, relax. God planned it this way, so that the blood supply of these muscles would be constantly replenished, and so that pain would be avoided by having the uterine muscles alternately work and rest. The cervix is thinned out and stretched slowly, little by little, to allow the baby's head to be eased through it—rather the way one might stretch a rubber band to slip a ball through.

"During this period you have to relax all muscles *completely.* You see, you feel pain in labor whenever the muscles of the abdominal wall are kept tense while the uterus is rising during contractions. When a mother does this—usually without realizing she's doing it—the aching in these abdominal muscles increases with each contraction and soon spreads throughout the muscles of the pelvic area, making them ache, across the muscles of the lower back and hips, and even down into her thighs, so she literally 'aches all over' during the remainder of the labor, with increasing intensity. Each time a woman grabs onto something when a contraction begins and grits her teeth against the pain, her pain increases. But if you learn to relax properly, letting all muscles become 'limp,' this brings miraculous relief, no matter how intense the contractions. I let myself become so limp I felt as if I was falling through the bed! With Paulie I had a long first stage—almost fifteen and a half hours, but during this whole time I was so relaxed that the contractions didn't hurt. I could feel my uterus drawing up into power-ful contractions as labor progressed, but I just allowed my awareness to encourage its powerful rise and kept my body limp. I found that if I resisted the strength of the contractions the *least bit,* it would begin to hurt.''

Carolyn had forgotten all about her mending by now, and a small torn blouse lay untouched in her lap. ''Near the end of this stage comes the *transition period,* she continued. ''This is when the baby's head is finally being pushed on through the cervix into the birth canal. These contractions are the longest and the most powerful ones of the whole labor. But by keeping the muscles of my abdomen completely limp as the uterus contracted, I was able to experience the changing sensations without being afraid.''

Mary leaned forward in her chair. ''But how can you do that?'' she asked breathlessly.

Carolyn smiled. ''Well, you see the important thing is to have no muscular resistance to the rise of the uterine contractions. In early labor when one is doing light activity, it is enough to stop when a contraction begins, lean over the back of a chair or something and release all tension in the abdominal muscles until the contraction passes. I spent part of my labor in a rocking chair. During a contrac-tion I would stop rocking and go limp all over, my head falling for-ward and my feet resting on a step stool, until the contraction passed. As labor progressed, I was only comfortable lying down. It's important to be lying in the correct position, either curled up slightly on the left side, or propped up in the bed in the 'recliner chair' position with pillows under one's knees. A woman should *never* lie on her back in labor. I was comfortable lying on my side, with my knees drawn up and my head bent forward. It was easier for me to keep my abdomen relaxed during contractions in this position.

''Then, in this relaxed position, as labor progresses, a woman auto-matically begins to breathe a little faster. The uterus is working harder and needs more oxygen, so deeper, even, in-and-out breaths are needed. It's like the breathing one does when taking a brisk walk, except that only the uterus is working. All the rest of the body must stay limp. The only thing to remember about breathing is to *slow it down*, if you start tensing up or breathing too fast.

"At this time the baby's head is pressed against the lower spine, and this can cause a backache. Ralph rubbed my back and it was a big help. But this transition period is very short, Mary. It lasts only for a half hour or so, or an hour and a half at the most if the contractions are not very close together.

"After these few minutes the baby's head slipped through the cervix into the birth canal, and I felt much better. (This is the beginning of the *second stage of labor*.) My backache disappeared. The contractions came farther apart, so I rested limply between them. I felt the urge to bear down with each contraction, and was surprised to find that this not only didn't hurt, but felt good!

"At this time I wanted to sit up, so that gravity could help me press the baby down more easily. I tried sitting on the edge of a stool, with Ralph behind me for support, and pushed this way for a while. But then I felt like getting back on the bed, so Ralph put pillows at the head of the bed and helped me get comfortable propped up against them. He rolled pillows under my knees so that my legs could stay relaxed and drawn up between contractions.

"When a contraction began I took a deep breath in, let it out, took another deep breath and breathed out *slowly* through my mouth and throat while I leaned over and pushed, holding onto my knees for support. Ralph positioned himself behind me on the bed so that I was totally supported while pushing. It was strengthening to feel his strong arms around me. Ralph reminded me (as Dr. Gordon had taught us) to push firmly but not too hard, to take new breaths whenever I felt like it and to stop pushing whenever I wanted. He said that if it hurt to push, I should listen to my body and not push until it was more comfortable to do so. Long, hard pushing or pushing too soon are no more effective than pushing while breathing out slowly, just at the peak of the contraction. After a few contractions, I learned how to get in tune with what my body was doing, and I could tell my pushing was more effective. One reason hard pushing and long breath-holding is unwise is because the vaginal opening needs time to thin out and open as gently as the cervix did, since forcing it open too fast might make it tear. Also, pushing until purple in the face depletes the oxygen to baby and mother and increases her blood pressure. It simply is not necessary.

"This is the really exciting time in labor, Mary! After about an hour and a half the baby's head began to press against my rectum, and I thought I had to have a bowel movement. I didn't realize that this was my baby! As the head came further down this sensation completely disappeared, and I began to get a prickly 'pins and needles' sensation as the baby's head bulged against the *perineum*—that's the outlet—and I knew my baby was about to be born. This sensation of fullness is like something you've never felt before! Some women get badly frightened and tighten up the outlet, making it hurt, or tear. I was able to keep my outlet relaxed, to "allow" it to stretch further, until the prickly, burning sensation began to disappear. Dr. Gordon had explained that this is because the pressure of the baby against the perineum blocks the circulation somewhat as it widens. Anyway, I couldn't feel anything there. Do you know how it feels when circulation is gradually cut off when your foot falls asleep—how first it feels tingly and finally numb?

Mary nodded, fascinated with what she was learning.

"The outlet is 'asleep' during the actual birth, so all I felt was the bulging pressure of the baby's head which had dilated the birth canal to its fullest capacity. And then I felt the exciting fast passage of his little body moving from the vagina as the birth was completed. The pleasant physical sensations within the birth canal and the emotional climax of this moment were too exciting to describe! Dr. Gordon told Ralph to have me pant in and out as the head was born, so that the baby would be born slowly and I would not tear. Ralph supported the baby's head as he was born. Then I pushed the baby's body out—and there was Paulie!"

Carolyn paused and gazed out the window with a faraway look, recalling that most happy moment, which she had experienced three times. Then she finished her story.

"Ralph handed the baby to me and I placed him against my breast. Ralph pulled a blanket over us both. Baby and I snuggled under the blanket while I delivered the afterbirth. (The blanket was around my middle at this point!) Having baby against my breast helped my uterus contract again, and after only two or three contractions the placenta and sac in which the baby had lived slipped out. (The *placenta* is the organ that nourishes the baby, and the *amniotic sac* is the bag of waters in which baby lives. The *umbilical cord* links the baby to the placenta for nourishment.)

"I felt I had just taken part in the greatest miracle in the world! I felt like both laughing and crying, though I didn't really show it, as I don't like to display my emotions. But Ralph! He was jubilant!

"Dr. Gordon examined the afterbirth carefully to be sure it was all there and checked to see if I needed any stitches. (I didn't). He explained how to massage my abdomen every few minutes to be sure I could feel the uterus firm underneath. It must stay contracted to prevent hemorrhaging. I had fixed a light lunch during early labor, and now the three of us enjoyed it together. After making sure I was all right, the doctor left.

"Was there much difference between your first labor and the others?" Mary asked.

"No," Carolyn said, "not in the sensations themselves. With Paulie each stage was longer and I did get more tired. With Julie and Greg the first stage of labor seemed shorter, perhaps because I was more confident and kept working around the house. In fact, I was able to handle my contractions so well during labor with Greg that I put a pie in the oven during the transition period, when I finally had to leave the kitchen and go into the bedroom. The second stage lasted only a few minutes. Dr. Gordon was already there, and we had spread sterile coverings on the floor so that I could give birth while squatting, leaning back against the wall for support."

She thought back a moment, smiling to herself. "The pie got a little burned before Ralph remembered to take it out. Dr. Gordon said he enjoyed coming to my birthings because he always got a feast besides!

"But let me tell you about the second stage with Paulie. I was propped up on the bed to push, and made such awful noises while pressing down and breathing out at the same time, that I sounded rather like a dying cow!"

Mary laughed appreciatively.

"I was really embarrassed to be making so much noise, because I wasn't in pain. I tried to explain this to Ralph, and he just held me closer in his arms and said, 'I believe you, honey. You've convinced me. But did you know you're making me work hard too?' I looked back over my shoulder and made a face at him for his teasing, but then another contraction came on, so we had to get back to work.

"I was more tired after Paulie's birth, but felt jubilant. After a few hours rest I felt wonderful. And after Julie's and Greg's births I felt so strong each time that I could have picked up my baby and walked a mile!"

"I'm not sure I'd want a home birth," Mary mused, "at least not the first time, though I want a happy experience like yours."

"I understand how you feel, Mary."

"Carolyn, what made you want a natural birth in the first place? I know why *I* want it, because I've always felt in my heart that God made me the way I am, and I'm not afraid to trust him that he made me the right way. But most people don't understand how I feel."

"There was no one thing, really," Carolyn answered thoughtfully. "I've felt like you, ever since I was in my teens, but I never had anyone I could talk to about it. Then, one experience of Ralph's and mine really set me to thinking seriously about childbirth. A student from Indonesia spent the day with us, and in the course of our conversation he began to tell us about childbirth customs in his country.

"He said that the Indonesian women just leave their work in the fields for an hour or so to squat and bear their children and shortly afterward are back at work again. But one time he overheard some of their white missionary friends *laughing* among themselves over the way the 'ignorant' Indonesian women gave birth to their babies.

"He seemed very bitter about this. He said he saw no reason why the Indonesian women, who are healthy and muscular from their work in the fields, should go home to bear their children and suffer like the missionary women. He told us that the Indonesian women he knew accept childbirth as a perfectly normal process, and it doesn't seem to trouble them.

"That conversation set me to thinking," Carolyn said. "What about the 'curse of Eve' tradition? If God meant for *all* women to suffer in giving birth, why did the Indonesian women escape it but not the missionary women? Then, one day when I was doing visitation for our church, I stopped at the house of a Chinese family."

Mary sat listening in rapt attention.

"Several of the children in this family were in our Sunday school. The mother looked so young I could hardly believe that she had *ten* children! Her last baby was only a week old, and while the other little ones tumbled about on the floor, one child who had been in my class climbed into my lap and put her arms around me as the mother told me all about her latest birth experience.

" 'Usually it's nothing,' she told me, 'you know, just a *push, push* —like a *one, two.*' She said she could deliver her babies by herself and had always gone about her daily work the day after a child was born.

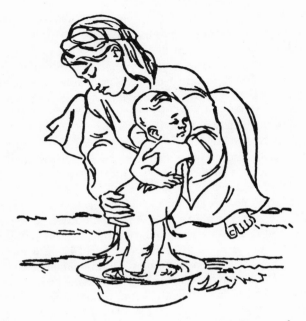

Vietnamese mother squatting to give her baby a road-side bath. Notice how she sits right on her heels, her knees wide apart, like the correct position for giving birth. This drawing is a copy of a photograph.

But she had always called in a midwife—just in case something should go wrong.

"Two of her babies were born before the midwife arrived, and she had delivered them and taken care of them by herself. She was most annoyed that she'd still had to pay the midwife the regular fee just the same!

"But this time, she said, she was glad the midwife came as the baby was 'a-reverse.' At first I didn't understand what she meant, but she gestured with her hands as if she were holding something and turning it over. Then I realized she meant that she'd had a breech baby—its little bottom presented first, instead of its head.

"She told how her husband had been assisting at the birth. Once the midwife asked him to put the lubricating cream on her sterile gloves, but he squirted so much from the tube that her hands kept slipping as she tried to turn the baby's position to make the birth easier. The mother beamed as she told how they had all laughed over this and how the midwife had had to change her gloves so that she could try again.

"I could hardly believe my ears! Here she had been in the midst of a most difficult delivery, and yet she said that she had been *laughing!* So I asked her if she had ever had any anesthesia.

"She was completely puzzled by the word at first. Then she understood and shook her head. Mary, I can't tell you how I felt that day! Here she'd had a breech baby and had to work so hard that she said she'd been too tired to take over her full household responsibilities until the baby was three days old!

"Her cheerful, normal attitude toward giving birth made a profound impression on me. I couldn't help thinking of Sarah in the Bible—bearing a child when she was an old, old woman, who yet said, 'God hath made me to laugh, so that all that hear will laugh with me.'

"My interest was really aroused now," Carolyn continued. "It was right after my visit with the Chinese lady that I turned completely away from any confidence in 'orthodox' obstetrics and began to study the natural childbirth philosophy in earnest. I began to look for more items about how native women bear their children. I read, for example, that Laotian women bear their babies more easily than we do, although some of their customs don't add to the mother's comfort—like having their husbands blow in their ears throughout their labor, so the baby will have enough air!"

Just then Julie appeared in the doorway, pink-cheeked and warm from her nap. She climbed into Carolyn's lap and tugged at her blouse, murmuring, "Nummies, Mama." Carolyn settled her at the breast, and Julie watched Mary shyly out of the corner of her eye as she nursed briefly.

"But aren't you still nursing baby Greg?" Mary asked incredulously. "How can you nurse them *both?*"

"Julie isn't ready to wean yet," Carolyn smiled. "I have plenty of milk for both babies. You see, Julie nurses very little. She wants it mainly for comfort, not for food. She only nurses once or twice a day—after a nap, before bedtime, or when she's hurt. And since the milk supply is directly related to how much a mother nurses, my body easily produces enough." Buttoning her blouse a moment later she said to Julie, "Why not sit on Mary's lap, honey, while I go see if baby brother is waking up?"

Julie hid her face as Mary picked her up but didn't resist. A moment later Carolyn came back into the room turning the pages of a book. "I began thumbing through books on anthropology," she said, "to try to find some explanation for women suffering in our culture but not in many of the others. Margaret Mead, the well-known anthropologist, says the majority of women suffer severe pain in childbirth, *or* accept giving birth matter-of-factly, depending on the culture in which they live. She says that pain, when it occurs, is not due to the physiology of the birth process, but to the attitudes toward birth that a woman has 'learned' from her culture. Listen to this!" Carolyn sat down and began to read from the page she had marked:

So child-birth may be experienced according to the phrasing given it by the culture, as an experience that is dangerous and painful, interesting and engrossing, matter-of-fact and mildly hazardous. . . . Whether they are allowed to see births or not, men contribute their share to the way in which child-birth is viewed, and I have seen male informants writhe on the floor, in magnificent pantomime of a painful delivery, who have never themselves seen or heard a woman in labour. . . . Men who feel copulation as aggressive may have different phantasies about the dire effects on their wives of their dreadful uncontrolled aggressive desires from men who feel copulation as pleasant, who may share in a cultural phrasing which insists that the child "sleeps quietly until it is time to be born, then puts its hands above its head and comes out." . . .

It cannot be argued that child-birth is both an unbearable pain and a bearable pain, both a situation from which all women naturally shrink in dread and a situation towards which all women naturally move readily and happily, both a danger to be avoided and a consummation devoutly to be desired. At least one aspect must be regarded as learned. . . . There seems some reason to believe that the male imagination, undisciplined and uninformed by immediate bodily clues or immediate bodily experiences, may have contributed disproportionately to the cultural superstructure of belief and practice regarding childbearing. It is perhaps not without significance that in those Polynesian societies where the male participates in his wife's delivery as a husband, not as a magician or a priest, there is an extremely simple, uncomplicated attitude towards birth; women do not scream, but instead work, and men need no self-imposed expiatory activities afterwards.[1]

"Why, then," Mary exclaimed, understanding the point, "whether or not a woman experiences severe pain in childbirth depends on whether or not she has been conditioned by the culture she lives in to expect it!'' She thought a moment, frowning. ''But what about the teaching of the Bible? Doesn't it say that God has condemned *all* the women of the world to suffer in childbirth because of Eve?''

''This'll surprise you, Mary,'' Carolyn said emphatically, ''but the Bible doesn't say that at all! I brought this problem up with Pastor Dirkson. He looked up the meaning of all the Hebrew and Greek words used about childbirth in the Bible, and he discovered that there is nothing there that says women are meant to suffer pain when they bear a child. I want you and John to go ask him about this. He can explain it much better than I can.

''Incidentally, it's interesting that it's we mothers who can really promote natural childbirth. Doctors have seen so many women suffer that they hesitate to believe a birth is possible without it. And preachers—well, how can they go around telling women they shouldn't be suffering in childbirth when they are? But we women can spread the word because we *know!*''

''Carolyn,'' Mary said, as she put Julie down and rose to leave, ''I just can't tell you how much this day has meant for me! I thought I was the only woman in the world who felt the way I do about having babies—but now I know I have lots of company!''

NOTE

1. Margaret Mead, *Male and Female* (New York: Morrow, 1949), pp. 236–238. Reprinted by permission.

7. A Kindness in His Justice

Oh that men would praise the Lord for his goodness, and for his wonderful works to the children of men!
—*Psalm 107:8, KJV*

Mary and John were not aware of the threadbare carpet on the living room floor of the parsonage, worn thin by the feet of many seekers after counsel and hope. Nor did they notice the many patiently mended little places in the faded curtains hanging over the old-fashioned bay window. But they were aware of the crackling fire in the fireplace shedding a warmth throughout the room and of something undefinable in the peaceful atmosphere of this home that made them feel at ease.

"This is delicious nut bread, Mrs. Dirkson," Mary remarked.

"Thank you, Mary," replied the pastor's wife. "I've learned to make it from scratch using wheat germ and other whole grains. It takes longer, but tastes so much better and is much more nutritious. Would you care for another glass of milk with it?"

"No thanks," Mary replied, and then added ruefully, "I'm afraid I'm not a very good cook. John likes to cook better than I do, and does a lot of it."

"She's being modest," John defended her. "I haven't complained, have I, Mary? The only thing I've really missed is cheese soufflé like Aunt Em makes."

"I don't know much about soufflés," Mary admitted, "So I've been afraid to try—but someday I'll surprise you!"

"I'll be glad to show you how, Mary," Mrs. Dirkson offered, "if you'll come over some morning. It's not hard once you've learned how." Just then Pastor Dirkson came in the back door. "Come on in the living room, Carl," his wife called. "John and Mary are already here."

The pastor hung up his coat and came into the room. "Sorry I've kept you waiting," he said, nodding a greeting to them both. He took a chair near the fire, leaning forward to warm his hands. "I paid Mrs.

Arkwright a call this evening, but it's hard to break away from her, so I'm later than I'd intended to be. Poor soul—she's so lonely.''

"Mother goes over to see her quite often," Mary said. "I suppose I could stop by once in a while, too."

"She'd certainly appreciate a visit, Mary. No more thank you, Ruth. Come join us," he said as he finished the slice of nut bread his wife had served him. He pulled out a chair for her beside him and reached for his Bible. "I understand you've come to see me about the same problem that worried Carolyn Thebes. Is that right?"

"Yes," John replied. "Mary told me about her visit with Carolyn the other day, and this question about the Bible saying that God cursed all women with pain in childbirth really came out into the open. Carolyn said she'd gone over this problem with you and wanted us to come talk to you about it.

"We had quite a discussion with Mary's folks one day," John went on, "about the three basic causes for suffering. We felt that these three were, first, the sinful acts of people which as often as not cause suffering of the innocent; second, calamities of nature; and, third, the presence of an evil force at work in our world. But we don't know where the 'curse of Eve' would fit into this summary."

"That's a good summary, John," the pastor told him. "I assume that by the 'curse of Eve,' you mean that women have been given an unfair punishment of physical pain, while man has been allowed to get by with the lighter punishment of tilling the ground?"

John nodded, so Pastor Dirkson told him, "God didn't discriminate unfairly against women at the outset of our Bible. I've studied every passage in the Bible pertaining to childbirth and checked the English translations against the original languages, and I've found that *there is not one single verse in the entire Bible that mentions any 'curse' on Eve or on all womankind.* On the contrary, a 'curse' is only mentioned as being on those women who did *not* bear a child. In the Bible, the mother of children is portrayed as a woman blessed by God, the barren woman as a woman whom God had judged. Even centuries later, after the time of Christ, this concept was still prevalent among Jews and Christians alike. In an apocryphal account of Anna, the mother of Mary, there's an example of this. Anna's maid berates her in this way:

I cannot wish you a greater curse than you are under, in that God hath shut up your womb, that you should not be a mother in Israel."[1]

The pastor was warming to his subject now, guilty at times of "sermonizing" in his conversation.

"The common interpretation of the 'curse of Eve' is based on one lone verse in the Bible, found in the third chapter of Genesis where the sin of Adam and Eve is recorded. But think back to Eden a moment. After Adam and Eve had sinned, did a wrathful God come storming into the garden in a rage to wreak vengeance on their heads?

"Not at all! A compassionate Creator came calling them, searching for the sinners. It was human beings who had broken fellowship with God, who were no longer at ease in God's holy presence, and who had hidden themselves!

"The revelation of God's great love for sinners begins in Eden. The message of Calvary begins in Eden. God's longing for the sinner to be restored to fellowship with himself ultimately led to his great sacrifice of his own Son, to pay the penalty for humanity's sin. And as a loving God came calling, seeking to reestablish communion with the sinners in the garden, so he's still calling all humankind, longing to restore to fellowship with himself all who'll accept his forgiveness through Calvary. This is the central message of the Bible, the very core of Christianity:

For God so loved the world that he gave his one and only Son, that whoever believes in him shall not perish but have everlasting life.
For as in Adam all die, even so in Christ shall all be made alive.

"But God, though he loved Adam and Eve, and through them the whole human race, and though he provided a means for their forgiveness, still found it necessary to impose a discipline upon them in this temporal life. Why don't we look at Genesis 3:16 and 17."

John opened his own Bible to this passage, sharing it with Mary. The pastor began reading from the King James Version, pointing out the underlying Hebrew word:

"Unto the woman he said, I will greatly multiply thy *sorrow* (*etsev*) and thy conception; in *sorrow* (*etsev*) thou shalt bring forth children.

"Do you notice that the word 'curse' is not used here, and neither is the word 'pain'? But now, let's compare what God says to Eve with what he says to Adam in the following verse:

And unto Adam he said, . . . cursed is the ground for thy sake; in *sorrow* (*etsev*) shalt thou eat of it all the days of thy life."

"The Hebrew words are the same for the man and the woman!" Mary exclaimed.

"Yes, they are. But have you never noticed that the English words, 'sorrow' for Eve and 'sorrow' for Adam are also the same? Notice, too, in the context, that the word 'cursed' is used of the *ground* and of the *serpent,* but not of Adam or Eve. Look now, in the margin[2] of your Bible, at the alternate translation for 'sorrow' in reference to Adam. What is it?"

"It says 'toil,' " Mary answered, looking over John's arm to read the smaller print. "That means hard work. Why, pastor!" she exclaimed again, "that's exactly what Carolyn told me giving birth is like. She said it's hard work! But why is the word 'toil' not in the margin for the woman too, since the Hebrew word is the same for her as for Adam?"

"There's no good reason, Mary," Mrs. Dirkson commented, "except that translators are influenced by the attitudes of the cultures they live in."

"Yes," the pastor agreed. "You see, translators sometimes unconsciously give words a very different meaning from that intended by the original author, simply because they live in different eras, different cultures, and have from childhood looked at many phases of life from different philosophical points of view. This is one reason we must never discontinue the study of the Bible in the original languages."

"Carolyn and I talked about the attitude toward childbirth being different in different cultures," Mary said, seeing his point.

"Yes, that's very true. In the last hundred years especially, biblical scholars have become more and more aware of certain cultural differences between life in Bible times and life in our Western culture. But, unfortunately, they haven't had enough knowledge of anthropology to realize that there are cultural differences in other areas, in attitudes toward childbearing for example. Thus Bible translators and scholars have mistakenly assumed that childbirth is the same the world over and that every mention of it in the Bible meant to the Hebrew women exactly what it means to the women in their own culture.

"But what about the culture of Moses' day and the experiences of the women of that time? We should remember that the Hebrews were what we would call a more primitive race. They were an agricultural, nomadic people, and the sense of family was very strong. Large families are considered a blessing in most agricultural societies, and the

Hebrews considered a woman who had given birth to many children to be highly honored.''

"Carolyn also explained to me that many primitive women give birth more easily and matter-of-factly than in our culture,'' Mary interrupted him.

"That's another good point. Samuel Zwemer, an early missionary to the Arabs, says that Arab women didn't have painful deliveries until *after* their society had been adversely affected by Western culture. Even when trekking across the desert, an Arab woman simply dropped behind the caravan when her labor began. After giving birth to her infant in the sand she would walk, sometimes for many hours, to overtake the caravan, carrying her baby. The experiences of the Hebrew women of the Pentateuch were surely similar to these, since they were of the same Semitic origin and culture.

"Now let's come back to this Hebrew word *etsev* in Genesis, keeping the Hebrew culture in mind. A Hebrew rabbi, Samson Hirsch, who lived a hundred years ago, carefully explains the meaning of this word. He says that *etsev* refers *only* to a mental state, specifically, to that of 'renunciation,' or a 'giving up' of oneself, as in toil.[3]

"Rabbi Hirsch is careful to point out to the Jewish people of his generation that God used the same word, *etsev,* for Eve as for Adam! He says too that God disciplined them not *because* they had sinned but *'for their sakes.'* Eve was to toil to bring forth the fruit of the body, Adam was to toil to bring forth the fruit of the ground, that they might learn to appreciate the good gifts that had been so freely given them before.''

"It's still true, isn't it,'' John observed, "that we don't really appreciate the things we get for nothing, without lifting a finger?''

"Yes, it is, John. This discipline of working for what we receive is really a blessing in disguise.

"Now Rabbi Hirsch also points out most emphatically that the Jews have *never* believed that there was any 'curse' on Adam and Eve but only on the ground and on the serpent. The earliest Christians also make this same distinction.

"But there is something else I'd like you to notice, before we turn to one passage in the New Testament. Ruth, would you please hand me my copy of the Revised Standard Version?'' His wife handed it to him. "Listen:

To the woman he said, 'I will greatly multiply your *pain* (*etsev*) in childbearing: in *pain* (*etsev*) you shall bring forth children, . . .'

And to Adam he said, . . . 'cursed is the ground because of you; in *toil* (*etsev*) shall you eat of it all the days of your life.'

"What right did they have to do that!" John exclaimed indignantly, "—translating *pain* for the woman and *toil* for the man, when the Hebrew word is the same for them both!"

Pastor Dirkson smiled. "Remember what I said to you about translators 'reading into' a word from another language their own understanding of it, because of cultural differences? That's exactly what's been done here. The common belief in our culture is that the birth of a child always causes its mother great pain. One modern paraphrase has the words 'intense pain and suffering' for the woman, but for the man translates this same word as 'struggle' and 'sweat'!⁴ Only one of the newer translations that I've seen translates this accurately as 'labor.'⁵

"Now, there's a verse in the New Testament about childbirth that I'd like you to look at a moment—or shall we wait and take this up another time?"

"Oh, no," Mary said eagerly, "please, let's go on."

"All right. This is a statement made by our Lord in John 16:21 and 22." He waited until John had found the passage in his Bible before reading:

"A woman when she is in travail hath sorrow, because her hour is come: but as soon as she is delivered of the child, she remembereth no more the anguish, for joy that a man has been born into the world.

And ye now therefore have sorrow: but I will see you again, and your hearts will rejoice, and your joy no man taketh from you."

"I don't understand these verses . . ." Mary admitted.

"Neither do I, Mary," John told her. "I'm hoping the pastor will help explain them."

"This verse is poorly translated," Pastor Dirkson said, "as you will realize in a moment. The words translated 'in travail' are from the Greek word *tiktō*, which simply means 'to bring forth a child.' For example, this same word is used in Luke of the birth of Christ:

And she *brought forth* (*tiktō*) her first born son, and wrapped him in swaddling clothes. . . .

"The word 'sorrow' is from the Greek word *lupē*, which, like *etsev*, refers only to a state of the emotions.[6] Historical records just prior to Christ's time reveal that a birth during this period in history generally took only two to three hours, so we can be certain that Christ is not speaking of the 'sorrow' of a prolonged, painful, delivery.''

"Could he be referring to the sorrow of exertion in giving birth?'' Mary asked.

"It seems possible, Mary,'' the pastor nodded. "After all, giving birth is a task requiring complete, sober absorption. *Lupē* might also refer here to the mother's anxiety in her labor, until the task had been successfully accomplished.

"In this passage Jesus is using a parallel similar to that in Genesis between man and woman, only here, he compares a woman's experience of giving birth to the disciples' coming experience of waiting in sorrow for his release from the grave. But the comparison is not primarily of the sorrow, but of the *joy* that is to follow.

"It's most revealing that Christ is aware of the tremendous joy or elation a mother experiences immediately after a normal birth. This is not just a state of being happy that it's all over and the child has arrived safely, but it is an exhilaration that sweeps from her mind all thought of whatever anxiety or weariness of toil she may have experienced— 'she remembereth it no more.' This exciting climax to the birth experience is a most important part of it and gives it the needed balance. We see in this, as in so many other things, the wise and loving plan of our great Creator. In Christ's day, because women neither experienced real suffering in a normal birth, nor were their minds dulled by drugs at this final moment of birth, they *did* experience this sense of exaltation immediately afterward, as he tells us.

"But there's one more word in this verse that's mistranslated. It's the word 'anguish' from the Greek word *thlipsis*, which means simply 'applying pressure, compressing together, or squeezing,' as in squeezing out the grapes, or in pushing someone out of his or her place.''[7]

"Then you mean that Jesus said the mother no longer remembers pushing the baby out of his or her place!'' exclaimed Mary excitedly.

"Yes, Mary. That's exactly what Jesus said. In Latin translations of this verse *thlipsis* is translated as *pressurae,* meaning, the 'pressures' of childbirth. This is a common word to use of childbirth for these people, as for example in the apocryphal account of the birth of Christ where Mary says to Joseph:

Take me down from off the ass, for that which is in me *presses* to come forth. . . . Then said Mary again to Joseph, Take me down, for that which is within me *mightily presses* me.[8]

"Do you see how she felt her baby being pressed, pushed down, by the uterus? Now, let's translate John 16:21 literally and see what impression it makes:

A woman when she is *giving birth* (*tiktō*) has *sorrow* (*lupē*) because her hour is come: but as soon as she has given birth to the child, she no longer remembers the *pressures* (*thlipsis*), for joy that a child has been born into the world."

"That's a beautiful verse!" Mrs. Dirkson commented, as she went over to the fire to stir up the embers. The coals sputtered and then burst into flame again.

"It is indeed beautiful," her husband agreed. "But what is the real emphasis of this whole passage?"

All were silent a moment, thinking, until John suggested, "Isn't Jesus trying to comfort his disciples? He knows he's going to die, and he's trying to get them to look beyond the sorrow they'll experience at his death to the great joy they'll know when his resurrection takes place."

"Good, John," the pastor said, pleased. "Jesus draws from an example they all know—the excited joy of a new mother just after the birth of her child—to comfort their hearts. He pictures the mother giving birth, no doubt groaning in her bearing-down efforts to push her child out of his place within her body. Suddenly her task is completed, as her child breaks forth from the dark womb into life. With a glad cry, and unbelieving tears of laughter, she takes into her arms the wonderful reward of her labor—her very own live, perfect baby!

"Jesus is drawing from a moment of the most intense joy in human experience, to illustrate the intense joy his disciples will know, when he himself breaks forth from the dark tomb into new life—in the power and glory of the resurrection!"

"I've gained a new respect for the Bible tonight," John remarked thoughtfully. "We surely thank you for the time you've taken to explain these things, pastor. I suppose there's more you could tell us about this?"

"Oh, yes, a great deal more," he smiled, "but we'll save that for another time." He walked with John and Mary to the door after they had slipped into their wraps and held it open for them.

"Good night, Mrs. Dirkson," Mary called back, "and thank you for the refreshments."

"You're most welcome, both of you. Good night."

Long after John had gone to sleep that night, Mary lay awake in the dark thinking over what she had learned that evening. She felt fully released from the anxiety in her mind that God had condemned her to pain—an anxious burden that women like herself had carried for centuries. The words and melody of a lovely hymn came to her mind, and as it echoed over and over, she gradually drifted away into the most peaceful slumber that she had ever known.

> There's a wideness in God's mercy,
> Like the wideness of the sea;
> There's a kindness in His justice,
> Which is more than liberty.

> For the love of God is broader
> Than the measure of man's mind;
> And the heart of the Eternal
> Is most wonderfully kind.

> If our love were but more simple
> We would take Him at His word,
> And our lives would be all sunshine
> In the sweetness of our Lord.[9]

NOTES

1. *Protevangelion of James* 2:6, 7.
2. *The Oxford Self-Pronouncing Bible,* Teacher's Edition, King James Version.
3. Rabbi Samson Raphael Hirsch, *The Pentateuch* (a translation and commentary), vol. I, Genesis, rendered into English by the publisher (London: Isaac Levy, 1959).
4. *The Living Bible.*
5. *The New English Bible.*
6. W. F. Arndt and F. W. Gingrich, eds., *A Greek-English Lexicon of the New Testament, and Other Early Christian Literature* (Chicago: University of Chicago Press, 1957).
7. Ibid.
8. *Protevangelion of James* 12:10–12.
9. Frederick Faber, "There's a Wideness in God's Mercy."

8. Smaller Than a Hand

He shall feed his flock like a shepherd: he shall gather the lambs with his arm, and carry them in his bosom, and shall gently lead those that are with young.

—Isaiah 40:11, KJV

The clapboards of the tiny frame house clung tenaciously together. The overgrown weeds in the scraggly yard lent an air of desertion, but a curtain shifted at the window as Mary and her mother came up the walk. It was evident that someone lived in this forlorn little brown house.

"I must get Dad over here some Saturday to nail up those loose boards," Mrs. Johnson remarked to her daughter.

"John can come trim the yard when Dad comes," Mary said, generously offering her husband's services, too, without his knowing it. "It's a good thing it rains so much here, isn't it, Mother? At least it keeps the yard green."

As Mary lifted her hand, she was startled by the door opening suddenly, before she'd had time to touch the doorbell.

"I saw you folks a-comin' up the walk," Mrs. Arkwright told them. "I sit by the window and watch, most days, for someone to come see me. I get so lonely now with Mr. Arkwright gone!" She brushed an invisible tear from her cheek with her gnarled hand as she led them into the little house, which smelled faintly of stale grease and fried onions.

Mary wrinkled her nose at the musty odors as she and her mother sat down. It's funny, she thought to herself, as she looked around the room—that I don't remember this place as being so dirty. All I can remember is that Jo Lynn and I always were given a piece of candy from that blue bowl when we came with Mother to visit. I suppose there were dust balls under the furniture and that the window sills were gray with dirt then, too, and we just didn't notice it.

"It's a lovely day today, isn't it?" Mary's mother said pleasantly to Mrs. Arkwright, after they had been seated.

"I'm very well, thank you," the old lady replied, misunderstanding, "except I git a bit more pain in my shoulders with this cold weather. My, Mary! how you've grown!" She looked Mary up and down unabashedly. "You're quite the young lady now, ain't you though!"

"I'm *married* now," said Mary, not too politely, annoyed at being spoken to like a child.

"Eh?"

"*I'm married now,*" Mary answered, speaking louder.

"Eh? Eh? What's that?" Mrs. Arkwright looked questioningly at Mary's mother.

"SHE'S MARRIED NOW," Mrs. Johnson shouted, and Mrs. Arkwright nodded happily.

"Married! Well, I declare! Seems just the other day you and Jo Lynn was a-skippin' up the walk to see me. Married! D'you have any kiddies yet?"

"We're going to have a baby next spring," Mary replied loudly.

"How nice! A baby! Well, I declare! Is it a boy or a girl?"

"No—ah, we don't know," said Mary lamely, then, gathering her courage she said, more loudly still, "It hasn't been BORN yet."

"A boy!" exclaimed Mrs. Arkwright with delight. "Now ain't that nice!" She stopped rocking as Mrs. Johnson leaned over and shouted in her ear.

"THE BABY HASN'T BEEN BORN YET."

"Oh, not born yet. Well, I declare. Excuse me a minute," she said, fumbling with her hearing aid, "I don't believe this thing's workin' just right. I can't seem to hear you." She eased herself out of the rocker and limped into the next room, calling back over her shoulder, "I'll see if I can find a better battery."

"You'd think she'd know, Mother," Mary whispered, "I *am* wearing a maternity dress."

"You're still quite slender though, Mary," her mother soothed her ruffled feelings. "Mrs. Arkwright lost track of styles long ago. She doesn't know a maternity dress from any other unless a woman is very obviously pregnant."

They could hear an eerie collection of squeaks, whistles, and static coming from the next room, as Mrs. Arkwright shuffled through a drawer full of hearing-aid batteries and tested them.

"She's trying to find a good battery," Mary's mother explained.

"She never knows the new ones from the old, so she has to test them all."

"But doesn't the county keep her supplied with good ones?" Mary asked.

"Yes, but you see, she never throws the old ones away, as she's so afraid she'll run out of them altogether someday. But this way she gets them all mixed up. She'll probably come back with an older one than she had before."

After what seemed an interminable length of time, Mrs. Arkwright reappeared, apparently satisfied with the battery she had chosen. She was carrying a yellowed bit of cloth in her hands. "I've got something for your baby," she told Mary. "I love babies! This little dress was left from our Betsy who died of the dipytheria." She smoothed out the little dress with her stiffened, arthritic fingers, as she placed it in Mary's lap. "There's nobody I'd ruther give it to than you, Mary. Your mother's always been so good to me."

Mary nodded a gracious thank you to her, having been notified by a look in her mother's eye that she dare not refuse the gift. As she opened the musty folds, she saw it had been lovely once, painstakingly embroidered, with tatted lace around the sleeves and hem. She folded it again and laid it gently in her lap.

"Would you care to have some tea?" Mrs. Arkwright offered.

"No, thank you," Mary answered, but her mother was already saying,

"YES, WE WOULD ENJOY IT."

Mrs. Arkwright hobbled out into the little kitchen to put the water on to boil, obviously pleased that they would stay.

"Mother, why did you say that?!" Mary scolded. "You know we can't stay much longer. I have to be home when John gets there, so we'll be on time for the doctor's appointment."

"This won't take long, Mary. Did you see how happy she was when we said we'd love to have tea with her? You see, it gives such pleasure to people like her to be able to do some little thing for others, because they have so few chances to repay the many favors done for them."

After another lengthy delay, Mrs. Arkwright returned with a tray. She set it down on the table near Mrs. Johnson. Although she filled the cups as carefully as she could, her hands trembled so much that a little tea splashed out of each one.

"It's kind of you folks to bring me the berry pie. I thought you might's well share it, as I don't eat so very much. These here are wildberries, ain't they?"

Mrs. Johnson nodded in the affirmative.

"Thank you for the tea, Mrs. Arkwright," Mary shouted, when they had finished their repast. "We really must be getting home in a little while."

"Go home with you a little while?" Mrs. Arkwright cried, her face creasing into a thousand tiny wrinkles as she beamed at Mary. "Why, if you ain't the sweetest thing! I'd be delighted! Just a minute. I'll go get my wraps."

"Mother!" Mary cried in dismay, as Mrs. Arkwright fumbled in the closet for her coat, "what'll I do now?!"

Mrs. Johnson couldn't help smiling. "Don't worry, dear. Leave her off at my house instead while you and John go to the doctor. You can take her home again on your way back. It'll do her good to get out."

"Are you too warm, Mary?" John questioned her in concern. She was lying on the examining table waiting for the doctor to come in, and John had noticed that her cheeks were very flushed.

"I'm all right," she said, "I'm just a little unnerved from the visit with Mrs. Arkwright. She's such a *character!*" The doctor entered the examining room while she was speaking.

"Did I hear Mrs. Arkwright's name?" he asked as he greeted them. He too noticed Mary's flushed look. "She's a character, all right, Mary, but she's kindhearted and a very wise woman. She prefers her own home remedies most of the time. Diagnoses her own troubles, too—usually quite accurately I might add. I wish more of my patients didn't think that a prescription for every little thing is the only answer and paid more attention to maintaining their own health."

Mary relaxed a bit as the doctor talked. "You're looking well, Mary," he observed, as he touched her hand gently for a moment. As he had expected, it was cold and her palms were moist with perspiration. Her tension was obvious to him.

"I've never felt better," she replied, "but I still haven't felt the baby move. It's about time for that, isn't it?."

"Soon now, I should think. Usually the baby quickens around the eighteenth week of pregnancy. I should be able to hear the heartbeat today, though.'' He placed his stethoscope over her abdomen and listened intently, moving it two or three times. "It's there, all right. Want to listen, John?''

John awkwardly placed the stethoscope on the spot the doctor indicated. He listened carefully and moved the instrument gingerly a time or two without success.

"You'll be able to hear it next month,'' Dr. Gordon reassured him, "when the heartbeat's stronger. We'll let Mary listen then, too.''

"How big is the baby now?'' John asked, handing the stethoscope back to the doctor.

"Hold out your hand,'' was the reply. As John did so, the doctor said, "The baby would fit into the curve of your hand. At four months, it's between six and seven inches long and weighs about four and a quarter ounces.''

"Smaller than a hand,'' John said wonderingly, looking at his own. In imagination he could feel the weight of the little body snuggled into his palm.

"Now Mary,'' the doctor said, turning back to her, "let's see how well you've learned to relax. Take a deep relaxed breath, please, and let it out slowly.''

Try as she would, Mary could not; she began to blush even more. The harder she tried to breathe slowly and deeply in the diaphragm, the more rapidly she breathed in and out with her upper chest.

"I honestly have been practicing, doctor,'' she said, dismayed.

"Can you relax your hand?'' he asked, lifting it by the wrist. Her hand swung stiffly back and forth as he shook it gently. "Let it hang loosely,'' he told her, and she relaxed it a bit more. "It's still too tense. Let it go *completely limp,* so I can shake it like an old dishrag.'' Mary obeyed, and as her hand relaxed, she unconsciously took her first slow deep breath also.

"Good!'' he encouraged her. "Now we're getting somewhere.'' Mary began breathing more deeply and more rhythmically, relaxing her tensions more and more.

"You have the right idea, Mary,'' Dr. Gordon encouraged her, "but you must learn to release your tensions much more quickly. Sit up a moment now, and I'll explain what I mean.'' He took her hand and helped her to a sitting position.

"I purposely tested Mary's ability to relax first today,'' he explained to them both, "to illustrate what tension is, so you can recognize it. I realized as soon as I came into the room, by the unusual color in her cheeks, by her cold, moist hands, and by her rapid breathing—we call it hyperventilating—that Mary was in a mild state of anxiety, although outwardly she acted very calm. If you were to go into labor with just this much tension, Mary, and be unable to release it, you'd soon be in pain, because tension inhibits the normal progress of the birth.

"Here's an exaggerated example of what tension does. Suppose you're crossing the street with a small child who suddenly darts away from you, just as an ambulance comes screeching around the corner, sirens going full blast. In that instant, the blood rushes to your head, your heart beats faster, you breathe rapidly, and many of your normal body processes, such as digestion, are temporarily inhibited. A mild state of tension produces all these same symptoms, only in a modified form.

"But why are you tense today, Mary? You've known me all your life. You're not afraid of me?"

"No," she said.

"But you're a little anxious about the examination today?"

Mary nodded.

"You're not alone in this," he smiled reassuringly. "Most young women coming in for a first internal examination feel just as you do. They aren't sure just what the doctor will do, they're embarrassed at the thought of a vaginal examination, and they tense to cover their anxiety with an appearance of poise. Is this how you feel?"

"Well, yes," Mary admitted, "I can't help being a little nervous about it."

"I'm glad you're honest with me, Mary. Let your bit of anxiety today be an object lesson for you; this is *the same state of tension* in which nearly all women about to have their first babies enter the unfamiliar surroundings of a modern hospital. Remember what I said to you about the natural shyness of a young woman, John?"

John nodded, understanding.

"Tension due to the simple embarrassment of a young wife in labor can be a tremendous pain-producing factor. The primitive woman giving birth out in the fields or in her own little hut, as well as the woman in our society giving birth in her own home, suffers no such embarrassment. And a young woman can overcome her reticence and gain the poise and self-confidence she needs for this experience if she's prepared beforehand, even if she is to give birth in the hospital. Now

Mary,'' he added, "I'll explain what I'm going to do today, so you needn't feel anxious or embarrassed.

"We'll do a routine physical first, such as I've often done for you. Then we'll measure the bones of your pelvis to see if they're of adequate size to permit a normal delivery. Then I'll examine you internally by means of an instrument like this.'' He picked up a small instrument and handed it to her.

"This is called a speculum," he said, as she turned it over in her hands, "and it's used to hold the vaginal walls apart so that I can examine the cervix inside your body. I do very much the same thing when I use a tongue depressor to hold down your tongue when I look at your throat. The cervix, you know, is the little doorway into the uterus, so it's important for me to know that it's in good condition. If you take deep abdominal breaths, as you've been doing, and keep the vaginal walls relaxed, the speculum won't cause you any discomfort.''

Mary looked relieved. "Well, is that all there is to it? I'm glad you told me. Will you examine the cervix each time I come in from now on?''

"No, just this first time, and possibly on a few occasions near the end of your pregnancy.''

"There's one other thing that really worries me, doctor,'' Mary said, as she handed the speculum to John to look over. "How do I know that my baby will be all right? I've heard so many things about stillborn babies and babies born with defects.''

"That'll take time to answer,'' he replied, as he proceeded with the examination, "so let's wait and discuss it in my office a bit later.''

"Now to come back to your question, Mary . . .'' Dr. Gordon said, as he slipped into his chair behind the desk. John and Mary had been waiting in his office for several minutes while he had been busy with

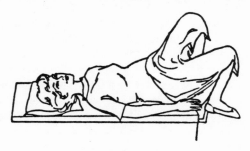

Patient in position for a pelvic examination.

other patients. The doctor looked weary as he ran his fingers through his graying hair, wondering how he should go about telling these young people what they wanted to know.

"I have some more instructions for you today, Mary," he said first, as he handed her another small folder. "Please study them carefully and do as they say."

"I certainly will," she said earnestly.

"Now, you should both realize," he began, "that there is always a possibility of abnormality in a new baby. At the same time, I would reassure you that you are both doing a great deal toward making it possible for your baby to be normal and healthy by preparing for a natural birth.

"Do you know that there are *seventeen* other countries in the world that have a lower death rate for babies than in the United States?[1] In most of these other nations, natural childbirth is more widely practiced than in our country. Twenty years ago we were losing twice as many babies per thousand live births as in Sweden. In 1980 we were *still* losing twice as many babies as Sweden! Even though our infant mortality is half what it was twenty years ago, these other nations have had a far more remarkable improvement than the United States. Of the twenty-five nations for which statistics are recorded, only seven reporting nations lose more babies than the United States each year."

"Why, doctor!" exclaimed Mary. "I thought the United States was way ahead of all other countries in the field of medicine!"

"This is true of many of our medical specialties, Mary," he said, "but it's a fact that in infant mortality our nation is still behind. Infant deaths due to childbirth are one of the major causes of mortality in this country. But what is even more sad is the number of babies who live who are damaged each year during birth due to the tranquilizers, analgesic drugs, and local and general anesthetics given the mothers. The number of children suffering from cerebral palsy has not diminished in twenty years,[2] and it is impossible to count the number of children who have suffered at least minimal brain impairment, or who are hyperactive. Unfortunately, the use of medications during labor and birth is not diminishing. In 1977 it was estimated that at least 95 percent of births in U.S. hospitals were medicated, even though careful research has shown that psychoactive medications given during childbirth cause an average IQ loss of four points.[3] Not only that, but inhalation anesthesia is still being used for about a third of all deliveries, which is a major cause of maternal deaths as well.[4] And it has been said that 90 percent of all deaths from obstetric anesthesia are preventable.[5] There is even evidence that both maternal and neonatal deaths are underreported[6] and may be double what the reports say.[7]

"Recently many doctors changed from using inhalation anesthesia to nerve block anesthetics for the birth, believing this was safer for the baby. But we now know that there is no such thing as a placental barrier, so that *anything* given the mother reaches the baby and can depress the infant's wellbeing. The condition of the baby is assessed at one minute after birth and again at five minutes on the basis of five signs: heart rate, respiration, muscle tone, reflex response, and color. This is called the Apgar scoring system, with the scores ranging between 1 and 10. A 0 score would be a dead baby. A 10 score means a baby in excellent condition. But a baby may show a splendid Apgar rating at birth and yet later become sluggish in breathing or in sucking instincts, because the toxins leave his or her system much more slowly than they do the mother's."[8]

"That's a disgrace!" John exploded.

"Indeed it is," Dr. Gordon agreed. "And this is not the 1940s or 1950s. These sad things are occurring needlessly in these last two decades of the twentieth century! How many of our children are there who are not mentally defective, but whose intelligence is below normal, who are poor readers, who are hyperactive, but who might have been bright and normal if they had not received some slight damage to their higher brain cells because of the drugs and anesthetics used as they were being born, or because of the medications unnecessarily given during pregnancy?"

"Another thing that saddens me is the depression of so many new mothers who've been drugged, following the birth of their children. Some doctors claim that this is a 'natural' result of the effort and excitement of giving birth, but we don't feel depressed after the excitement of strenuous exercise, do we?"

"Certainly not!" John agreed. "You feel physically tired but emotionally refreshed."

"There's no proven physiological reason for the depression of so many new mothers in the United States.[9] Their depression often springs from an inner resentment, which they can't identify.[10] A mother may even secretly reject her child, although she guiltily struggles to conceal this fact, even from herself.

"Doctor," Mary said, as seriously as she had ever spoken in her life, "I want to learn all I can about how to give birth as naturally as possible, for my baby's sake."

"I know you do, Mary, and I'll do all I know how to help you. I am committed to birthing that is as physiologic as possible, and I encourage babies to be born at home when all is well. Have you given this any consideration?"

"Yes," John answered for them both. "We've talked about it, but we're not quite comfortable with the responsibilities involved, at least not yet."

"That's all right," Dr. Gordon replied. "We now have an alternative birthing room at the hospital, in order to make the birth there as homelike as possible. Would you prefer that?"

"Oh, that would be wonderful!" Mary sighed.

"Both of you should remember, though, that there *is* a proper use of analgesics and anesthetics in childbirth in the very small percentage of births in which there is a genuine problem. In an emergency these measures can be lifesaving to mother and child alike. Even Dr. Dick-Read—that great humanitarian who was the pioneer of the natural childbirth movement—found it necessary to perform a cesarean or to assist a birth by other means in about 3 to 5 percent of his patients. That's about one out of every twenty or twenty-five births.

"I realize that, Dr. Gordon," Mary assured him. "And I'm grateful that I can trust you not to intervene unless it's really necessary."

"I can see you're going to be a prize patient!" Dr. Gordon gave her a warm smile and added, "I'll explain any procedures to you both that may have to be performed and will carry them out only with your understanding and consent."

"I have one more question," Mary said. "I've read some things about *induced labor*—stimulating labor artificially. Is there any advantage to that, or is it dangerous?"

"It is dangerous, Mary, if unwisely carried out, as in any other attempts to 'improve' upon a natural function. It seems to increase the incidence of fetal distress and contribute to the phenomenal increase in the number of cesarean births, which now occur in one out of every three to five births in many American hospitals.[11] It is also of considerable risk to the mother unless monitored very closely. I am speaking of induction or augmentation of labor through commonly used agents like pitocin. The medical literature is full of warnings against its injudicious use. As a matter of policy, I am opposed to the routine use of any procedure that was developed as an aid for use in special cases. This includes such things as ultrasound and amniocentesis during pregnancy, the use of intravenous and continual electronic monitoring during labor, as well as routine induction and augmentation of labor. There are risks with all these procedures and they need to be reserved for those special circumstances when they may be lifesaving.

"Apart from a medical standpoint, however, the reason I hesitate to stimulate labor artificially is that it makes the contractions so much more uncomfortable for the mother, and this in turn stresses the baby. The contractions of an induced labor are not the same as normal contractions. They are stronger, harder, and seem to rise and fall more quickly. The woman in labor has a much more difficult time controlling her relaxation and breathing, and the contractions may be quite painful. Oxygen to her baby is reduced because of her increased discomfort and tension. If for some serious reason induction seems necessary, I'll discuss it with you both thoroughly at the time so that we can arrive at a mutual decision.

"Well," Dr. Gordon said, pausing, "Do you have any other questions?"

Mary shook her head, and the doctor rose. "Thanks to your cooperation," he said, "you can expect your experience of giving birth to be a much safer and happier one. It is a privilege to have such intelligent young people as my clients."

Mary and John animatedly discussed the information they had gained from the doctor all through supper that evening. Mary began filling the sink with warm water when they finished, while John cleared the table.

Suddenly she cried in dismay, "John! We forgot all about Mrs. Arkwright! We were supposed to take her home!"

NOTES

1. Myron E. Wegman, M.D., "Annual Summary of Vital Statistics—1980," *Pediatrics*, vol. 68, no. 6, December 1981.
2. *International Medical News Service*, Los Angeles, December 1, 1977.
3. Yvonne Brackbill, Ph.D., "Lasting Behavioral Effects of Obstetric Medication on Children," a longitudinal study of 50,000 children, and released by the National Institute of Health in 1978. The NIH delayed release of the information for some

time, "censored key portions" and "watered-down" some of the conclusions in its report, according to Dr. Brackbill.

4. Ibid.
5. "90 percent of Obstetric Anesthesia Deaths Called Preventable," *Ob. Gyn. News,* vol. 2, no. 13, 1978.
6. *Morbidity and Mortality Weekly Report* (Atlanta, GA: Center for Disease Control), vol. 28, no. 22, June 8, 1979.
7. "The Risk of Childbearing Re-Evaluated," *American Journal of Public Health,* vol. 17, no. 7, July 1981.
8. "Neonatal Depression Tied to Meperidine," *Ob. Gyn News,* vol. 15, no. 4; "Effects of Local Anesthesia on Neonate Quickly Evaluated," *Ob. Gyn. News,* vol. 5, no. 21, 1971. Demerol is a form of Meperidine, the most widely used analgesic in childbirth.
9. Virginia Larsen, M.D., *Attitudes and Stresses Affecting Perinatal Adjustment* (Fort Steilacoom, WA: Mental Health Research Institute, 1966).
10. James Clark Moloney, M.D., "Post-Partum Depression," *Child-Family Digest,* February 1952.
11. "Maternal Deaths Associated with Induction of Labor," *Obstetrical and Gynecological Survey,* vol. 24; 1969 p. 1363; "Neonatalogists Seen Concerned About Iatrogenic Prematurity," *Ob. Gyn. News,* vol. 10, no. 14, 1970; "Induced Deliveries Tied to Problems for Babies," *Washington Post,* November 7, 1977.

9. Bring a Torch, Jeanette, Isabella

Lo, children are an heritage of the Lord: and the fruit of the womb is his reward.

—*Psalm 127:3, KJV*

Mary stirred in her sleep, turned restlessly again, and suddenly was wide awake. There it was! She lay perfectly still, waiting, waiting. There! Again! Soft as the brush of a butterfly's wing, fragile as a dewdrop trembling on a leaf, she felt her baby move. A flush of warm excitement infused her whole being. There it is again! Rising up on one elbow, she looked to see if John was awake. Watching him a moment, she was disappointed that he was breathing evenly in a sound slumber. She hesitated, but couldn't restrain herself from reaching over and shaking his shoulder gently.

"John," she whispered softly, "wake up! I can feel the baby! He's moving! John!" He mumbled in his sleep and turned over. She shook him again, a little impatiently this time.

"The baby's moving, John. Wake up, honey!"

"'Zat so?" he said sleepily. "How nice." He tried to doze off again, but she was persistent.

"Give me your hand, honey, so you can feel him, too." She took his hand and placed it over where she'd felt the baby. "Here, put it right here. Did you feel that? No, no, not there—over here." She shifted his hand from place to place, but he couldn't feel anything.

"Your hand's always in the wrong place when the baby moves," she said, exasperated. "Here—over here now." But it was hopeless. The baby's movements were too slight for John to detect, so she gave up trying and let him drift back to sleep.

But Mary lay awake, her eyes wide open in the dark, anticipating with delight each delicate flutter of the tiny limbs within her body. A new life inside mine, she thought reverently. Only God could make such a miracle possible! Thank you, God, she whispered to him softly.

He seemed to be standing there beside her, so close, so close, that if she reached out she could touch his hand in the soft darkness of this glad night.

As the first timid rays of the lazy winter sun crept stealthily around the sides and under the hem of Mary's bright yellow and brown kitchen curtains, the aroma of bran muffins baking in the oven drew John more quickly than usual from his ritual with comb and razor.

"M-m-m-m. Smells good in here. Are we celebrating something?" He gathered Mary into his arms and gave her an energetic honeymoon hug.

"No," she said, smoothing down her hair when he let her go, "I just felt like making something special this morning. The muffins are about done, if you want to sit down." She opened the oven door to take a peek, then closed it for a moment longer while she poured the juice.

"You're not cross with me for waking you last night, are you, John?" she asked. If he had been cross, he hardly would have remembered it under the spell of the delicious breakfast set on a bright cloth before him, with his radiant young wife beaming at him from across the table.

"Not a bit, honey," he fibbed, as he reached for a muffin. "You said something about the baby, I remember."

"John!" she scolded. "Don't you remember? The baby was *moving* —first time I've ever felt him. I guess he's sleeping now—I haven't felt even a whisper of a motion this morning." A faraway look came into her eyes as her thoughts turned inward for a moment.

"That's wonderful, Mary," John said. His interest was genuine, now that he was wide awake.

"I was thinking, last night," Mary chatted gaily as they ate, "that I'm not just going to *be* a mother—I already *am* a mother, with a really true baby! Isn't that exciting?"

"Sure is," John agreed, sharing her enthusiasm. "Even though I don't exactly feel like a father yet, I know I already am. We need to pray for our baby every day, honey. And," he teased, "I like being married to the prettiest 'really truly' mother in the whole world!"

Breakfast over, John pulled on his coat and picked up the stack of papers he had graded the night before. Mary still looked so irresistible that he stopped to kiss her again, until she laughingly pushed him away and waved him out the door so he would be on time for his classes.

Mary flew happily through her work that morning. Even the futile efforts of the sun trying to penetrate the sodden clouds didn't dampen her spirits. She finished the breakfast dishes and gave the stove an extra polish before straightening the bedroom and making the bed. As soon as she finished cleaning the front room of their little home, she reached for the second folder the doctor had given her at the office several days before and sat down.

With a new, sobering sense of responsibility, Mary studied its pages again, determined to follow the doctor's instructions conscientiously, for the baby's sake, for John's sake, and for her own.

PRENATAL INSTRUCTIONS

Diet

Maintain a balanced diet of the following groups of basic foods:

Leafy green and yellow vegetables, raw or lightly cooked
Fruit, citrus fruit, tomatoes, fresh whenever possible
Root vegetables, herbs, legumes (peas, lentils, beans), soy flour
Milk, cheeses, yogurt, skimmed milk powder, butter, cottage cheese
Lean meats, poultry, fish, organ meats, (such as liver), eggs
Whole grain breads, flours, and cereals (unsugared), wheat germ
Nuts of all kinds
A spoonful of salad oil each day in cooking or dressings

• Two eggs a day and a quart of low-fat milk, plus lean meat, fish, or fowl at least once a day will insure an adequate protein intake. (About 100 grams of protein a day are needed during pregnancy.) Inadequate protein is a prime cause of birth defects and the toxemia of late pregnancy.

• Brewers' yeast increases needed B vitamins and helps combat fatigue. Vitamin supplements and iron may be prescribed. Vitamins A, C and E, zinc and folic acid are especially helpful.

• Avoid sweets, fats, pastries, soft drinks, and other nonnutritional, processed or refined foods, food coloring and other food additivies.

• Avoid caffeine, nicotine, alcohol, amphetamines, and all medications including aspirin, sleeping pills, tranquilizers, cough medicines, antihistamines, diuretics, antibiotics, nausea pills, and so on.

Discuss any medication your doctor may prescribe with him or her and ask to know the contents, so that together you can weigh the benefits against the risks.

• Do not take diet pills or go on crash diets to avoid weight gain. A healthy woman will gain twenty to thirty-five pounds during her pregnancy and perhaps more. The number of pounds is not nearly as important as the *kind* of food that puts them on. The weight gain should be from wholesome foods in as natural a state as possible, not from junk foods. "Watch nutrition, not the scales" is the rule.

• Nausea in early pregnancy may be related to low blood sugar or a vitamin-B deficiency. Small amounts of protein foods eaten frequently and at bedtime may help. Remember, baby is drawing nourishment *all* the time, not just at your mealtimes.

Relaxation

When comfortable in either of the following positions, allow all muscles to become completely limp, and relax completely. Do not move for twenty minutes. Get up slowly.

I. After the fifth month of pregnancy (before, if you wish) relax in the lateral or in "three-quarter" position: lie on your left side, your head and right shoulder resting on a pillow; put the left arm behind you, curved slightly at the elbow, and bend the left knee; draw the right knee partway up, toward your chest; place a pillow under the right knee so that your abdomen barely touches the floor or the bed. If you are not comfortable, try a larger or smaller pillow under the right knee. Be sure to have none of your weight on your abdomen. It wouldn't hurt the baby, but would be less comfortable for you. Keep your abdomen sagging limply beneath you like a hammock. Use this position for sleep at night also during the later months of pregnancy.

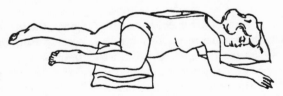

II. Later in pregnancy, in addition to the lateral position, practice relaxing in the "recliner-chair" or "lounge-chair" position, with the chair back at a 45-degree angle, the knees resting on supports, and pillows or arm rests under the arms. (See "recliner-chair resting position" p. 170.) If you don't have a recliner or lounge chair, turn a straight-back chair upside down on the floor, place pillows against its back, and lean against that, with pillows or rolled blankets for support under your knees and arms.

Exercises

I. *Muscular Control of the Vagina and Perineum*

This exercise is *very important*. Tighten all the muscles of the pelvic floor (including urethra, vagina, and anus) by drawing them in as one would clench a fist. Hold these muscles tightly for a count of three. Slowly, slowly, "let go" until the muscles are completely slack. Do this twelve to twenty times in a row, at least twice each day.

II. *Stretching the Leg Muscles Inside the Upper Thigh*

A. Lie on your back, bend the knees, keeping feet flat on the floor, and move your heels halfway back toward the hips. Let your knees fall widely apart. Stretch them in an effort to touch the floor on each side. Bring your knees together, then let them fall outward again. Do this several times each day.

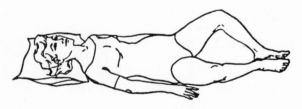

B. An easier way to stretch these inner thigh muscles is to sit on the floor, soles of the feet together, and then "bounce" the knees outward with your palms on the inside of the knees, pushing them out.

C. Or, sit on the floor, knees together in front of you. Have your husband apply *gentle* pressure to the outside of the knees as you try to push them outward against his resistance.

III. *Loosening the Joints of the Lower Spine and Pelvis*

A. Pelvic rock

1. Lie on your back on the floor, place hands on hips, and try to

touch the floor with the small of your back. Notice how this "rocks" your bony pelvis.

2. Stand, feet together six inches from wall, with your back against the wall. Try to touch wall with the small of your back. Do this several times. Notice how this moves the pelvis back and forth.

3. On hands and knees, thighs at right angles to the floor, rock the pelvis *only,* keeping upper back level and head in the same position. Push buttocks up, rock them down, tightening their muscles as you do so, and tightening the muscles of the upper thighs and pelvic floor. Up, down, and *tighten.* Repeat several times.

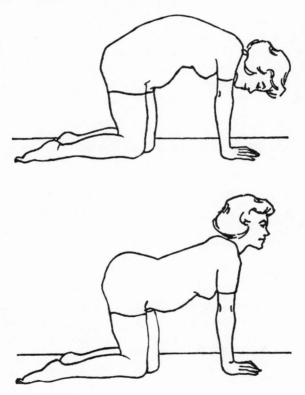

B. Relieving backache

Get on your hands and knees, as for position 3 pelvic rock. Arch the upper back, relax neck, and let head drop forward.

Slowly raise your head, relaxing the muscles across the middle back as you do so, until all tension is gone in the tired muscles, letting it "sag" gently. Repeat whenever your back is achy and tired.

C. Squatting

1. Sit on your heels, knees wide apart, like a primitive woman. (See figure p. 96.) Lean against a wall for balance, if necessary.

2. Sit "Indian style" or "tailor style" frequently, with knees out, feet crossed, and drawn up close to the body.

IV. *Practicing Good Posture*

Stand against a door and try to touch it with the small of your back. Place your hands under your ribs on each side of the chest. Now pretend you are lifting the rib cage *up*. As you do this, you will automatically straighten your shoulders, tuck your hips under, and raise your chin. Take a walk each day, using this good posture. (Be careful to avoid chilling or becoming overtired.) Hold your head high as if proud to be pregnant. You *are* proud, aren't you?

Breathing

There are three natural breathing patterns to learn to recognize.

I. *"Sleep" Breathing*

The muscles of the abdomen and lower chest rise and fall gently when this is done properly, as in sleep. Take a breath deep into the diaphragm. Hold for a count of three, then exhale slowly. Repeat, relaxing more completely with each exhalation.

II. *"Work" Breathing*

Expand the chest and diaphragm while taking slightly deeper breaths. If breathing starts speeding up during activity, or during labor, consciously *slow it down*. Use this breathing during any activity to help avoid shortness of breath and fatigue. Be sure to breathe out completely after each breath that is drawn in.

III. *Pushing Breaths*

Take a full, deep breath. Exhale, blowing out until the chest seems completely empty. This is a "cleansing breath." Take another breath, drawing it in deeply, then begin letting it out *very* slowly, through a slightly open mouth and throat as *if* bearing down. This is the breathing used while pressing the baby out. While pushing, whenever you need more air, take another breath, breathe out *slowly,* mouth and throat slightly open. This makes a soft groaning or moaning sound as air escapes past the larynx. Practice the pushing breath a number of times (without bearing down!) until you are comfortable with how it is done, following each set with a cleansing breath.

IV. *Panting*

Breathe rapidly with little short breaths in the upper chest, mouth open. You will be asked to do this only when you must not bear down, as during the final moments of the baby's birth, so his head will emerge slowly and you will not tear. Concentrate on breathing *out*: "a—HU, a—HU, a—HU."

Summary

Drink enough water; eat small, well-balanced meals. Set aside thirty minutes each day to *faithfully* do the following:

• Lie on back, practice slow, deep breathing for three or four minutes.

• Turn onto left side, slip pillow under left knee and thigh and relax completely for twenty minutes.

• Before getting up, turn on back, practice stretching inner leg muscles a few times (Exercise II).

• Get onto hands and knees, arch and lower back a few times (Exercise III).

• Stand up slowly. Practice pushing breaths.

• Use "work" breathing while doing tasks around the house.

• Practice vaginal exercise frequently, while sitting, standing, or lying down.

• Sit "Indian style" while watching TV, reading, et cetera.

• Practice "squatting" while dusting furniture or "picking up."

• Practice good posture and diaphragm breathing during a daily walk.

Mary finished reading the folder, put it down on the floor open at the summary, and lay down on her back. She practiced the slow, deep-sleep breathing ten times, and then turned over to relax, but found she had no pillow for her knee.

Getting up again, she chose three flexible pillows—one for her head and two to experiment with, to find which was the more comfortable, for her right knee and thigh. She chose the smaller one, as her abdomen was still fairly small. She lay down and let her whole body sag.

The first few minutes she felt restless, but did not move, taking deep, lazy "sleeping" breaths. Eventually she became completely relaxed and was floating off on a cloud somewhere when she heard the mailman come up the walk and drop some mail in their box. She did not flicker an eyelash, however, or stir a muscle until the timer on her kitchen clock signaled that her time was up.

Then she turned on her back, drew up her knees, and practiced dropping them to the outside simultaneously. She did this only four or five times, as it really made the muscles "pull" on the inside of her thighs, showing how weak these muscles were.

Before getting up, she got onto her hands and knees and alternately arched and dropped her back half a dozen times. Then, tremendously pleased with her own self-control at not having jumped up at once to get the mail—although she had been tempted—she got up slowly and walked to the door.

There was a letter from Aunt Em, and Mary sat down to read it.

December 5

Dear John and Mary,

We have thought of you both so many times since you visited us last summer, and have prayed that God would bless your lives together as he has blessed ours.

George had a slight stroke the day after Thanksgiving. He has had a bit of paralysis on his left side since then, but we are grateful that he has no other aftereffects.

As the Christmas season approaches, we trust it will be a most blessed time for you—your first Christmas together. May God fill you with a realization of the beauty and joy of the event of that first Christmas time—the birth of our Savior and Lord.

With love,
Aunt Emma

The evergreens in yard after yard put on their only blossoms of the year—shiny red, blue, yellow, pink, and gold lights—as the heightened anticipation of another Christmas grew keener. Day after day the little town increased its adorning to celebrate the birth of the Christ Child. Silver bells and streamers framed the streets. Passers-by greeted one another gaily and hummed along with the age-old carols echoing from the stores along the avenue. Even nature cooperated in the festivities, silently adding delicate white trimming to shrubs and treetops, houses, lawns, and fences.

It seemed to Mary that there had never been a lovelier Advent season. Her thoughts turned again and again to another Mary, with an affinity she had never felt before. The maiden of old trusted God and obeyed him, Mary thought to herself, but how she must have been misunderstood and ridiculed by friends and relatives for her condition. How hard it must have been to be pregnant and not married—beginning to look big, as I am, and not have anyone understand. I wonder if her own mother believed her. How could she explain—"Mother, I am pregnant, but it is God who made me so. You see, an angel came and told me how it would be. . . ."

No one would believe her! And how could she explain to Joseph, her beloved? Mary felt in her own soul the agony of misunderstanding experienced by that other Mary, whose growing body could no longer conceal the secret of her heart. No wonder she had rushed to Elizabeth, to a woman who walked with God, who would listen and believe her story.

What did Elizabeth say to her? Such happy words. "Blessed art thou among women," she had proclaimed, "and blessed is the fruit of thy womb."

The "fruit of the womb"—how often that lovely phrase is used in the Bible of a tiny baby like mine, Mary realized. Christ, too, before his birth, was called the "fruit of the womb"—a "fruit" like my own child. Jesus could have come some other way, as Adam had, but he chose instead to come to live on earth by way of a woman's body.

Mary's heart must have overflowed with joy at Elizabeth's words, although she probably little realized that her Child would share redemptively every experience of a human being, beginning with conception, prenatal life, and birth, going on through infancy, childhood, adolescence, maturity, and death, then rising to life again that all might live through him. Mary only knew that she was pregnant and that the angel had said her child was to be the Messiah. Blessed by Elizabeth's words, she sang in reply,

My soul doth magnify the Lord,
And my spirit hath rejoiced in God my Savior. . . .
For He that is mighty hath done to me great things;
And holy is His name. . . .

"Are you quite sure you don't want to go along, Mary?" her mother asked, as the carolers prepared to leave the Johnsons' on Christmas Eve.

"No, Mother. You need my help if the carolers are all coming here afterward. Jo Lynn can show John all the places that we usually stop to carol."

"You sure you don't mind, Mary?" Jo Lynn asked in surprise.

"Not a bit!" Mary replied. "Have a good time now."

John and Mary exchanged a secret glance that said more than any spoken words of devotion ever could. She blew him a kiss as he and Jo Lynn went out the door. She felt a growing security in John's love, a bond that drew them closer with every passing day. Jo Lynn is so young, so ignorant of life, Mary thought smugly to herself. How could I ever have been jealous of her?

Mrs. Johnson had not failed to notice her daughter's new poise. She realized that if Mary had not always been so sensitive, Jo Lynn wouldn't have been such a tease. She began slicing the fruitcake which Mary arranged in even rows on a tray. While they worked, she told her mother some of the things she had been learning and how much she looked forward to having her baby naturally, because she believed that God meant giving birth to be a blessed experience for a mother.

Mrs. Johnson thought back to her own experiences, but the memories were so unpleasant that she deliberately turned her attention to something else. She was worried about Mary's idealism. She knew from sad experience that giving birth simply wasn't like that. How hard it was going to be for her to see her daughter disappointed. But Mary seemed so confident, so happy—she decided it was better to keep her doubts to herself.

Mr. Johnson had started a crackling fire to warm the numb feet and hands of the carolers when they returned. The fragrant cocoa was steaming on the stove, and the table was laden with Christmas Eve delicacies when the first stray notes of "Hark, the Herald Angels Sing" reached their ears from far down the street.

"Here they come!" exclaimed Mary happily, moving near the win-

dow to hear more clearly. She stood just behind the living-room drap-
eries where she could not be seen, as the carolers sang their last refrain
before streaming up onto the porch and into the cheerful hospitality of
the Johnsons' home:

> Bring a torch, Jeannette, Isabella,
> Bring a torch, it is dark in the stall;
> Jesus awaits, good folks of the village,
> Run quickly, I hear Mary's soft call,
> Ah!—Ah!—Beautiful is the mother,
> Ah!—Ah!—Beautiful is her child!

10. Words of Life and Beauty

*Open my eyes that I may see
wonderful things in your law.*
—Psalm 119:18, NIV

Several weeks elapsed before John and Mary were able to meet with the pastor to discuss childbirth and the Bible again. John hurried over to the parsonage one Friday evening after an early basketball game. Mary was already there as she had spent the afternoon with Mrs. Dirkson.

Pastor Dirkson invited them into his study, where his reference material was readily available. He seated himself at his desk after the others had made themselves comfortable, arranged some notes on the desk before him, and leaned back in his chair.

"Let's review, first of all, the two passages that we discussed last time," he suggested. "What does the Genesis passage teach us about motherhood?"

"Well, I'd say," John began, since the women didn't answer, "that it teaches that we don't accomplish anything in this life without giving something of ourselves in return. In other words, Eve was to renounce herself—give of her own strength—in her efforts to bring forth a child."

"That's true," Mrs. Dirkson interrupted earnestly, "but the Bible says that Eve recognized her children as coming from God, and she doesn't say anything about toiling in birth."

"Wasn't Eve punished for her sin at all then?" Mary asked.

"I've always thought," Mrs. Dirkson replied, "that Eve first fully realized the awful consequences of her sin and must have suffered an agony of remorse when she witnessed one son slain and her firstborn son the murderer!"

"Do you remember how God comforted her?" her husband asked.

"Yes, Carl. God gave her the privilege of giving birth again! I've often seen, in my mind, the warm, sweet body of little Seth nestled in Eve's arms, as she kissed him over and over through her tears of repentance and grief. She tells us herself that God sent her this little baby to comfort her heart because of Abel's death.''

"Then could it possibly be," Mary suggested thoughtfully, "that Genesis 3:16 means that Eve was to be disciplined by giving of herself through all the years of her life rather than just by the one discipline of giving birth?''

"I believe so, Mary," the pastor told her, "for, you see, Adam's 'renunciation' wasn't that of a day but of a lifetime. Paul tells us in 1 Timothy 2:15 that all Christian women, like Eve, should work out their salvation 'through *motherhood,* if only women *continue* in faith, love and holiness, with a sober mind' (NEB). The key word in Paul's statement is *continue.* This is an *ongoing* process in a woman's life. She's to continue to give of herself in all the Christian graces, especially as an example before the eyes of her children.

"Rabbi Hirsch shows how the Jews believed that Genesis 3:16 applies to a woman's whole life, for he says:

Of the 'renunciation' of the man, the wife is, to the greatest part free. Not by the sweat of her brow has she to gain her bread. . . . The whole life of a woman, from earliest girlhood, is a life of sacrifice, giving herself up for others. . . . There is no higher happiness for a woman than to have children.''[1]

"Well, of course!" Mary noted. "Most little girls want to get married and have children when they grow up. But," she added thoughtfully, "my baby will be John's child too. I want him to be as involved as I am in our child.''

Pastor Dirkson nodded in agreement. "Yes, Mary, and that's in this verse too. You see, an alternate translation, which I believe is the correct one and nearest to Paul's meaning, says: 'Yet she will be saved through motherhood—*if only husband and wife continue in mutual fidelity, love, and holiness, with a sober mind* (NEB footnote).''

"That's great," John smiled. "I was beginning to feel left out! Regardless of what earlier cultures may have done, I want to share in parenting from the time we know a baby is on the way. That seems to me what being a 'father' is all about.

"But hey, here's an interesting thing!" he exclaimed, as a thought struck him. "The verse in John that you talked about last time sort of complements the one in Genesis, doesn't it? Genesis 3:16 tells only of a mother's sorrow of renunciation, but Jesus goes beyond this to tell of a mother's great *joy,* the reward of her efforts, especially just after she's given of herself in childbirth.''

"It's true of all of us then, isn't it," Pastor Dirkson said smiling, "that it is 'more blessed to give than to receive'? And parents who share in the burden of self-giving for their children will share in its joys. But we must go on.

"Apart from the verses we've just discussed, all the others about childbirth in the Bible fall into two categories. First, there are specific instances of women in the Hebrew culture giving birth, and, second, there are illustrations of some aspect of the birth of a child that were used by the prophets and Paul in teaching the people.

"Unfortunately, several of these passages have been so distorted in our English translations that they give very *in*accurate pictures of the childbirth customs of the ancient Hebrew women in their more primitive, more oriental culture. Do you remember what we said their attitude toward birth was?''

"The most important thing," Mrs. Dirkson suggested, "was their belief that a mother was blessed by God if he gave her the privilege of giving birth to and of nursing her own babies. She was considered 'cursed' only if she didn't have children.''

"This is most important, Ruth," her husband said. "The Jews thought so highly of motherhood that Jerusalem itself was compared to a mother who comforts her babies, who carries them on her side, and bounces them happily on her knees. So any translations involving the birth of a child must fit into this cultural belief that it was a blessing to the mother.

"To show you how some of these verses have been mistranslated, let me explain what the Hebrew and Greek words for childbirth are. There are five of these words, all of which, when applied to a birth, mean simply 'bringing forth,' or 'begetting,' or 'making,' and so forth. Frequently, however, we find these words mistranslated as 'travail,' 'sorrow,' 'pain,' 'pangs,' and in the newer translations even as 'writhe'!

"These Bible words are *yalad* and *chul,* in the Old Testament, and *tiktō, gennaō, and ōdinō,* in the New Testament. We'll discuss these five words one at a time.

"*Yalad,* for example, is used not only of a mother giving birth, but also of a *father* having sons 'born' to him, as Isaac was '*born* (*yalad*) to Abraham,' and as sons were '*born* (*yalad*) to Jacob.' *Yalad* is used of fathers in this way dozens of times in the genealogies: this man begat (*yalad*) a son, and he begat (*yalad*) a son, and so forth.

"*Yalad* is even used sometimes of God's acts in creation, as when he says to Job:

Knowest thou . . . who hath *begotten* (*yalad*) the drops of dew?

"It is only when *yalad* is used of a woman that it is ever translated as 'travail.' "

John was obviously disturbed. "This is more unfair than what was done to *etsev*!" he exploded. "It doesn't seem to have any justification at all!"

"It has no justification from a linguistic standpoint," the pastor told him. "But look now at what has been done to the second Hebrew word for giving birth, *chul*. Do you remember the Hebrew fondness for parallelism—how they liked to have two words meaning essentially the same thing, so they could use them in parallel phrases? They used *yalad* and *chul* interchangeably in this way.

"Not only is *chul* used of a mother, but it is also used of God's part in a birth, and in his creating of all things. He is spoken of as '*shaping* (*chul*)' the unborn child in the womb, or of 'making the hinds to *calve* (*chul*),' or as '*making* (*chul*)' a man, or as '*forming* (*chul*)' the earth. *Chul* and *yalad* are sometimes used interchangeably of God's acts of creation, as in this verse found in Deuteronomy 32:18:

"Of the Rock that *begat* (*yalad*) thee thou are unmindful, and hast forgotten God that *formed* (*chul*) thee."

"If these words are used interchangeably of God, can you give us an example of their being used for a mother, too?" John asked.

"Indeed I can," Pastor Dirkson replied. "How about this passage from Micah 4:9, 10, in the Revised Standard Version?

Has your counselor perished,
    that *pangs* (*chul*) have seized you like a woman in *travail* (*yalad*).
Writhe (*chul*) and groan, O daughter of Zion,
    like a woman in *travail* (*yalad*)."

John shifted angrily in his chair, but Pastor Dirkson reminded him that mistranslations such as this were unintentional. They were mistakes, made because the translators had been blinded by their own culture.

"Let's look at the New Testament words for childbirth now," he suggested, after John had calmed down. "As I mentioned before, these words are *tiktō, gennaō,* and *ōdinō.* All three of these words are used interchangeably of childbirth, all three are used at one time or another in the Septuagint to translate *yalad,* and all three are used to translate *chul.* This shows how closely all five of these words are interrelated.

"We discussed *tiktō* in connection with John 16:21 last time. It is occasionally mistranslated as 'travail,' but it is usually translated correctly as 'to bring forth' a child.

"*Gennaō* is used of a mother giving birth, or of a father 'begetting,' as was *yalad.* In the genealogies of Matthew 1, for example, *gennaō* is used of the father begetting a son, over and over. It is also a word used of God as a parent, as were *yalad* and *chul.* For instance in Hebrews 1:5:

For unto which of the angels said he at any time, Thou art my Son, this day have I *begotten (gennaō)* thee?

"The fifth word used of childbirth, *ōdinō,* is the New Testament word most often mistranslated as the 'pain' or 'travail' of a mother. But we know this isn't correct, because it is used interchangeably with the other words for childbirth, and also because the early Christians translated it into Latin as *parturio,* from which we get our English word 'parturition,' which simply refers to the *process* of giving birth. *Ōdinō* is best translated as 'labor,' that is, the *act* of bringing to birth, as Paul says in Galatians 4:19:

My little children, of whom I *labor (ōdinō)* in birth again, until Christ be formed in you.

"Now this isn't to say," Pastor Dirkson explained, "that pain wasn't ever present in a birth in Bible days. For example, we might say, 'Janet had a baby yesterday.' We're making a simple statement of fact—as these Hebrew and Greek words do—we're not explaining what *kind* of a birth experience Janet had.

"In the few times in the Bible in which it mentions that difficulty arose for a woman giving birth, *additional* words are used to make this fact clear. And, in every case, these additional words make it clear that the mother is suffering from exhaustion—from not being able to *work* any longer, as it says in Isaiah 37:3:

The children are brought to the birth, and there is not *strength* to bring forth.

"This confirms our belief that the ancient Hebrews thought of childbirth primarily as a 'work' process. Let's look at the story of Rachel for an example. Here a word is added to show that her labor was 'stiff, difficult, fierce' when Benjamin was born."

"Rachel died in childbirth, didn't she?" Mary asked.

"Yes, Mary. But remember that Rachel had wanted children. In fact, she was so jealous of her sister Leah's having children that one can almost see her stamp her foot as she demands of Jacob petulantly, 'Give me children, or else I die!'

"God heard her prayer when she turned to him and gave her a son. At Joseph's birth she was so delighted that she cried, 'May the Lord add to me another son!' Notice that this was a *request* Rachel made.

"But with Rachel's second labor all wasn't well. She couldn't have known beforehand that her second child would be born with much greater toil than the first. Something was obviously wrong, for the midwife tells her before the child's birth, 'This one, too, is a son for you.'

"Since the midwife was aware of the sex of the child before his birth, he was obviously in an abnormal position, and Rachel toiled in vain to give birth to him, until she was weeping and exhausted. As she felt the last shreds of her energy slipping away, and her child not yet born, the midwife tries to encourage her by saying, 'Come now, Rachel, don't be afraid. Push just a little more, and we'll have this boy delivered, too.'

"Rachel succeeded in giving Benjamin birth, but she was too weakened to recover and she died. I wonder if you realize that Rachel's is the only death caused by childbirth that's recorded in the entire Bible?"

"Why, no," John said. "I thought there were many."

Pastor Dirkson explained, shaking his head, "One other death at childbirth is recorded, but it wasn't caused from the birth itself, but from the shock of bad news occurring right at this time. And this mother, too, died after the birth of her second child. (1 Sam. 4:21; 14:3.) Do you remember the story of Eli?"

"Wasn't he the high priest when Hannah brought her boy Samuel to the temple?" Mary asked.

"Yes. He was a godly man, but his sons were wicked, and on one occasion they took the ark of God with them into battle. The ark was stolen by the Philistines. Eli's sons were killed in battle, and when Eli heard the news, he fell over in his chair, and died of a broken neck.

"Eli's daughter-in-law was pregnant, and when this evil news was brought to her, her labor began prematurely, at seven months, according to Jewish tradition. The Bible relates that she didn't even know when her child had been born because she was so absorbed with her grief.

"The midwives tried to get her attention and to comfort her by saying. 'Look! Look here! Your child has already been born. You have another little son! Look!' But 'she answered them not, neither did she regard it.' And she died of grief, sobbing over and over,

> The ark of God is taken!
> The glory is departed from Israel!
> The ark of God is taken!''

"This surely opens my eyes to some things, pastor," John said. "I've always thought of childbirth in the Bible as being associated with pain, death, or woe."

"Many of us, John," the pastor said, "have been as guilty of misinterpreting passages about childbirth through careless reading as translators have been. Childbirth in the Bible is primarily spoken of as a beautiful event, even in our English Bibles, but we've somehow overlooked this fact. And in all the actual records of a birth, apart from the two we just mentioned, the association is a happy one. The mothers often seem especially aware of God at this time and of his great goodness to them.

"We can still interpret correctly the examples of childbirth used for illustration by the prophets and by Paul, even when they're inaccurately translated. Remember that the comparison isn't 'pain,' or 'anguish' in every case, as the English indicates; look for the phenomenon or aspect of a birth experience in the Hebrew culture that is being used for comparison.

"Is it, for example, the groan or gasp of effort that accompanies the work of bearing down? Is it the posture—crouching or kneeling and bending over the abdomen, as if aiding a contraction? Is it absorption in the task, so that one neither sees nor hears what is going on around one? Is it the fact that birth occurs when it is unexpected, or is it the certainty that a woman with a child in her womb must some day give birth to him? and so on.

"Some of these comparisons are unhappy ones. In Jeremiah, the prophet of the leisure classes of court society, for example, we find examples of gasping, being out of breath, or of hands so weak from the labor of birth that they can no longer grasp a support. You see, the Bible reveals people as they were. And although most Hebrew women seem to have had normal birth experiences, a few did not, which is true in any culture."

"What I'd like to know," John mused, "is how this idea of a curse of 'pain' on Eve came to be believed at all, if it's not anywhere in the Bible, or even in the early theology of the Jews."

"I'd be glad to show you some of the ways this concept developed." Pastor Dirkson offered, "if you'd care to come back next week."

"I'd surely like to," John replied. "Wouldn't you, Mary?" She nodded, so he suggested, "How about Thursday night? We have a late game next Friday, so I couldn't make it then."

Mrs. Dirkson explained that special choir rehearsals for the Easter cantata were to begin the following Thursday, but that they were welcome to come afterward, and all agreed.

NOTE

1. Rabbi Samson Raphael Hirsch, *The Pentateuch* (a translation and commentary), vol. I, Genesis, rendered into English by the publisher (London: Isaac Levy, 1959), p. 83.

11. Through a Glass, Darkly

*At present all I know is a little fraction of the truth, but the time
will come when I shall know it as fully as God now knows me!*
—*1 Corinthians 13:13*, PHILLIPS

Mary put away the last of the pots and pans and wiped up the remaining traces of grated cheese. She could never manage to bake, it seemed, without messing up the whole kitchen. She hoped John would be pleased with her cheese soufflé. Of course it had burned a bit on the bottom—but maybe he wouldn't notice. It fell as it cooked too, at least compared to the lovely, high fluff of Mrs. Dirkson's, when she had made one to show Mary how it was done.

She stepped back to take one last critical look at her handiwork before setting a salad on the table. There wasn't time for anything else. She slipped into the bedroom to brighten her weary features just as John arrived.

"Hi! Anybody home?" he called cheerily as he walked in the door. Mary laid down her brush and went to greet him. He came up beside her, where he could reach around her for a quick hug, and she tipped her head obligingly so he could kiss her.

As they sat together over their evening meal, John related the events of the day. Mary was unusually tired, so she said little. After they had finished dinner Mary poured him a cup of tea and took her place again, folding her napkin carefully over and over in her lap, still waiting expectantly for some comment on the soufflé she had made for him.

John sipped his tea quietly, then looked up and asked, "How about another cup?" To his astonishment, she rose abruptly from her chair, burst into tears, and flung herself out of the room. Bewildered, he got up from the table and followed her.

"Honey, what's the matter?" he asked anxiously. "Did I say or do something to hurt you?"

"No," she sobbed, "it's just—here I slaved all afternoon because you've been wanting a cheese soufflé like Aunt Em's, and then," she daubed at her eyes, "you don't even say *one word* about it! I know I'm not the world's greatest cook, but, . . ." Mary burst into a fresh flood of tears, feeling sheepish over her emotion but unable to control it.

John thought to himself that the soufflé wasn't exactly like one of Aunt Em's, but he knew better than to say so!

"Mary," he tried to console her, "I'm an ungrateful wretch, and I'm terribly sorry. It was thoughtful of you to take so much time to please me, and I love you for it. Forgive me, honey? Remember what Uncle George said about the two bears?"

Mary was quieter now, listening.

"Bear, and forbear," John said softly. "I'll try to bear your burdens —share them with you more, honey—if you'll forbear this time and forgive me for being thoughtless. Okay?"

Mary nodded, her head against his shoulder. Suddenly a thought occurred to John. "Mary," he asked, "did you do your relaxing today?" She shook her head.

"Yesterday?" she shook her head again.

"The day before?"

"No," she admitted sheepishly.

"Now look, honey," he said, his voice rising, "I'd rather have you take care of your own health and our baby's than to go fussing over me!"

"But, . . ." She tried to explain, but he interrupted her excuses.

"You know what Dr. Gordon said—that most women in our society are too tense, and that if you want a comfortable birth you won't have it just by wishing for it! Remember that he said it would be safer for you and the baby, too, if you'd do as he said."

Mary listened abjectly as he lectured on with locker-room enthusiasm.

"When I take my boys out for spring training, I say to them, 'Any of you guys can get out there and run, see? But that's not enough for me! I want you to do your best *every day* in obeying the training rules. *Understand?* You won't win the race on the day of the meet but in all the weeks of patient training and discipline that come beforehand. *Understand?*'

"It's the same with you, Mary. Any mother can give birth, but that's not enough! Because I love you, I want you to have the happiest, safest, and best possible experience, and I want you to be as faithful in training for it as I expect my boys to be in training for a meet!''

"*Understand?*" Mary mimicked him, smiling now, "All right, preacher. I promise."

"Take time for yourself these days, honey, and don't worry so much about me," John added. "Why don't you go in and relax right now before we go over to the Dirksons'? I'll call you when time's up."

Mary took her two pillows and lay down on the living-room floor to relax. Because she'd been upset, it took her nearly five minutes to let her whole body become limp. But because she had learned to relax well, in spite of several days' lapse, she was soon able to release all her physical and emotional tensions. Shortly after she became relaxed, she fell asleep, since she was exhausted. It seemed as if only a few minutes had elapsed before John was shaking her gently, saying it was time for them to get ready to go.

"Tonight," Pastor Dirkson began, as they sat in his study once more, "as we discuss this subject for the last time, I'll attempt to show you how this evil teaching that God damned all women with pain developed. We've already seen that this teaching isn't biblical and that it isn't a part of Jewish theology. Some of our theologians have thought that it was carried over into the church from the tradition of the Pharisees, but this isn't true. In fact, because the Jews have never believed that God wants women to suffer pain in childbirth, they haven't hesitated to relieve this pain whenever it has occurred, as far as their knowledge has made this possible. One present-day rabbi says:

In rabbinic writings the question is never raised [i.e., of refusing to relieve pain in childbirth]; as has been remarked, 'the prohibition of analgesics would contradict Jewish theology.' Indeed, the sympathy of Jewish law for the sufferings accompanying childbirth is so strong that some of its leading exponents justify the recourse to contraceptive sterilization by mothers who fear the pain of further births."[1]

"But Christians don't oppose the use of analgesics either," John pointed out.

"Not today," the pastor explained, "but the church strongly opposed the relief of pain in childbirth in the last century, because they taught that a woman's cries and screams of pain in childbirth pleased the ears of God! Did you know, for example, that in France two women were once burned to death by the church—the one for accepting relief for her pain in childbirth, and the other for giving it to her?''[2]

"How perfectly awful!" Mary gasped.

"But during the same period in which these two women were martyred by the church, a great deal was being done to reduce man's struggle with his 'curse' of tilling the ground, with the development of the tools and machinery of the industrial age. The church was completely inconsistent in this. They saw no reason to oppose the development of labor-saving devices, on the grounds that it would thwart God's punishment of 'toil' on man and interfere with stalwart Christian character. But of the woman, it was declared that any relief of pain in childbirth was completely unjustifiable, because God had decreed that she should suffer. These church leaders said . . ." Pastor Dirkson paused, open a book on his desk to a passage he had marked, and read:

"Let . . . our women be trained to have courage and resilience, and to the proper appreciation of their high vocation and duties; then I guarantee that they will not cry out for chloroform under the pangs of labor, but cling with redoubled love and sacrifice to the beings whom they bring into existence in pain."[3]

"But why should it be more important for women to endure suffering than for men?" John asked. "I don't understand this."

"I'll show you in a moment, John, how women were singled out as needing special punishment from God. Actually, the whole concept of physical pain making a person more godly was widely believed in one period of church history—so much so that pain was frequently self-inflicted in order to make oneself 'holy.' The body was regarded as intrinsically evil and in need of being 'mortified,' as the flagellants did when they whipped themselves.

"Here again the church teaching differed from the Jews', which never suggested that 'there is virtue or some desirable *beau ideal* in bodily anguish.'[4] And of course, this is also a distortion of the New Testament teaching that Christians may have to endure sufferings because of their faith but that God will bring blessing in spite of, and during, these sufferings of persecution by others. This idea of physical pain leading to godliness continued to be applied to married women, even though no longer applied to men, until very recently.

"But let's go back now to the origin of Christianity and see if we can spot where this teaching began. In the first-century church there is no evidence that women were singled out for a special curse. As a matter of fact, early Christians write in most lofty terms of the parturient Christian woman.

"A second-century Christian, Clement of Alexandria, tells us that motherhood is such an exalted state that it can be compared to the motherhood of the church over the believers.[5] And he compares the milk of a nursing mother, which he says is given to her for her infant by God, to the heavenly 'manna, the celestial food of angels that flowed down from heaven on the ancient Hebrews.'[6]

"Still another early Christian demonstrates that God doesn't inflict pain on humankind and that Christians need not abuse their physical bodies by pain in order to become godly, for he says:

What is pain but the interruption of harmony?
. . . There is therefore no pain where there is harmony."[7]

"He sounds like a twentieth-century Christian," John observed. "Remember our discussion about the causes for suffering, Mary?" Mary smiled that she did indeed remember.

Pastor Dirkson opened another of the volumes on the desk in front of him. "After the beginning of the third century A.D.," he said, "we find a change of attitude beginning among Christians—a change that degrades womanhood, looks on the intercourse of marriage as sinful lust, on motherhood as a necessary evil, and on the birth of a child as the shameful consequence of sin. With such a degrading attitude toward women, the idea that God had singled her out for special punishment began to form. The first expression of this attitude is found in the following passage." He pulled the open volume closer and began to read:

"No one of you at all, best beloved sisters, from the time that she had first known the Lord, and learned the truth concerning her own [that is, woman's] condition, would have desired too gladsome a style of dress; so as not rather to go about in humble garb, and to effect meanness of appearance, walking about as Eve mourning and repentant, in order that by every garb of penitence she might the more fully expiate that which she derives from Eve. . . . And do you know that you are each an Eve? The sentence of God on this sex of yours lives in this age: the guilt must of necessity live too. *You* are the devil's gateway: *you* are the unsealer of that forbidden tree: *you* are the first deserter of the divine law: *you* are she who persuaded him whom the devil was not valiant enough to attack. *You* destroyed so easily God's image, man. On account of *your* desert, that is, death—even the Son of God had to die!"[8]

Mary shuddered. "I can almost feel the long, bony finger of that old man pointing at me now!"

Pastor Dirkson turned a few more pages of his book. "This same writer," he said, "tells us that the birth of children is the evil result of marriage and that marriage is in the same class as fornication and adultery. He says that the curse of 'Sodom and Gomorrah' will fall with 'woe' upon the woman who commits the sin of marrying and that God will punish her with 'the burdensome fruit of marriage heaving in the womb, [or] in the bosom.' "9

"This is incredible!" John exclaimed, interrupting.

"Adam's punishment is no longer mentioned side by side with Eve's as in Jewish and early Christian writings. A woman now stands alone, as an inferior, ignoble creature, created for man's downfall, punished by 'the sorrows and the groans of women'10 and by being her husband's slave, if she marries. By twisting biblical truths, these church leaders taught that married women were under a special curse, and that only the virgin could escape the 'curse of Eve.' Not only that, but they taught that a woman who did *not* marry was *no longer inferior to man!* They said, '. . . with that of men your lot and your condition is equal.'11 They even went so far as to say:

Virginity has no children, but what is more, it has contempt for offspring. . . ."12

"How could anyone think of a tiny baby as *contemptible?!*" Mary protested.

Pastor Dirkson shook his head. "Of course," he added, "this was also a twisting of the early church's teaching that virginity, for a man or a woman, was a holy calling—one of 'standing constantly before God' as his special servant. The right motive makes a great difference! By the fourth century, Mary, there were even mothers who deserted their own children to attempt to prove their holiness!13 This is completely contrary to New Testament teaching, and completely contrary to Jewish teaching. In fact, the rabbi who has a large family has always been regarded with great respect. *Not* to marry was regarded by the Jews in centuries past as a sin. The Talmud states that the man who remains unmarried 'is not even a Man,'14 and that—" The pastor shuffled through his notes, looking for the quotation he wanted. "Here it is:

If a man remain unmarried after the age of twenty, his life is a constant transgression. The Holy One—Blessed be He!—waits until that period to see if one enters the matrimonial state, and curses his bones if he remain single.[15]

"During the Reformation there was a reaction to the church's teachings about marriage. We find pastors of that time marrying, but the change in attitude was only partial. Married women still occupied a lowly position in the social order. In fact, in the Thomas Matthew Bible (1537) husbands are even advised to beat their wives if necessary! Matthew based this on the teaching of 1 Peter 3:3:

Sara obeyed Abraham and called hym Lorde, whose daughters ye are as longe as ye doe well and be not afraid of every shadowe.

"Down at the bottom of the page we find this inspirational footnote:

He dwelleth wyth his wyfe according to knowledge, that taketh her as a necessarye healper and not as a bond slave. And yf she be not obedient, and healpful unto him endevoureth to beate the feare of God into her heade, that thereby she maye be compelled to learne the dutie and to do it."

"It sounds as though Sir Thomas Matthew must have had a difficult wife," John laughed, shaking his head. "I wonder if his drastic treatment worked."

"Better not try it," Mary warned him, smiling.

"Not only did women have a low position in society," Pastor Dirkson said, "but it was actually not until this time—during the sixteenth and seventeenth centuries—that the concept of 'pain in childbirth' was included in the 'curse of Eve' teaching. Previously only the 'sorrow' and 'groans of toil' in childbirth, the 'sorrow' of the bereavement of children, and subjection to one's husband were mentioned.

"For example, according to German scholars, the word most often associated with pain in labor, Wehen, can't be traced farther back than the Middle Ages, and Wehmutter, meaning 'mother's pains' (the contemporary word for 'midwife'), can't be found before 1540.[16]

"Also, in medieval times the church had a service for new mothers called the 'Purification of Women,' patterned after Mary's having brought the baby Jesus to the temple for her purification. In this ceremony, one of two beautiful Psalms was read to the new mother—either Psalm 121 or Psalm 128.

"After the English church broke with Rome, this service was included in *The Book of Common Prayer*[17] and has been commonly called the 'Churching of Women.' The prayer book was written during the rule of Edward VI, in 1549, and revised in 1552. In these two versions of the prayer book Psalm 128 was left out, but Psalm 121 was still used.

"But *a century later* pain in childbirth was so widely believed to be inevitable that Psalm 116 was used instead. This is a prayer of thanksgiving after being delivered from suffering; it has nothing to do with the birth of a child."

Pastor Dirkson opened a copy of the prayer book and explained, "From 1662 on, with few changes since, when a woman brought a baby to church after its birth this service was read to her:

Forasmuch as it hath pleased Almighty God of His Goodness to give you safe deliverance, and hath preserved you in the great danger of childbirth; you shall therefore give hearty thanks unto God and say. . .

[from Psalm 116] The snares of death compassed me round and the pains of hell gat hold upon me. I found trouble and heaviness, and I called upon the name of the Lord. . . . I was in misery and he helped me. . . . Thou has delivered my soul from death.

"After the woman had repeated this passage, the following prayer was read to her:

Oh, Almighty God, we give Thee humble thanks for that Thou hast vouchsafed to deliver this woman, Thy servant, from the great pain and peril of childbirth."

Pastor Dirkson closed the book, took off his glasses, laid them on his desk, and leaned back in his chair. "As a matter of fact," he said, "childbirth *was* a time of great pain and peril when this was written, and theologians assumed that this was true of childbirth anywhere in the world in all ages. Were there any reasons why pain might be more common at this time than in preceding centuries?"

"Well," John mused, "hard-working peasant people give birth more easily, as a rule, than the less active city people. And people left the farms in large numbers during this time to live in the cities."

"That was surely one factor. And events like the Black Death, which wiped out a third of Europe's population in the fifteenth century, the diseases and filth prevalent in the cities, all made childbirth a hazardous affair.

"But the fact that pain existed doesn't explain why it became a part of church doctrine. This was a period of many changes in the church—

a period of reaction to the excesses of the Roman church which included, in the Calvinistic and Puritan movements, a rejection of anything pleasant to the senses, whether artistry, or music, or pageantry, or physical pleasures. So, although the clergy now married, a taint still remained on the functions of a *married woman*—a taint that could only be expiated by the sufferings of childbirth. Only the prostitute or mistress—never the godly wife!—ever enjoyed intercourse in such a society. Childbirth, since it involved a woman's sexual organs, shared an association with the clandestine nature of intercourse, so that the idea that childbirth was a physical experience that a woman might even enjoy would have been unthinkable in such a society.

"One time a young bride timidly approached her famous preacher husband and informed him that she was expecting a child. With fire in his eye, he told her never to mention such a subject to him again. And she never did, although she bore him several children."

"It's only in recent decades, isn't it," John mused, "that we've come to realize that sex in marriage is normal and wholesome, and something to be enjoyed by both husband and wife."

"Yes, John. But remember that not all Christians have shared such unwholesome attitudes in any period of church history. But the damage of such attitudes was widespread. Today, we do have more reasonable attitudes toward sex, and toward an expectant mother, too, and I think this is one reason our society is finally beginning to move toward a more wholesome attitude about the birth process as well.

"The really sad thing to me is that although the church has abandoned other false teachings such as flagellism, the burning of heretics, searching out witches, and the evils of marriage, it has been slower than the rest of our culture in accepting childbirth as normal. This false teaching of God's curse of pain on all mothers has been growing stronger, not weaker. We see this in the fact that where the King James translates words referring to childbirth as 'sorrow,' more recently— that is, within the last fifty years and less—translators have been changing these same words to read as 'pangs,' 'anguish,' 'writhing,' and even 'agony'! Can you think of any reason for this?"

"I've heard of the terrible death rate of the nineteenth century due to puerperal fever," John replied, "when up to a third of the mothers died from childbirth in some years."

"Yes. You see, along with this terrible death rate, a great fear of dying in childbirth developed. This great fear caused a woman to become so tense during labor that she resisted the normal progress of the birth and created agonizing experiences of suffering for herself. In this way, a vicious cycle was maintained. Probably no period in the history of the world has seen so much suffering connected with childbirth as the last century. This suffering led medical men to search for ways to relieve it, and anesthesia was discovered. But, you see, since the time its use began until Dr. Dick-Read began his research over sixty years ago, few in our culture had even bothered to look for *normal* causes for pain in the normal physiological function of the birth of a child, because of the church's teaching that the mother's pain was due to the 'curse of Eve,' in other words, due to the vindictiveness of God!

"Dr. Dick-Read couldn't accept this philosophy. His personal belief that God was a God of love gave him the incentive to begin, and to continue, his search for the real causes of childbirth pain. I'll give you a sample of what he says about his approach in his book *Childbirth Without Fear.*" The pastor picked up his reading glasses with one accustomed hand as he selected a book from those ranged across the entire back edge of his massive desk. "Here's the passage I want," he said. "Listen to this:

My close association with the birth of a child has led me to believe there is a limitation to science, and the extending boundaries of human knowledge have only reached the foothills of the towering mountains of Omniscience. This philosophy of childbirth is written, therefore, in terms of a belief in God. . . ."[18]

"We human beings are surely ignorant, aren't we?" John commented wryly. "The Bible reveals God as a wonderful Creator and a God of love all the time—but we haven't believed it in relation to a birth. Thanks so much, Pastor, for all the time you've given to help us learn the truth."

NOTES

1. Rabbi Immanuel Jakobovits, *Jewish Medical Ethics: A Comparative and Historical Study of the Jewish Religious Attitude to Medicine and Its Practice* (New York: Philosophical Library, 1959), pp. 103, 104.
2. E. S. Cowles, *Religion and Medicine in the Church* (New York: Macmillan, 1925), p. 18.

3. C. Capellmann, *Pastoral-Medizin* (1878), quoted in Jakobovits, *Jewish Medical Ethics*, pp. 103, 104.
4. Jakobovits, *Jewish Medical Ethics*.
5. Clement of Alexandria, "The Instructor," Book I, Chap. VI, in *The Ante-Nicene Fathers* (Grand Rapids, MI: Eerdmans, 1951), vol. 2, pp. 419ff.
6. Ibid.
7. Clement of Rome, "The Clementine Homilies," Book XIX, Chap. XX, in *The Ante-Nicene Fathers*, vol. 8, pp. 173ff.
8. Tertullian, "On the Apparel of Woman," Book I, Chap. I, in *The Ante-Nicene Fathers*, vol. 4, p. 14.
9. Tertullian, *To His Wife*, Book I, Chap. V, and *On Exhortation to Chastity*, Chap. IX, p. 436. Op. cit.
10. Cyprian, "The Treatise of Cyprian," Treatise II, in *The Ante-Nicene Fathers*, vol. 5, p. 436.
11. Ibid.
12. Ibid., Treatise IX.
13. F. W. Farrar, *Lives of the Fathers* (Edinburgh: Black, 1889), vol. 2, pp. 302, 303.
14. *The Talmud* (London: Soncino Press, 1936), Bereshith 17.
15. Maurice Harris, *Translations from the Talmud, Midrashim, and Kabbala* (New York: Dunne, 1901), p. 141.
16. Herr Ernst Burkhardt, who translated Dr. Dick-Read's *Childbirth Without Fear* into German, and Dr. Rudolf Hellmann, of Hamburg, in his paper *"Schmerz oder Erlebnis der Entbindung,"* January 1959, quoted in Dick-Read, *Childbirth Without Fear*, 3rd rev. ed., pp. 98, 99.
17. *The Book of Common Prayer*, used in the Church of England and in the Protestant Episcopal churches of the United States.
18. Grantly Dick-Read, M.D., *Childbirth Without Fear*, 4th rev. ed. (New York: Harper & Row, 1972), p. 36.

12. God Is My Rock

He who dwells in the shelter of the Most High
will rest in the shadow of the Almighty.
I will say of the Lord, "He is my refuge and my fortress,
my God, in whom I trust."

—*Psalm 91:1, 2, NIV*

Spring slipped softly into the countryside, touching the trees and shrubs with her fairy's wand until they were masses of pink and white blossoms, framed in the dainty green of new leaves. No crashing storms announced her arrival—no sudden transformation from a barren brown and white landscape to one covered with a mantle of green. All winter long the many evergreen trees retained their color. All winter long the lawns were green under the gentle rains.

Beautiful spring. One's gaze is arrested by the stunning rose, lavender, and pink-shaded rhododendrons, each flower so large that two hands cupped together could not contain all its fragrant petals. Masses of roses, azaleas, and daffodils fill the yards with the softest of pastels. Because spring tiptoes in with utmost delicacy, she can paint landscapes of the most fragile beauty. A sudden transformation to such loveliness from barren soil would be almost too much for the senses to bear.

Mary had always loved the spring, and now, this year, each opening blossom, each little bud expanded almost to the bursting point with new life within, reminded her of her own budding fruit. Never before had she felt such a kinship with all nature. Never before had she been so keenly aware of God's constant presence. She felt a peace and serenity in the knowledge of his nearness that was deeper and more meaningful than she had ever experienced before. Now that the "fruit of her womb" was almost ripe, her faith in the God who had caused it to grow there was complete.

John noticed this new serenity in Mary. He thought, as he observed his wife day after day, that perhaps many women had longed to look forward to giving birth as a natural, beautiful experience given by a loving Creator, but had hesitated to follow the leading of their hearts because they thought that this was contrary to the teaching of the Bible. He felt profoundly grateful to their pastor for his counsel in this matter.

Mary's pen, never far away, was frequently at hand now, as she tried, day after day, to express in words the beauty that filled the world around her.

One day she and John had driven out into the country and had seen frisky baby lambs gamboling on the soft grass of farm after farm. How they had laughed at one wee fellow, trying to enjoy a snack from his mother. His short legs could not keep pace with hers when he tried to reach his dinner. Skipping quickly up in front of her, he placed himself across her path and leaned against her with all his might so she would stand still. But as soon as he stopped leaning against her forelegs and ran back for his drink, she ambled on again, and he had to go without his meal.

"Apparently his mother doesn't believe in demand feeding!" John had chuckled.

The late March day had been perfect—with billowing white clouds gliding leisurely across an azure sky. Mary had tried to jot down some of her impressions of the scenery when they arrived home, but somehow, along with her inner peace and serenity, there was a restless stirring of anticipation, matched by the restless limbs of her growing baby, and she could not bring herself to concentrate on words.

One early April day as she sat on the couch watching the soothing touch of a spring rain on the beauty outside her window, she thought of Helen Keller, blind, deaf, and dumb, and she began a poem again—

> You say she's blind?—
>> She who walks a country lane
>> And lifts her face to greet the rain,
> Or wanders through a garden fair
>> Inhaling all the fragrance there?
>
> You say she's deaf?—
>> Who, standing near the ocean's roar
>>> Can feel its pounding from the shore,
>> Or hear . . .

But Mary could not finish it. Her expectancy had infused her with this strange paradox of feelings—restlessness, at the very time she was experiencing such peace and trust in God! This time, as she put down her pen and paper, she knew she would not try to write again until her baby was in her arms. Hearing the click of the mailbox, Mary roused herself from her reverie.

Shifting her weight a little in order to work herself up off the couch, she finally got to her feet and walked to the door. Returning to the room with a letter from Aunt Em in her hand, she felt a strange, uneasy premonition. She hesitated for a moment, then opened the letter and read it.

Tues., April 2

Dear John and Mary,
I am sitting by the bedside of my dear George, as he comes to the end of his struggle for life. He is very weak and may leave us at any moment. A nurse friend is here with me and has been such a help.
A week ago yesterday George suffered a cerebral spasm and has been losing ground constantly. We think he has not suffered, and for this we thank God sincerely. . . .

Mary's eyes filled with tears as she read, and she could barely see to finish Aunt Em's letter.

Wed., April 3

Now I am alone. George passed quietly away in his sleep last night as we watched over him. . . . As the world judges, he has not been successful, but our intimate and family life has been unsurpassed in happiness and love. I have so many wonderful memories and pray God for the courage to go on alone now. I know that my loved one is with his God, and that he will know ''neither pain, nor sickness, nor sorrow,'' any more. I am determined not to weep selfish tears for my own loss, but only to rejoice for his happiness.

Lovingly,
Aunt Emma

P.S. Mary, last night George motioned toward his top dresser drawer. I followed where he pointed. Opening the drawer, I saw a slip of paper lying on some old notebooks. I brought it over to him, and, guessing what he wanted, asked, ''Is this for Mary?'' He nodded, pleased that I had understood, and closed his eyes, exhausted. He never opened them again.

The slip of paper had fallen to the floor unnoticed. Mary left it where it fell and hurried to the phone to call John. He came home as quickly as he could make arrangements, to find his wife in tears, Aunt Em's letter still in her hand. Guessing the contents before he opened it, he read the letter and then attempted to comfort Mary.

"You needn't worry about Aunt Em, honey," he assured her. "She has such deep faith in God. He'll give her strength to carry on alone."

"I know," Mary sobbed in his arms, "but—it seemed that I was just getting to know Uncle George. He was the dearest old man! At the same time it seemed to me as if I'd known him all my life. Isn't that odd?"

"No, it's not odd," John said thoughtfully. "The more I think about it, the more I realize that you and Uncle George are kindred spirits. You're alike in many ways. Probably that's why you felt so drawn to him from the very first. By the way, where is this slip of paper Aunt Em mentions?" He looked around the room.

"Why, I don't know," Mary said, wiping her eyes. "I must have dropped it."

"Here it is." John picked it up off the floor and opened it. "It's a poem for you, Mary. Uncle George must have wanted you to have it."

Mary looked over John's arm and saw that Aunt Emma had written a note of explanation at the top of the page. "George's poem was inspired by the sight of an enormous white rock, sculptured by the ocean's waves into the shape of a great throne."

"He must have written that years ago," John exclaimed. "I remember one summer when they took me with them to the coast. Uncle George was constantly reminding me to notice this or notice that, how beautiful it was. I'll read this to you, honey." He smoothed out the creases against his knee, and read:

> The Psalmist saw a throne like this,
>   And cried in reverential bliss—
> O God, of great eternal power,
>   Thou art my Rock, and my High Tower!
>
> A fortress Thou, O God, above;
>   Thee will I trust, and Thee I'll love.
> On Thee I'll call, and Thee I'll praise,

To Thee my hands with reverence raise.
When in distress I'll cry to Thee,
 For Thou, O God, wilt succor me.

Upon my knees I'll worship Thee
 Sing forth Thy praise continually.
O God, of great and mighty power—
 Thou art my Rock, and my High Tower!

Mary's tears had dried on her cheeks as she listened. "Uncle George is in the shadow of that Rock now, isn't he?—more completely than at any time he was living here."

"Yes," said John. "It's a wonderful thing to be a Christian, isn't it? To know that when this life ends, our fullest life is just beginning."

That evening, as Mary and John took their daily walk, Uncle George and Aunt Emma were still very much in their thoughts. John patiently slowed his steps to Mary's and walked beside his very pregnant wife with a sense of protectiveness and pride. They stopped often along the quiet streets to look up through the lacy network of new leaves on old trees, silhouetted against the sky, with the moon, dimmed by passing clouds, shining softly through. All around them was evidence of the constant love and mercy of God. They realized anew that the beauty of this life, which comes from God, is but a shadow of the beauty of the life to come, where is needed "no candle, neither light of the sun; for the Lord God giveth them light. . . ." And they realized again that after night comes morning; and after winter, spring; and after death, the resurrection.

13. In Quietness and in Confidence

He will keep in perfect peace the one who trusts in him, whose thoughts turn often to the Lord.

—Isaiah 26:3, AUTHOR'S PARAPHRASE

Easter had come and gone. Each passing day seemed longer to Mary than the one before. She tried to forget the calendar and keep busy, but her eager anticipation of the arrival of her baby occupied her thoughts and left little room for enthusiasm over any other project.

Space was at a premium in their little bedroom, with the bassinet and baby's dresser fitted into the only empty corners of the room. The dresser drawers were bulging with the many gifts Mary's friends had given her at a shower, and she had gone over each item many times, fingering the woven softness of sacques and booties or the silken delicacy of bonnets and blankets.

Thursday morning as Mary washed the few breakfast dishes, she glanced frequently out the window at the bright April landscape, hoping that April might not slip over into May before her baby had arrived. She was glad that she and John had had a chance to visit the maternity section of the hospital and see a film on the birth of a baby. John had also gone with her on her last visit to the doctor, although he hadn't gone with her every time. On impulse, Mary dried her hands suddenly, went into the bedroom and returned with the instructions the doctor had given her to study a couple of months before.

These reminded her to report at once any persistent headache, swelling, puffiness, or sudden weight gain, and any bleeding or premature breaking of the waters (fluid from the sac in which the baby had been growing). They told her of the three signs of labor she was to watch for and report to him:

SIGNS OF LABOR

1. A pinkish discharge from the vagina, known as "the show." This is the "plug" that has kept the cervix closed in pregnancy.

2. Leaking of fluid from the sac, which may rupture suddenly with a rush of fluid, or from which the water may leak slowly.
3. The beginning of contractions. These are felt as *a slight tightening and pressure in the lower abdomen just above the pelvic bone.* A slight pressure may also be felt on the lower back, making one sit up a bit straighter.

If this tightening low in the abdomen is felt occurring at intervals of ten to fifteen or twenty minutes, it is time to call the doctor. Being relaxed and confident, having prepared for a natural birth, *do not think that you are not really in labor because the contractions are not painful,* or you may become further along in labor than you realize, which will result in confusion and hurry in the last moments.

Dr. Gordon had told them that when he first began training his patients for natural childbirth, he found many of them coming to the hospital far advanced in labor, so that he really had to rush to deliver their babies in time. Neither he nor the mothers had realized that they were so near birth, because they had had no discomfort. He told Mary not to go to bed and relax completely once active labor had begun, unless she planned to have her baby at home. If her choice was to go to the hospital, light activity was better. The slight tension this involves would make her more aware of contractions, so that she would know when to go to the hospital. If she learned the signs of labor well, she needn't worry about knowing when to go. Occasionally even the best laid plans go awry, however, so he asked Mary to memorize the rules to follow in case of emergency birth.

She held the sheet in her hand, but looked out the kitchen window absently as she went over the instructions from memory:

EMERGENCY UNASSISTED BIRTH INSTRUCTIONS

1. Remain quiet and confident. Millions of women before you have borne their babies in this natural manner.
2. Brace yourself in a semisitting position on a padded surface (such as a folded blanket, covered by newspapers or a clean sheet), your back supported by large pillows or by a wall. *Do not lie down on your back!*
3. Draw up your knees, grasp them with your hands, take a deep breath, and bear down gently with each contraction. (These instructions assume that the first stage of labor and the transition

period have passed and that the baby has descended into the birth canal, ready to be born.)

4. As you feel the baby's head about to be born, *stop pushing,* and pant with short breaths in the upper chest, so the baby will be born slowly by uterine contraction alone.

5. Support the baby's head with your hand as it emerges and support the body as the shoulders emerge. The baby will rotate as he is born until he is facing you. Draw him up toward you over the pubic bone as the rest of his body emerges.

6. Break the bag of waters and remove baby immediately if he is born in it, so he will not drown as he draws his first breath. Lay baby over your abdomen, his head lower than his body, and clear his air passages so he can breathe by wiping away any mucus.

7. If baby doesn't breathe at once (he nearly always does, after a spontaneous birth), keep his head low and spank his heels. If this doesn't work, do mouth-to-mouth breathing, through a clean handkerchief, if available. Cover both his mouth and nose with your mouth and with *very tiny puffs* blow into baby's lungs rhythmically for as long as necessary. This must be done *very gently* in order not to harm the baby's lungs.

8. Wrap baby warmly in whatever is handy, put him to the breast at once if the cord is long enough (*never pull on it!*), and cough gently with each contraction to aid in expelling the afterbirth. Be patient—this may take five minutes to an hour.

9. Wrap up the afterbirth with the baby (he won't mind!) without tying or cutting the cord, until scissors and string can be sterilized for doing so, or until medical help is available.

10. Keep the uterus round and hard to prevent bleeding by massaging your abdomen *firmly* from time to time. Let baby nurse frequently, and you may get up and walk around as soon and as frequently as you wish.

Mary was satisfied that she knew the rules well without looking at them; she put the papers away, knowing she was prepared for any contingency. After finishing the few dishes she had left, she picked up a baby jacket she was making, sat down in a comfortable chair, and as she knit continued to think back over the things the doctor had explained on the last office visit.

Dr. Gordon said that he had invited a certified nurse-midwife, Doris Elleson, to become a partner in his practice, and that she would be delivering many of the babies. He would be available for medical backup in the event of any kind of problem. Miss Elleson would be setting up childbirth classes in his office as soon as she arrived; these classes would help ensure that all his patients and their husbands received adequate preparation. "You and John have been easy to teach," he said, "but it is really better if a couple can have several sessions in a group with other couples, with ample time to ask questions and practice relaxation under careful supervision. Miss Elleson will be here before your next office visit," he added, "and I want you to meet her so you can decide if you would be comfortable with her at the birth, or if you want me. It is up to you."

John and Mary had decided to birth their baby in the hospital's alternate birthing room, rather than at home or in the hospital's standard delivery room. After meeting Miss Elleson, they decided to invite her to be at the birth. Mary felt confident in the doctor's recommendation of her ability and knew this would also relieve some of his burden of overwork from a rapidly growing practice.

Mary put her knitting needles down, picked up another ball of yarn, tied it on, and, as she began knitting again, continued her careful rehearsal of the coming birth. She would be able to labor and give birth in the same bed. John would be with her the entire time. In fact, the room had a double bed so that he could lie down with her at any time, if they wanted. The room had two comfortable chairs, one of them a rocking chair. Mary knew she would be more comfortable spending part of the time rocking rather than in bed. She was also free to walk around the halls as much as she wanted. The baby would stay in the room with them after the birth. If all went well, they would be discharged within a few hours after the birth. If the birth occurred during the latter part of the day, they might choose to be transferred to the maternity ward overnight before discharge. They could not stay overnight in the birthing room, as some other laboring mother might need it.

The doctor had explained that Mary was to be propped up in a semisitting position for the birth, because women have instinctively used variations of this position for centuries. They have apparently found it the most comfortable and the one in which they can push to best advantage. The doctor explained that it takes much less energy to push an object down than it does to push it upward and out. Even animals wisely use the aid of gravity in delivering their young.

"You won't be tied down in any way during the birth, Mary," he assured her. "Dr. Dick-Read says that he has *never* tied down a pair of arms and legs![1] John can support you so that you can bend your head forward and draw your knees upward and out while bearing down. By grasping your knees either just underneath them or in front of them, and bending your elbows slightly outward, you will have plenty of leverage for pressing the baby downward. You'll be able to rest by moving your legs as is necessary for your comfort and by relaxing against your husband or against some other support between contractions."

Dr. Gordon had said he hoped that it would be possible for Mary's baby to be born without her having to have an *episiotomy*—a surgical incision made in the perineum to widen the orifice for the final stage of birth. "A friend of mine who has attended the delivery of from six hundred to seven hundred babies in Africa told me," he said, "that she had never seen a third-degree laceration, and that fewer than ten times had she felt it necessary to perform an episiotomy. Her record is better than mine," he admitted to them, smiling, "but her success has given me incentive to learn how to control the actual birth better, so that the mother will be spared the unnatural discomfort of the stitches afterward. If I or Miss Elleson feel it necessary to make an incision, Mary, you won't feel it. One doctor has told his patients that he'll even refund their fees if they can tell when he makes the incisions. They can't! This is because the perineum is insensitive during the birth, although feeling returns to it almost immediately afterward."

"Many of our friends," John had interrupted, "when they hear that Mary's to have an unmedicated birth without a lot of pain, shrug their shoulders and say, 'Oh, that's only hypnotism.' What do you say about that, Doctor?"

"Of course it's not hypnotism. Is God responsible for pain in the normal physiological function of birth?" he asked them. "We know the Bible doesn't teach this. But how then can a Christian be unwilling to believe that pain in childbirth can be prevented by following commonsense preparation during pregnancy?

"In our mechanically minded American society, we doctors have tended to look with microscopic concern at all the physical details of a

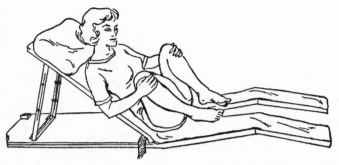

Natural-childbirth patient bearing down in raised position. In the absence of something to push her feet against, she may grip her knees as shown, pulling them widely apart as she bears down.

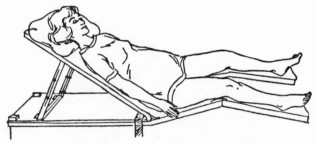

Natural-childbirth patient resting in raised position. It is important to have the knees supported slightly above the level of the hips in order to relax the legs completely. This is the "recliner-chair" position for relaxation during pregnancy also.

birth, but we've only recently been learning what the midwife has known all along—that childbirth is a great deal more than just a physical event. It's an experience of tremendous emotional and sexual significance in a woman's life. Do you remember what I told you about this in our discussion before your marriage?''

Both John and Mary replied that they did.

"This physical and emotional pleasure," the doctor said, "like the pleasant stimulation a mother receives in suckling her child later, is as pure and right in God's sight as the physical pleasure she derives from

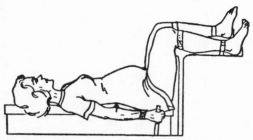

Wrong position for bearing down. Notice how the mother arches her back in order to push. This position for bearing down is not only exhausting and ineffective but causes severe backache the next day.

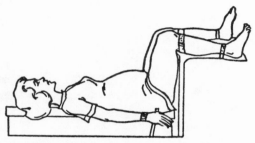

Obstetric patient in wrong position on delivery table attempting to rest between contractions. Notice that she is completely unable to change position.

stroking the tiny limbs of her baby with her fingers, or feeling the soft whisper of baby's breath against her cheek. It is our Creator who has made a mother so."

Mary glanced at the clock. Only ten o'clock—the morning was passing slowly. She decided to walk over to Carolyn's for a few minutes and ask her about a few more things still on her mind. She put her knitting away and slipped into a jacket.

The air was mild and fragrant. Mary walked slowly, enjoying every minute of it. The words of a little poem that John had found and brought to her one day came to her mind, and she held her head a little higher, confident and happy, as the charming words repeated themselves in her mind:

> She carries life in her body
>> as a girl in a dry country carries
>> a pitcher of water cupped in her hands
>> delighting
>> the thirsty eyes of the dwellers
>> in those parched lands.
>
> She is as quiet and as certain
>> as Earth in reluctant spring,
>> which waits for a night of warm showers
>> dissolving
>> the last delay of winter
>> and dazzling the dawn with flowers.[2]

"Come on out to the backyard, Mary," Carolyn greeted her as she stood at the door. "Greg's in his playpen, and Julie and Paul are digging in the sand." She led Mary through the house and on out to the backyard, where they could watch the children playing. Carolyn thoughtfully brought out a straight-backed chair for Mary, before jack-knifing herself into one of the garden chairs.

"You look good, Mary," she told her. "Is everything okay?"

"Sure is," Mary smiled, "except that I'm getting impatient. I can't sleep on my back any more—the baby's too heavy on my spine. And Dr. Gordon said the pressure also interferes with the circulation of blood, which isn't good for my baby."

"It isn't good for you either, Mary, "Carolyn added. "It can raise your blood pressure, cause swelling in your legs and increase any tendency to varicose veins. But don't you use the side position you've learned for relaxing? That's what I did. It was the only way I could sleep without having to shift positions every little while and keep Ralph awake."

"The only trouble with that," Mary confided, "is that when I'm sprawled out with my knee up on an extra pillow in the bed, there's hardly room for John! He's pushed over into one narrow strip of bed. I've told him I wouldn't mind if he'd sleep on the couch, but he says he doesn't mind being crowded."

"Of course *you* didn't offer to sleep on the couch, did you?" Carolyn teased her.

"No, it's too narrow," Mary laughed. "I'd have to lie on my back, and I'm not supposed to do that." She hesitated a moment, and then said, "I'd like to ask you about a couple more things, Carolyn."

"Okay, shoot," Carolyn said agreeably.

Mary sat up a bit straighter as a little foot reminded her that things were getting pretty crowded in her baby's warm nest. "What do the nurses mean when they talk about 'prepping'?" she asked.

"Well, some doctors have a nurse prep the patient by clipping or shaving some of the pubic hair, but Dr. Gordon doesn't feel it is necessary. And he only asks for an enema to be given if there is hard matter in the bowel or rectum, which is not only uncomfortable, but can also impair the baby's descent. Usually the contractions of early labor stimulate the bowels to move, so that no enema is needed. From time to time you will be examined vaginally to see how far the cervix is opened, though this must be done with exquisite concern for sterile technique, as it is a possible source of infection to the mother. Two fingers are inserted into the vagina and then spread apart, to determine how many centimeters the cervix has opened, how well the cervix is effacing (thinning out), and how well the baby's head is descending."

"I've heard those vaginal exams are really awful," Mary said worriedly.

"It's not too uncomfortable, Mary, unless it's done during a contraction—and you can ask them to wait until the contraction is over, unless there is a special need to determine what is happening *during* a contraction. For example, it's important to know that the cervix has completed dilation before beginning to push. But don't worry about the exams and don't tighten up and resist them because of embarrassment, because then it is more uncomfortable. There's really no need to be embarrassed—the nurses do them so often they don't think any more about it than I do about changing my babies. Their minds are more likely to be on what they ought to fix for supper or what they should wear to go out that evening. Anyway, Dr. Gordon has taught the nurses to tell how far along the mother is by observing her actions, so they make internal examinations much less frequently."

"Then I'll just relax as best I can when they're necessary."

"That's the spirit, Mary. They'll explain the reasons for everything being done. And if they don't, *ask*. Excuse me a minute!"

Carolyn jumped up to pick Julie off the fence. She scolded her daughter, set her back in the sandbox, and put the baby's toys back in his playpen before returning to her chair. Baby Greg solemnly began dropping his toys outside his playpen again, one by one, as soon as her back was turned.

Carolyn curled up in her chair, casting a weather eye at her young daughter again. "Julie!" she warned. Julie obediently climbed back into the sandbox with Paul, deciding to wait for a more opportune moment, when her mother wasn't watching, to climb back up the fence.

"Let's see. Where were we?" Carolyn pondered. "Oh, yes. I wanted to tell you that there are a couple of things that may be uncomfortable. One is the injection of the anesthetic needle into the perineum if any stitches are needed afterward. You should know," Carolyn warned, "that many doctors routinely give the injection *before* the birth and cut the perineum (the episiotomy), which is unfortunate, because it robs the woman of the sensations of birth. They make this incision 'for fear that' she might tear far too often, rather than when it is truly and obviously necessary.

"The second discomfort may be after the birth, when uterine contractions may feel 'crampy' as the uterus shrinks back to a smaller size. This usually occurs when the baby is put to breast, or the uterus is massaged to keep it contracted. But it is extremely important that it stay firm, to prevent bleeding other than the normal light flow in the days after birth.

"You are really blessed to have the supervision of a good doctor like Dr. Gordon. He doesn't do an episiotomy routinely. By the way, are you going to have him at the birth or the new nurse-midwife, Doris Elleson?

"We've decided to have Doris. Dr. Gordon called us to come over to meet her in his office the other day, and we feel very confident in her skills. We were really comfortable with her as a person too. And we have definitely decided we want the birthing room at the hospital. But, what if I had a breech baby? Is a natural birth still possible?"

"Yes, it is, though unfortunately most breeches are now delivered routinely by cesarean. Many doctors are not even taught in medical school how to deliver breeches vaginally. And cesarean is a major operation with risks to both mothers and babies. A study in one university hospital reported twice as many infant deaths with cesarean section as with vaginal breech births.[3] You can trust Dr. Gordon, Mary, for the kind of birth experience you want, even if the baby is breech or posterior (baby's face up rather than down). An individual judgment will be made based on several factors, including the size of the baby, the position of the presenting part, how well the labor is progressing, and so on. Certified nurse-midwives know how to deliver a breech baby vaginally. If surgery seems indicated, Dr. Gordon would perform the cesarean.

"But you should know that it is often possible to 'turn' a breech baby in the weeks before birth. It involves lying on one's back for ten minutes on a hard surface, with the hips raised by pillows to a level of nine to twelve inches above the mother's head. This should be done twice a day, on an empty stomach. Just before lunch and dinner is a good time. It should be started at about the thirtieth week of pregnancy and continued for several weeks. There is an old saying, 'If you can't turn the baby, turn the mother!' This is a safe way to 'turn the mother,' hips above her head, so that the baby will turn before her due date comes. Some say that with this position babies do turn about 90 percent of the time,[4] so that the baby is born in the normal head-down position.

"The main differences for the mother in a breech birth may be that it usually takes longer, since the baby's bottom doesn't dilate either the cervix or the perineum as efficiently as the head. Of course, a longer labor is no more uncomfortable if you know how to relax properly. There's often much more backache with a breech, though, especially during transition, so someone may need to massage the mother's sacrum during more of her labor when she's lying down.

"If the labor seems especially 'heavy,' it is helpful to try different positions, such as kneeling, on hands and knees as for the pelvic rock, or standing, leaning the upper body over some support while the attendant waits behind the mother to 'catch' the baby. The squatting position widens the pelvic outlet by as much as 15 percent. In fact, it has been stated, *"When the mother is at risk or the baby is at risk, as in twin or breech deliveries for example, the standing-squat position for delivery is imperative."*[5] When a mother is supported in this position, the birth is easier and shorter because of the circulatory and mechanical advantages of this upright position. As soon as the breech is delivered, the whole body and head follow, helped by gravity."

"Carolyn, you've been such a help to me all along. I don't know how to thank you," Mary said earnestly as she rose to leave.

"My best thanks would be for you to have a happy experience like mine have been," Carolyn smiled, as she walked with her around the house. She waved goodbye as Mary went down the walk, before returning to her own little ones in the back yard.

NOTES

1. Grantly Dick-Read, M.D., *Childbirth Without Fear,* 4th rev. ed. (New York: Harper & Row, 1972), p. 289.
2. Written by Alexander Scott, printed in *A Book of Scotland,* ed. G. F. Maine (London: Collins, 1950), pp. 339, 340. Reprinted by permission.
3. "Says Many Breech Babies Can be Safely Delivered Vaginally," study reported in *International Medical News Service,* from *Ob. Gyn. News,* vol. 11, no. 23. The study was of 597 breech presentations in a major medical center.
4. "Postural Exercise Turns Fetus in Breech Position," reported in *International Medical News Service,* from *Ob. Gyn. News,* vol. 12, no. 1.
5. Michel Odent, M.D., "The Evolution of Obstetrics at Pithiviers," *Birth and the Family Journal.* vol. 8, no. 1, Spring 1981. Italics are in original article. Reprinted by permission.

14. The Gift of God

Every good gift and every perfect gift is from above, coming down from the Father of the heavenly lights, who does not change like shifting shadows.

—James 1:17, NIV

Once again Mary shifted in her sleep. The first streaks of dawn were appearing across the morning sky. She glanced at her watch—five o'clock, it said. She lay back, wondering why she felt restless. She placed her hand on her abdomen, feeling for a contraction, but there didn't seem to be one. Finally she drifted back to sleep.

"Are you all right, Mary?" John asked her at the breakfast table later. "You seemed restless last night." He looked at her anxiously, but she seemed relaxed and cheerful.

"I'm fine," she assured him, sitting up a little straighter in her chair as she felt a fleeting pressure on her lower back.

"You're sure you don't want me to stay home today?"

"Oh, no John."

"Be sure to call me if your labor starts, honey. The principal said he'd arrange for my classes if I had to leave during the school day."

"I will. Please, don't fret so about me."

"Promise?"

"I promise. I'll call you right away."

John kissed her goodbye and reluctantly started off to his classes. Mary picked up some of the breakfast dishes and carried them to the sink. Instinctively she stopped in the middle of the room, as she felt her lower abdomen tighten a bit. She glanced at the clock. Eight-twenty, it said. The feeling passed, and she went on with her work.

Eight-thirty. She had glanced at the clock again. Wouldn't it be exciting if my baby was to be born today? she thought dreamily, picturing him already cradled in the curve of her arm, or nestled against her shoulder. She was so glad that Doris Elleson had arrived in time to meet with her and John a couple of times. Doris had said how important John's role was and how he could help at various times through the labor and birth. She had said that yielding to his caresses was the best possible stimulus to effective labor, and she even encouraged John to "catch the baby" if all went well, if he chose to do so. Mary's heart skipped a beat at the thought of pressing her baby out into John's waiting hands. She wondered if she should call the doctor—although she was sure these little twinges couldn't be labor!

Eight-forty. This time Mary went to the phone. Dr. Gordon advised her to come over to the office to be checked, before deciding if she should go to the hospital.

Mary called John, who had just arrived at school. He was home again within a few minutes. They climbed into the car, and he began driving like mad toward the doctor's office.

"Please, don't drive so fast!" Mary gasped, stiffening because of a very uncomfortable contraction. She gripped the armrest of the car tensely, to keep from being jarred with every rise in the pavement. John slowed down and drove more carefully. In his mind he had pictured the baby as arriving any minute, and he was anxious to get to the office in time, in case they had to go right on to the hospital.

As they reached the approach to the office, another contraction began, unmistakable this time, and Mary again braced herself stiffly against it. As soon as it had passed, they left the car and walked into the office.

Dr. Gordon informed them that only slight dilation of the cervix had taken place and that Mary seemed to be in very early labor, the latent phase, which might go on for some time or even discontinue for a while. He suggested that they wait at home and check back with him or with Miss Elleson from time to time.

"Miss Elleson is at the hospital now," the doctor said, "and she will be with you throughout your labor. If there are any problems, she'll notify me to come. Otherwise, she is competent to handle the entire care through the birth. Since your labor will most likely be normal, you've made a wise decision in choosing her.

"Also," he continued, "the hospital has been informed that you will be using the alternative birth room. And they've been given written instructions that you're to be given no prep and no medication for pain unless you specifically ask for it. In addition, the baby will not be monitored electronically unless there is an indication that this might be necessary. And in that case," he added, "I would have been alerted, and either I or Miss Elleson would be continuously at your side also.

Here," he said, handing them a slip of paper, "take this with you to the hospital. It is a copy of my instructions to them, in case there are any questions from the staff.

"Now, Mary, when your contractions are five to ten minutes apart and about sixty seconds in length, it will be time to go to the hospital. A good sign will be when you can no longer converse through a contraction but need to 'center down' on what your body is doing by relaxing and breathing slowly. I'll be at my office all day, if you need to call."

"John, d'you know what?" Mary mused thoughtfully on the way home. "I wasn't the least bit relaxed on the way to the office, was I?"

"You sure weren't! You were hanging on for dear life!"

"No wonder those contractions were so uncomfortable!" she said soberly. "I was holding on so I wouldn't be jarred—but it made my contractions hurt. And I'm only in very early labor. I'm sure glad I've learned how to relax. I can see how *awful* labor could be if you started out all tensed up like that and didn't know how to relax!" Mary placed her hand absently over her abdomen and was surprised to find it hard as a rock beneath her touch.

"Why," she exclaimed in surprise, "I must be having a contraction right now, and I didn't even know it!"

"You've had a little time to quiet down," John smiled at her. He opened the car door for her, helped her out and up the walk, and closed the front door behind them. He held her close as he whispered softly in her ear, "Remember, honey, to trust the God who made you!" He stroked her hair and cheek as he added, "Just rest in his arms, and everything will be all right."

But to their great surprise, rather than increasing, Mary's labor began to slow down. John stayed at home with Mary, helping to time contractions. Twenty minutes apart, then ten, then thirty . . . After a couple of hours they gave it up. Mary lay down to rest while John fixed a light lunch for them.

By mid-afternoon Mary was greatly discouraged. Nothing seemed to be happening, and John suggested they go for a walk. Contractions started up again after they had walked a few blocks but then faded. Off and on. Off and on. Mary passed the mucus plug. She spent most of the time rocking in the rocking chair, in light activity, or lying on her side on the couch listening to their stereo or watching television with John. He didn't leave her for a moment.

After a light supper Mary insisted that John go to the ball game. Labor seemed to have stopped completely, and the team needed their head coach. John said he'd call home every half hour or so until his return. After the game he rushed home to find nothing had changed, and they went to bed, snuggled together. John kept stroking, touching, loving her, to stimulate her labor, until they fell asleep.

Mary slept lightly. Her senses were turned inward, even in her sleep, alert to her body, her baby. A contraction occurred now and then, her uterus "warming up" for the work ahead, but she dozed between them.

"John," she nudged toward morning. "John," she shook him. Startled, he sat up abruptly. He had been sleeping soundly. "I think we'd better start for the hospital, honey." They had laid everything out the night before and in a few moments were on their way.

They gave their names at the desk, and a nurse brought a wheelchair. Mary disdained it, however, preferring to walk. They went on up to the labor ward and a nurse took them into the birthing room. After seeing where Mary was to be, John returned to the desk to complete their registration. Mary undressed quickly and slipped into the hospital gown the nurse had given her. A few moments later Doris Elleson, cheerful and efficient, came in. After checking Mary's cervical dilatation she helped her get comfortably propped up in the bed in the recliner-chair position and slipped pillows under her knees. "You're three to four centimeters dilated, Mrs. Thomas," she explained, holding up two fingers to demonstrate the size of the opening.

Dismayed, Mary cried, "Is *that* all? I thought I was a lot farther along than that!"

"You're doing excellently," Miss Elleson encouraged her. "The cervix has thinned out nicely, and the baby's head fits well into the pelvic brim. By the way," she added, "please call me Doris. And is it all right if I call you Mary?"

When Mary nodded, she explained, "It's more restful to shift positions occasionally, but keep your joints—like knees and elbows—bent a little, as this helps you to relax. And be sure to keep your bladder and bowels empty, so that you can keep the birth outlet as loosely relaxed as possible. Whenever you feel like it, you can get up to rock in the rocking chair or walk up and down the halls. You have complete freedom to be in any position that's comfortable for you, in or out of the bed." She gave Mary a reassuring smile. "I'll let you rest now but will be back whenever you'd like me to come. Would you like to turn on your side before I leave and slip the extra pillow under your knee for a while?

"I'm comfortable just now, thank you."

After Doris had gone out, Mary studied the room as she waited for John to return. The walls were a soft pastel, and there were *pictures!* A contraction came on and she closed her eyes, took two or three deep breaths, and allowed herself to go limp. When the contraction had passed, she studied the pictures contentedly. One was the lovely "Madonna of the Streets," the other a chubby little girl asleep on her tummy, her knees tucked under her, her round little bottom making a hump under the blankets.

Mary turned her gaze toward the windows and discovered that they were framed with flowered material and that she could see the green tips of the trees in the courtyard below. The harmonious atmosphere of the room gave her a feeling of peace and of quiet anticipation.

Doris ushered John into the room to be with Mary. There was a recliner in the room with a magazine rack beside it, as well as the rocking chair. But he chose a straight-back chair instead and drew it up close to the bed. Kissing Mary he asked, "Is everything okay?"

"Yes, honey. Isn't this a pretty room? By the way," she said, "Miss Elleson wants us to call her Doris." Turning to Doris she said, "I feel as if I were in a guest room—not the hospital!"

"We want the mothers to feel that they're guests. They're certainly not invalids!" Doris said. She said down on the edge of the bed, keeping a hand on Mary's abdomen through a contraction. Her calm conversation and explanations were reassuring to both Mary and John. Whenever Mary was having a contraction, both Doris and John were silent until it passed. As one began, Mary took a few slow, relaxed breaths and let her whole body sag. Between contractions she chatted happily. Doris was pleased to see that she was relaxing properly and complimented her.

"Turn over onto your left side soon now, Mary, and see if you can relax enough to doze a while. The less you think about your uterus now, the more quickly it'll open the door for you. After a while," she explained, "the contractions will become much longer and closer together, as you know, and you'll feel more pressure on your lower spine. This is the transition period, during which you'll begin to feel the need to change from relaxing to pushing during the contractions.

"I know you'll remember to watch for this, too, John," she said, turning to him. "You can help Mary tell when it's near by timing the length of the contractions occasionally and by noticing when it gets harder for her to relax. If her back bothers her, you can help by pressing firmly with the heel of your hand where she shows you, and rotating your hand in a semicircular motion.

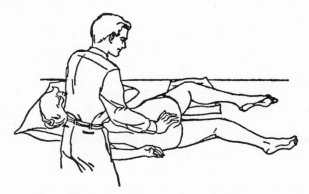

Husband massaging sacrum, using a semi-circular motion and pressing firmly with the heel of his hand.

"But the best thing you can do, John," she added, "is to be her lover, to kiss and caress her as if you were in your own bedroom at home. We professionals have been slow to realize that the affectionate caresses of the husband are tremendously effective stimuli to labor. Birth is a sexual event, and the husband's intimate touching causes a hormonal response that is the best possible 'prescription.' You can be guided by Mary's desires in this.

"I'm going to leave you two alone." Doris started toward the door as she explained, "I'll not come back into the room without knocking first, so your privacy won't be invaded. Don't hesitate to call me, though, whenever you want me." She slipped out and closed the door, hanging a sign on the front that said PLEASE KNOCK BEFORE ENTERING.

Mary let herself become limper and limper until she was barely aware of the contractions at all, although they were becoming stronger and more effective. Since the birthing room bed was a double bed, John lay down beside her, stroking her hair, her ears, her arms, her face, occasionally laying his hand on her abdomen to feel the strength and timing of the contractions. Time crept by at a snail's pace for him.

Mary opened her eyes finally, feeling refreshed. "I guess I didn't sleep much last night," she admitted. John held her closer, his caressing hand following the contours of her body in any way that pleased her.

After some time Miss Elleson tapped softly on the door. "May I come in?" John got off the bed and opened the door for her. She noticed at once that a flush had come into Mary's cheeks (a sign that the cervix is about three-fifths dilated), so she felt no need to make an internal examination to determine the progress of labor.

Mary pulled John's arm over and looked at his watch. "You ought to get something to eat," she said, worrying about him. "You didn't have breakfast and it's almost lunch time!"

"I'm staying right here!" he responded, so firmly that she didn't question it. Secretly she was relieved that he hadn't left her.

"Would you like a lunch tray sent up?" Doris asked John. He readily agreed. A few minutes later she returned with a tray for him and a glass of orange juice for Mary. She checked the baby's heartbeat, observed Mary through a couple of contractions, and then suggested that Mary get up and walk around for a while or rock in the chair. Mary was tired of lying in bed and glad for the suggestion.

Just as Mary started to get out of bed she was startled by the sac rupturing suddenly, and the clean bedding was flooded with water. Although she had known this would happen, it had surprised her by its suddenness, and she was also dismayed at having drenched the bedclothes.

"Oh, I'm sorry!" she apologized.

"Don't give it a thought, Mary." Doris stepped to the door and asked the nurses to bring some fresh bedding and some bed pads to place under Mary. "I'll need to check your cervix before you get up," she explained, "to be sure the baby's head is engaged properly so that the cord won't drop down first, what we call a *prolapse*." Once she had ascertained that the head was firmly engaged, she and John helped Mary to the rocker, covered it with towels, and helped her sit down.

It felt good to be rocking. Doris propped a footstool under her feet so that she could put her soles together and let her knees flop outward. She let her head droop forward as she rocked gently back and forth.

After almost an hour she stiffened. "My back! Please, rub it, honey!" John reached in between the chair back and Mary and tried to, but it was awkward. Mary decided to get back in bed.

Doris and John helped her onto the bed and onto her side. John began rubbing her back again, furiously, anxious to be of help. "You're about to shove me through the bed," Mary gasped, "and you don't need to—" she caught her breath "—rub my skin off!" She held her breath and waited for a long, powerful contraction to pass. "I can't relax," she complained, stiffening, as another strong contraction followed. She had obviously reached transition.

"Keep your abdominal wall relaxed, Mary," Doris said calmly. "Don't hold your breath, just breathe more deeply in and out, in and out, during the next contraction." She pressed her hand firmly on Mary's sacrum to show John how to make the hand pressure more effective and watched to be sure Mary did not begin breathing the shallow, rapid breaths that indicate tension. "Stay relaxed and breathe *deeply* now, in, out, in, out. That's it, not too fast." Mary found that following Miss Elleson's unobtrusive guidance kept her comfortable through the next few contractions.

"I feel like I want to sit up, Doris," Mary said. "May I?"

"Remember Mary, you are free to move into any position that is comfortable for you."

Doris raised the head of the bed again, and John helped Mary turn over and sit up. Doris rolled pillows into bolsters and put one under each of Mary's knees. Mary found this semisitting position far more comfortable at this stage of labor and again let her muscles become relaxed and limp. John kept the heel of his hand under the small of her back and breathed with her through the next several contractions, looking right into her eyes. "You're doing great!" he whispered, "I'm proud of you." An hour passed.

"I'm cold," Mary complained, "and I c-can't stop my l-legs from shaking." Doris quickly covered her more warmly, as John breathed with her during the next contraction. To her surprise, it ended abruptly, and she cried in relief, "There! That's better!" The baby's head had slipped on through the cervix into the birth canal, and she was immediately more comfortable. Emotionally keyed up from the excitement of the transition, she grabbed her knees and pushed with all her might.

"Wait, Mary," Doris chided gently. "Just relax and rest a bit. The contractions will come farther apart now. Push only when you feel one beginning, and if it hurts to push, don't push at all, but wait until it feels comfortable to do so.''

Mary relaxed against the pillow behind her on the raised bed. Opening her eyes, she was surprised to find John standing just beside her left arm, scrubbed and dressed in paper hospital regalia. She had momentarily forgotten all about him.

"You sure make a handsome intern!" she teased. He bowed deeply in mock acknowledgment of the compliment.

"Thank you, madam," he replied solemnly.

Just then Mary felt a contraction beginning. Again she gripped her knees and pressed firmly downward. She was amazed at how good it felt to be pressing the baby down! But again she became aware that Doris was saying something to her. As the contraction ended, Mary gave her her full attention.

"When a contraction begins, Mary," she was saying, "take a cleansing in-and-out breath; then take a deep breath, lean over and push gently, breathing *slowly* out through your throat and mouth as you push. Don't wait to take another breath any longer than is comfortable. Keep your birth outlet completely slack and limp as you push. Take another breath or two during the contraction if necessary. Press the baby down firmly, but don't strain. Have you read the Bible verse that says, 'Man that is born of a woman . . . comes forth as a flower'?''

Mary shook her head and listened, interested.

"Think of yourself as a flower too. In films that show a flower opening we see its petals unfold a bit, rest, open, rest, open, slowly, irresistibly, rhythmically, in the steady, even rhythm of all growing things. Mrs. Dick-Read says that a mother giving birth should think of herself as 'a rose unfolding.' " Her quiet tone was reassuring to Mary.

John had slipped his arm around Mary's shoulders. As each contraction began, he helped her lean over to push. She gripped her knees, pulled them up toward her shoulders, took a deep breath, let it out slowly in soft, moaning sighs as she pushed, took another, let it out slowly, slowly, and then sank back peacefully against John's shoulder when each contraction ended. She took two or three deep in-and-out breaths to replace her oxygen and cleanse her lungs and then relaxed limply against the pillows as she waited for the next contraction. She was grateful that she did not have to be moved to another room for the birth but could stay where she was. Dr. Gordon had explained earlier that throughout most of the world, mothers were permitted to stay in the same bed throughout labor and birth if all was going well.

"It's important to keep a mother propped up *enough,* John," Doris explained, "so that she doesn't have to do a 'sit-up' every time she needs to lean forward to push. You have her in the perfect position— about 70 degrees from the horizontal plane."

"Thanks, Doris," John said. "But be sure to tell me when I should come get ready to catch my baby."

"I will. It will be a while yet."

Another hour passed by quietly. Like a lovely flower, Mary thought. There's one! Deep breath—press down—keep breathing out—take a breath—press down—mouth open—. —Rest! —Press down! —Rest! —Press down. —Rest!

"Remember cleansing breaths after every contraction, Mary."

There was no unnecessary noise. Doris and John conversed quietly from time to time, but Mary didn't mind. She seemed oblivious to all that went on most of the time, but actually she was acutely aware of every slight sound or motion in the room. She just did not bother to respond.

She was perspiring freely now, and John tenderly wiped the perspiration from her forehead with some tissues from a box near by each time she rested after pressing down. Once he leaned over and whispered to her softly, "The 'renunciation of toil,' Mary?"

She nodded happily, turning her smiling face toward him without opening her eyes. ". . . labor of love," she murmured.

Again she felt the impulse to press down strongly, and this time as she did so she experienced a new sensation—a bulging feeling at the outlet of the birth canal. "Look here, Mary," someone was saying.

She opened her eyes and noticed that a nurse was holding a mirror so that she could see the top of a little head appearing. She roused from her half-stupor and cried excitedly, "The baby! Oh! Look, John! The baby! It has black hair!" John had the best view of all, as Doris had moved aside so he could deliver their child. His hands were scrubbed and gloved, and he was waiting for the baby, following Doris's gentle advice. Another nurse had come in to help them until the birth was complete.

Mary worked with a will now, with a mounting excitement, and soon began to feel a "pins and needles" sensation at the outlet. "It's such a bursting feeling," she gasped, short of breath, as the contraction passed. She appeared alarmed.

"Does it hurt?" Doris asked quietly.

"Yes," Mary started to say, then added, "No, well—it's—so *different,* so overwhelming!" Then she smiled and said thoughtfully, "I guess I'm just afraid it's *going* to hurt more and more!"

"Keep the outlet as limp as you can," Doris said quietly, "and the prickly feeling will be gone in a few seconds now. Don't push any more, but pant during contractions. Take little short breaths in your upper chest with your mouth open, breathing *out, out, out.*"

Mary did this during the next contraction. She found it difficult to keep from pushing. John had been massaging Mary's perineum and now supported it with his hand under Doris's unobtrusive direction.

"If you push now, you may tear," Doris explained. "In England, you know, a midwife considers it a disgrace if she lets a mother tear. She tells the mother to let her baby's head be born 'hair by hair.' "

"John, you're the funniest looking English midwife I ever saw!" Mary teased him unexpectedly, and they all laughed.

As another contraction began, Mary closed her eyes and panted, an exciting tension mounting in her head till it seemed about to burst with emotion. So hard not to push—such a tight, bulging—"There! There!" she cried happily, as the baby's head slipped out into daddy's hands.

"John! Look! The baby!" A tremendous awe had swept over John himself, as he felt the warm weight of his child's head cradled in his hands. He was silent, too choked up to speak. A moment later the baby's shoulders slipped through, and Mary reached down to lift out her own baby, her hands intertwining with John's. A tingling flush of hot warmth engulfed her whole body from head to toe as she felt her baby slipping smoothly through the vagina, and a few seconds later the young Mr. Thomas had made his debut into the world.

"Isn't he *beautiful,* John!" breathed Mary delightedly. "Isn't he a *beautiful* baby!"

John gazed in awe at the red, wrinkled face of their newborn son, the black hair plastered to the little head covered with its own brand of white baby cream. He saw the blue-white perfect little body in his hands slowly turning rosy warm. He felt too choked up to answer

Mary. As long as he lived, he would remember the feel of that small, warm body, fresh from his wife's womb.

As the cord stopped pulsing, he handed the baby to Mary. Doris placed two clamps on the cord a few inches apart, and handed John the scissors so he could cut the cord—which was a surprisingly pretty turquoise blue. Mary drew the baby to her breast. He was mewing like a tiny kitten. The nurse who was assisting threw a warm blanket over them both. And Baby Thomas, so recently thrust abruptly from the warm security of his mother's body into the cold world, stopped his whimpering and nestled contentedly in the warm security of his mother's loving arms, comforted by her familiar voice.

As Mary looked at the tiny bundle in her arms, such a wave of happiness swept over her that she could not keep the tears from streaming down her cheeks.

"Why, Mary! What's wrong!" John asked, alarmed.

"It's—nothing," Mary sobbed. "It's just that—I've never been so happy!"

As John daubed uselessly at her tears with his handkerchief, he surreptitiously brushed a tear from his own eye. A hush had come over the room, as he bent tenderly over his wife and newborn son. And for one long moment all were vividly aware of another Presence that filled the room—the eternal Spirit of the living God.

15. The "Little Bitsa Baby, in His Hand"

Can a woman forget the baby at her breast
and have no compassion on the child she has borne?
Though she may forget,
I will not forget you!

—*Isaiah 49:15,* NIV

"You certainly don't look as if you'd just had a baby!" one of the new mothers exclaimed, as a radiant Mary walked into the room she was to share.

"I don't feel like it either!" Mary answered happily. "It's like a dream our baby's here, isn't it, John?"

John smiled but made no reply. His active participation during the past hours had made the birth a vivid reality to him.

The nurse turned down the sheets of the bed and placed Mary's son beside her as soon as she was comfortable. "Any time you're tired," she instructed Mary, "just put your baby in this bassinet by your bed. If you need us for anything, turn on this light." She pinned the call light onto the side of the bed near Mary and asked, "Would you like me to put the baby in his bed now?"

"Oh, please, no," Mary pleaded. She was still too excited to want to rest.

"All right," the nurse said agreeably. Before she left the room she handed Mary a sheet of instructions covering both hospital regulations and how to care for herself.

After the nurse had gone, John pulled up a chair in order to see his new son better.

"Would you like to hold him, honey?" Mary asked.

"I'd love to," John said, taking the baby into his arms and holding him close. He was grateful for the hour the three of them had had alone together in the birthing room after the baby's birth. Doris had said that sometimes a mother and baby could leave a few hours after a natural birth. Some went home after twelve hours. But since it was now so late in the afternoon, Mary decided to stay overnight and go home first thing in the morning.

One of Mary's roommates spoke up. "The nurses will show you how to bathe the baby if you stay long enough in the morning. They don't like the baby bathed right after the birth, because the white covering on his skin (*vernix caseosa*) should be allowed to be absorbed into his skin. My pediatrician says this is the best protection against skin infection for the first few days of life. But you can watch my baby being bathed tomorrow if you like."

"I'd appreciate that," Mary said. "I've never been around tiny babies very much."

"Also," her friend continued, "this is a wonderful place to be with a new baby. We have our own dining hall and lounge, so we can be up as much as we like. Or they'll bring our meals to us if we prefer. And our husbands can come any time. The hospital only asks that they scrub their hands before holding their babies."

"Aren't there any visiting hours?" Mary asked her.

"Oh yes, for other visitors, because the babies aren't allowed in the room while they're here. But husbands can wander in and out any time they like."

"How nice," Mary sighed happily. "I wish you didn't have to leave at all, John, but I know my folks will be waiting for you to have supper with them after a while."

"I'll be back as soon as I can," he assured her, "and I'll bring your folks along."

"Were they excited when you told them about the baby?"

"*Were* they! Your mother sounded as if she was crying over the phone when I told her what an easy time you'd had and how happy you were. She was awfully worried about you, Mary."

"I know." Mary stroked the baby's petal-soft cheek with her finger as she said soberly, "I tried to tell Mother that God meant giving birth to be a beautiful experience, but she was afraid to believe it for me." Mary had scarcely lifted her eyes from God's sweet gift to her since he had been put beside her, but now she looked up at John, and he took courage to reach over and slip his finger into a tiny fist.

"Wow! You wouldn't think such a delicate thing could have such a grip!" he said proudly. "Boy, will he ever be able to clutch a bat!" He turned the blanket back to study the pink feet. "All eleven toes are there, all right."

"What?" Mary nearly sat upright in bed, astonished.

"I'm joking, hon. He's only got ten. By the way, your folks wanted to know what name we had decided on. I told them we'd talked about Susan, Jane, Robert, Peter, Nancy, Walter, Linda, Nelly, Tom, Kirk, Scott, Douglas, and on, and on, and on, but that you'd never been able to make up your mind!"

"Well, it won't be Susan, or Jane, or Nancy!" Mary smiled. "We really ought to decide, though," she said, more soberly. "What does he look like his name should be?"

John looked at his son thoughtfully for awhile. "It ought to be a distinguished name," he observed, "something like 'Gregory Piedmont Beadlehouser Thomas the First'?"

But Mary didn't laugh. "I like the name Gregory," she said, "only Carolyn has a Greg, too." A thoughtful look had come over her face. "John?"

"Yes?" he answered expectantly, sensing her earnestness.

"I have an idea." Mary paused, tore her loving gaze from her baby's face, and looked right into her husband's eyes. "I don't know what you'll think of it, honey," she told him seriously, "but I'd like to name our baby George."

After John left, Mary carefully read over the instructions the nurse had given her earlier. She was especially interested in the instructions for breastfeeding and for the exercises to use following childbirth.

EXERCISES AFTER CHILDBIRTH

1. Practice the vaginal contractions learned during pregnancy. This restores the muscles of the birth canal to their former tightness and resiliency. If there have been stitches, they will heal more quickly, with less soreness.

2. Lie on your stomach from time to time with large pillows under the hips, and a small one under your ankles. This position aids the uterus in returning to its normal place within the abdomen.

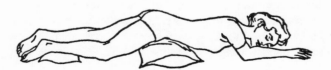

3. After returning home, once each day lie on your back, raise one leg ten inches off the ground without bending the knee, hold for a count of three, and lower slowly. Repeat with the other leg. Raise each leg two or three times each session, working up to ten times. This exercise helps restore a flat stomach.

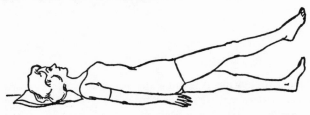

4. Practice good posture while sitting, standing, or walking, from the very first day.

BREASTFEEDING INSTRUCTIONS

1. Breastfeed baby often during the first twenty-four hours. This will cause the uterus to contract firmly and help prevent hemorrhage. It will also loosen the *colostrum* (the creamy-looking secretion that appears before the milk comes in on about the third day), so that the milk will be "let down" more easily when it first appears. (Animals instinctively suckle their offspring shortly after birth.)

2. To breastfeed baby, place him on the bed beside you, lying on his side with his head tilted back ever so slightly. Lie on your side with your breast near his mouth. Stroke one cheek lightly with a finger, or with the nipple, so the baby turns his head toward you and opens his mouth. Insert a good portion of the brown part of the nipple (the *areola*) into his mouth.

3. Let baby lie quietly beside you as he nurses. He should be handled as little as possible. With your index finger, keep the fleshy part of the breast pressed gently away from his nose, so he can breathe.

4. Breastfeed baby frequently the first day or two, a few minutes on each breast each time. Nursing every couple of hours or less keeps baby satisfied, helps the milk come in more quickly, and helps prevent engorgement and sore nipples.

5. Baby may not get enough liquid to need burping the first few

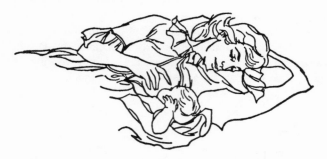

times, though he is getting the valuable colostrum. After the milk comes in, try burping him after each feeding, and sometimes halfway through. Rest the baby against your shoulder so that he is looking behind you (being sure to support the head and neck) and pat gently. Or, sit baby in your lap, leaning him forward slightly and cup his chin in your hand to support his wobbly head, patting his back until he "bubbles."

6. Baby may lose a few ounces of weight at first but will regain them rapidly when the milk begins to come in. (The milk looks thinner, more bluish than the colostrum, but don't worry—it's rich enough!) When the milk first appears, the breasts may become distended and overflow. Keep fresh, sterile pads over the nipples to absorb any excess milk. (The hospital supplies these. After you leave the hospital, you may purchase breast pads at the drug store, or you may prefer to use clean men's handkerchiefs, cut pieces of sanitary napkins, or flannel pads you make yourself.) As the initial swelling of the breasts recedes, some mothers fear that they've "lost their milk," but the supply is only adjusting to the demand. As baby gets older, the amount of milk produced will increase to meet his needs.

7. Wash the nipples with water only, as soap or astringent wipes are drying to the skin and may cause sore or cracked nipples. If any soreness occurs, report it at once, and a bland ointment may be prescribed to help them heal quickly.

8. The breasts should always be well supported from beneath by a nursing brassiere, with no pressure across the breasts or nipples.

9. Whether breastfeeding baby in bed or sitting up in a chair, always lift him *to* the breast so there is no downward pull on it.

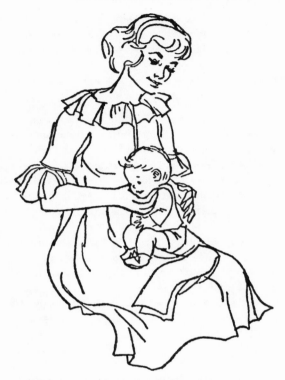

If the breast is pulled down to the baby, it may lose its shape permanently.

10. If a premature baby is too weak to suckle, he still needs his mother's milk. The milk can be expressed by hand directly into his mouth, or into a sterile container (after thoroughly scrubbing your hands). A baby doesn't actually "suck," but stimulates the "let-down" of the milk by the pressure of his gums, tongue, and palate around the nipple. This gentle squeezing action stimulates the milk flow, which is sometimes so rapid that the baby can hardly swallow fast enough at first! If this occurs, express a little milk first before putting baby on.

11. To express the milk manually, place the forefinger just below, and the thumb just above, the outer edges of the brown area surrounding the nipple. Press these fingers gently in a scissors

motion, at the same time pushing in toward the breast slightly. The milk will soon flow easily. A breast pump is often supplied by the hospital, but the manual method is usually more comfortable.

12. Continue to follow the rules of good nutrition used for pregnancy. Relax and enjoy your baby!

Mary finished combing her hair, pinned a flower in place, and returned to her bed, swinging her legs impatiently as she sat on the edge of it waiting for her parents. "Mother! Dad!" she cried happily, slipping down off the bed and hurrying forward to embrace them.

"Did you see Baby George before you came in?" she asked breathlessly, not waiting for an answer as she perched back up on the edge of the bed. "Isn't he a darling? Who does he look like? Don't you think he looks like John? Of course, John doesn't have such black hair."

"Just a minute, young lady," her father chided, holding up his hand in mock dismay. He was pleased that she looked so well and happy. "One question at a time please. So you think he looks like John, eh? You're supposed to say he looks like me. Babies are supposed to resemble their grandparents more than their parents, you know."

"I haven't decided who he looks like, but he's a darling!" her mother smiled. "I can hardly wait till you bring him home, so I can help spoil him!" Aside to Mary she whispered anxiously, "Doesn't it make your stitches sore to sit on the edge of the bed like that?"

"But I don't have any stitches, Mother," Mary explained, "so I'm not the least bit sore."

"You don't *have* any stitches?" Her mother sounded unbelieving.

Mary's dad wandered out into the hall to take another look at his new grandson. He read the sign on the nursery window again:

> Baby Thomas, boy
> Seven pounds, nine ounces
> Twenty-one inches
> Born April 29, 2:58 p.m.

He studied the small face through the window, trying to find some resemblance in the tiny features—perhaps to himself!

"I didn't need any stitches," Mary was explaining to her mother. "And maybe you won't believe me, but it was the most *wonderful* experience! I can still feel how my baby's head slipped out and how his little body followed!" She sat transfixed in the happy memory for a moment. Her mother was silent, not understanding, but knowing from Mary's obvious happiness that her daughter was telling the truth.

"I'm truly glad for you, dear," she said earnestly, meaning every word.

Mary turned around and motioned to her friends. "Mother, I ought to introduce my roommates. This is Janice Wells—she has a little girl, one of the prettiest babies here."

"How do you do," Mary's mother said kindly, and Janice smiled acknowledgment.

"Down at the end is Elaine Dieple," Mary said, with a sweep of her arm. "She has five children now."

Mrs. Johnson and Elaine exchanged greetings. "This is a lovely room you have here, rocking chairs and all," Mary's mother told them. "Things have surely changed since I had my babies!"

"They've changed even since I started my family," Elaine agreed, "and for the better, I might add. It's so much nicer having our babies with us."

"Maybe this isn't such a new way after all," Mary's mother smiled. "I read in the paper last year that in maternity wards in the Congo, each mother's bed has a little basket at the foot of it. When reporters walked through one of the wards one day, not a single baby was in his basket. They were all in bed with their mothers!"

Mary's father walked into the room in time to hear her last comment. "So you're returning to the jungles to have your babies, are you?" he kidded them. He pulled up a chair and made himself comfortable.

"Not exactly, Dad," Mary laughed. "But we can learn a lot from those who live closer to nature." Then she asked him eagerly, "Did you decide who the baby looks like?"

"Yes, I did," he grinned mischievously.

"Who? Tell me!"

"Well, little mother," he teased her. "I think he looks like his grandpa!"

It had been an exciting day. The nurses brought some juice, whole wheat crackers, and cheese for the mothers. Mary had been famished after the birth and was glad they had brought her supper early. She had really enjoyed her meal and couldn't believe she could be so hungry again! Janice Wells, in the bed next to her, said that all the hospital meals and snacks were really delicious and such a nice change from the constant planning and cooking at home.

Janice had a new baby girl, her second child. The baby was unusually beautiful for a newborn, with pink-white skin, lovely curling lashes, and dark hair so long its silken folds brushed against her dainty neck.

Janice, Elaine, and Mary had talked on into the evening on the universal topics of discussion in maternity wards everywhere—their labors, their babies, and the things they liked or didn't like about their doctors!

Elaine had had a natural birth, like Mary's. Janice had had a long, painful labor in spite of deep sedation and had had a saddle block (an injection in the lower spine that removes sensation from the pubic area and below) at birth. All three of them planned to nurse their babies.

Finally, Elaine and Janice turned out their lights, but before Mary turned out her light, she gently pulled her baby's bed close to take a last peek at him and to be sure—for the umpteenth time—that he was really breathing! He was sleeping quietly, so she carefully pushed him back, turned over onto her stomach, relaxed as completely as she could, and soon drifted into a peaceful, contented slumber. Her roommates were already asleep, and there were no sounds apart from the hushed rustling of normal night hospital activity.

Mary opened her eyes in the dark. Was that her baby? What was that muffled sound? She lay very still, listening. Soon she realized that the sound she heard came from the bed next to hers. She sat up a moment, listening to the soft crying, and then slipped into her robe and slippers and tiptoed over to Janice's side.

"Janice?" she whispered anxiously. "Can I help? Please don't cry!"

Janice didn't answer, but turned her wet cheek toward Mary to indicate that she'd heard and appreciated Mary's concern. Mary took Janice's hand in her own and held it in the dark, tears of pity welling up in her own eyes, as Janice wept helplessly for several minutes.

"Please, Janice—don't cry any more," she pleaded.

"I can't—help it," Janice sobbed. "I'm a dope!" she berated herself, searching in her own mind for a reason for her unhappiness. "I've always wanted a little girl, and everyone's been so nice, but—" she burst into fresh sobs, "I can't help crying. I don't know what's the matter with me!"

Gradually Janice became quieter as Mary comforted her. There were deep, deep questions in Mary's heart as she stroked her companion's arm in the dark, wondering why Janice should be so unhappy.

"You have a beautiful baby, Janice," she suggested hopefully. "Nothing should take that happiness away from you."

Janice was quieter now. "I know," she said. Gradually she became aware of someone's else's need besides her own. "Mary, you're a gem!" she told her, "but you shouldn't be up and around in the middle of the night like this. You go on back to bed now. I'll be all right. And thank you so much." She pressed Mary's hand gratefully.

Mary took another peek at her baby. He was stirring, so she drew him close and laid him beside her. She needed the reassurance of his presence just now. As she helped his tiny rosebud mouth find satisfaction, Mary thought how grateful she was for her experience in giving him birth! That experience would be framed in her memory like a jewel, forever. She wouldn't have traded places with Janice for anything! As she caressed her baby's downy head, she was so very happy that she'd had faith to believe that God "gives us richly all things to enjoy," not even excluding giving birth to a baby.

16. For of Such Is the Kingdom of God

You must let little children come to me, and you must never stop them. The kingdom of heaven belongs to little children like these!

—*Matthew 19:14, PHILLIPS*

"Aren't you about ready?" John called over his shoulder. "We're going to be late for church!"

"Just a minute! I'm changing the baby again." Mary was dressing the baby for the third time. "John," she reminded him, "you didn't take these blankets."

"More stuff!" he grumbled good-naturedly, coming back into the room to get them. "You'd think we were going to the North Pole!"

"A little baby *needs* a lot of things," Mary rationalized, deciding she'd better take an extra sweater for him, too. "Besides, Mom won't have anything at the house for him when we're there this afternoon."

John took the baby from Mary, and they hurried down the steps. A few moments later they reached the church.

"If it isn't the new baby!" Joanie greeted them, hurrying over to see him before they'd even entered. "Isn't he a darling," she cooed.

Every few steps someone else stopped the proud parents for a peek, until it seemed that they really would be late, even though they had arrived at the church on time.

Finally, they managed to slip away from the last eager admirer and seated themselves in the front pew with the other new mothers and fathers who were dedicating their babies on this Mother's Day Sunday. The thoughts of all the parents were hushed, after the bustling of preparation, by the familiar tones of the hymn, "Praise God from Whom All Blessings Flow." The majestic voice of the organ crescendoed the familiar melody into the sanctuary and it hung vibrating in radiant eloquence in the reverent air.

All blessings! John thought, looking at the tiny bundle he was holding in his arms. Glancing at Mary out of the corner of his eye, he thought she had never looked more beautiful. God had surely been good to him! Gradually he became aware of the preacher saying something and that the other parents were rising to their feet. He stood up, too. Each father held his baby, and each mother held a red rose that had been placed in her hands.

The dedication ceremony was short and simple. To everyone's surprise (and to the disappointment of a few people in the audience), not a baby cried. Afterward, some of the parents took their babies to the nursery, but since George was sleeping soundly, John and Mary simply moved a few pews farther back with him. The new grandmother hovered near, more than anxious to have the opportunity to take him out and rock him if he cried.

"With every great blessing," Pastor Dirkson told his congregation earnestly, "comes great responsibility. This is especially true of the blessing of a new baby brought into a home. For, as parents have, in renunciation of themselves, carefully prepared for the physical arrival of their child, so they must, in renunciation of all selfish desires, continue to give of themselves in the years to come, for his or her spiritual, as well as physical welfare.

"For a child is much more than a physical being. Each child is also an immortal soul! And as it is the Creator's plan to make possible, through a father and a mother, the physical life of a child, so it is his plan to make possible, through their dedicated lives, the child's awareness of and obedience to himself.

"For you see, the Bible teaches that God is like the first persons that a little child knows—the father and mother! In the gentleness of the father's strength the child is to learn of the pity of a mighty God for the weakness of man, as the Psalmist describes it:

As a father has compassion on his children,
so the Lord has compassion on those who fear him.

"From the loving providence of his or her father in meeting all his material needs, the child is to learn to trust also in the providence of his heavenly Father, of whom Jesus said:

Which of you, if his son asks for bread, will give him a stone? . . . If you, then, though you are evil, know how to give good gifts to your children, how much more will your Father in heaven give good gifts to those who ask him!

"From the constancy of his or her mother's steadfast love, which is never forgetful of his needs, the child is to learn of the greater constancy of the love of God:

> Can a mother forget the baby at her breast
> and have no compassion on the child she has borne?
> Though she may forget,
> I will not forget you!

"And from the mother's tender comforting, as she sooths away the tears in times of unhappiness, the child learns of the loving God who bears all our sorrows, and who can restore joy for any troubles. The Bible says: 'As one whom the mother comforts, so will I comfort you.'

"As the child grows older, both parents continue to share in guiding their little boy or girl to a growing awareness of responsibility to God . . .

> The fear of the Lord is the beginning of knowledge, . . .

> Listen, my child, to your father's instruction and do not forsake your mother's teaching.

"And both parents share in the daily teaching of the words of God found in Scripture to the child:

> Love the Lord your God with all your heart and with all your soul and with all your strength. These commandments that I give you today are to be upon your hearts. Impress them on your children. Talk about them when you sit at home and when you walk along the road, when you lie down and when you get up.

"Thus we realize that it was God's plan, when he ordained that new human beings should not come into the world as solitary creatures, but should be set 'in families,' that through this means they are to be brought into fellowship with the Creator. What a grave responsibility parents receive, with the gift from God of a tiny baby!

"But in the harmony and self-giving love of a godly home, in which a child is brought up by father and mother to know and trust the Creator who made him or her, we see the perfect wisdom of the unfolding pattern of God's design: father, mother, child!''

PART II

17. Evidence from Anthropology

Primitive Labors

There are two common misconceptions diametrically opposed to each other concerning childbirth among primitive peoples. The first is that "all primitive labors are painless"; the second is that "all womankind suffers agony in childbirth." Neither assumption is correct.

In every culture there are instances of difficulty such as abnormal presentation, disproportion, or uterine inertia. Attempts to relieve these conditions in primitive societies have frequently led to unbelievably cruel treatment of the suffering woman in order to force the child from her body. These attempts usually resulted in the death of the woman and her child. Furthermore, primitive women are usually ignorant of the physiology of conception, pregnancy, and birth. They are also often ignorant of the basic rules of good nutrition and personal hygiene and ways to relax during labor.

Obviously, "natural" childbirth is not "primitive" childbirth, as some have contended. The woman interested in a natural birth has the advantage of adequate prenatal training, and she has access to all present-day scientific aids if she has an abnormal condition that presents a problem. Analgesia, anesthesia, incision of the perineum, extraction of the baby by forceps, cesarean delivery, blood transfusions, and antibiotics are all available in the event that she needs them.

The astonishing fact remains, however, that despite all the disadvantages and the ignorant superstitions surrounding it, normal childbirth for women in most of the primitive societies was shorter, easier, and accepted more matter-of-factly, whether or not a certain amount of discomfort accompanied it. On this point, most anthropologists agree:

It is a strange thing that most of the anxiety over the crises of childbirth comes before the event, not at it. Magic, ritual, and tabu dominate the prenatal period, yet when the moment of birth is reached, the obstetrical problems are in normal cases handled with matter-of-fact effectiveness free of mumbo jumbo.[1]

Obviously, a careful study of the environmental and cultural factors that have contributed to easier childbirth among other peoples is useful. It is helpful to realize, for example, that the primitive woman developed flexibility in her pelvic and hip joints by crouching by her little fire to prepare the evening meal, and that she increased muscle tone and breath control in her long walk to the village well. These things made a tremendous difference to the facility and comfort with which she delivered her child, and her instinctive suckling of her newborn soon after the birth helped protect her from hemorrhaging.

Examples of easy deliveries in the more primitive cultures are numerous. Margaret Mead relates the following personal experience:

. . . One consideration in choosing that particular site was that Bangwin, our next-door neighbor, had a pregnant wife, and births are very hard to see in primitive society, where babies are likely to be born at 2 A.M. or when the mother is out fishing. True, in the end Bangwin's baby too was born when Tshamwole was out fishing.[2]

In a very different part of the world from Polynesia, Eskimo women often gave birth while migrating across the ice and snow. After the birth, the mother slipped the baby beneath her clothing at her bosom to keep it warm and resumed her journey. A very recent example of this was a fifteen-year-old Laplander who gave birth to her own twins one bitterly cold day while she was alone in the woods. She then walked *fifteen miles* to the nearest community, carrying her babies wrapped in fur bags. A doctor who examined them said that mother and babies were in excellent condition.

Thousands of additional examples could be given to demonstrate that *there is no anthropological evidence to support the theological dogma that women of all cultures have universally regarded childbirth as an "illness" or a "curse."*

On the contrary, it is probable that the joy of motherhood, which follows the satisfying orgasm of the birth experience, has enabled women in many cultures to adapt themselves successfully to unfortunate social conditions. A non-Christian woman from India expressed this philosophy by saying that bearing children had satisfied a deep personal need in her life, and that she believed that nature had been kinder to women than to men!

Cultural Differences

While it is true that women in most cultures have accepted the birth process matter-of-factly, Western culture is not the only one that deviates from this attitude. In societies where women attempt to identify themselves with the men, childbirth and motherhood are not well regarded. Among the warlike Aztecs with their highly developed culture, for example, there is evidence that the women disliked their role intensely. Among the Manus of New Guinea this was also true: the sex act was conducted prudishly, with a sense of shame, and all a woman's distinctive creative functions were undervalued.

In still other cultures quite the opposite is seen, and men have sought to identify themselves in some way with the birth process. Among the Basques in Spain the women would get up and go back to work after the birth of a child, while their husbands went to bed for a period of time. This custom is called the *couvade,* and it is found in many parts of the world. The practice of couvade has been found in South American cultures, in African tribes, in south India, in China, and among the Ainus of Japan.

In some cultures the mother remained separated for a period of time after childbirth, whether or not the father was also "lying-in." Her separation was usually akin to that required because of menstrual taboos rather than to any physiological inability to go back to her normal tasks. Many cultures have regarded menstruation superstitiously and treated it with religious restrictions. In these societies, the normal discharge following childbirth has been equated with menstruation and the woman is subjected to the same restrictions.

The Mountain Arapesh tribe of New Guinea provides good examples of menstrual taboos and a type of couvade:

Men have to stay away from the edge of the village where women bear their children, and wonder, with anguished curiosity that will never be satisfied, what it is like to bear children. Both boys and girls have to guard their growth so that they will be good parents. They will both be depleted by parenthood, a man no less than a woman. "You should have seen what a fine-looking man he was before he had all those children!" . . . To the female periodicities, both men and women adjust. During menstruation the woman rests in a small, badly built shelter over the edge of the hillside, and the man must fend for himself, care for the children, and abstain from entering his yam-garden, from which she is debarred. So during pregnancy he shares her taboos, and after child-birth he lies beside his newly-delivered wife, resting from the labour, from the hard work of child-bearing, which ages a man as much as it does a woman!³

Ancient Hebrew Culture

The first chapter of Exodus reveals that the women in Moses' day gave birth easily and often without assistance. Moses himself was born to his mother without her receiving assistance, or his presence would have been known (Exod. 2:2). The Hebrew midwives explained to Pharaoh that the Hebrew women were not like the indolent women of the Egyptian court and were often delivered of their children before the midwife could get to them.

The harder Pharaoh made the Hebrews work, the stronger they became, and the more easily did the women give birth to their babies. Although the statement of the midwives was made to explain to Pharaoh why they had not destroyed the male infants of the Hebrews, it must have been credible or it would not have been accepted.

Because the midwives feared God, "he gave them families" (Exod. 1:21, RSV). In other words, God *blessed* these women whose lives were committed to helping other women in childbirth by giving them the privilege of giving birth to many children themselves!

In Exodus 1:16 (RSV) mention is made of a "stool" or "birthstool" which the Hebrew women supposedly used when giving birth. But the Hebrews did not ordinarily use "stools" or "chairs" unless they were wealthy or persons of importance. Even in Christ's day people ordinarily reclined even at meals.

The Hebrew word translated "birthstool" is *ovnayim,* which means literally "two stones." The manner in which these stones were used is not certain, but mention of them indicates that the Hebrew births frequently took place as the women were working in the fields, as is common in other primitive cultures. The Levitical law requiring women to be "separated" for "purification" following childbirth had not yet been made, and the women probably resumed their tasks after the birth of the child.

A woman might have used these stones to lean against for support as she crouched, or knelt, to bear her child. Or, if someone was supporting her, she might have pushed against them with her feet to aid her expulsive efforts. But however she used them, it is highly unlikely that she sat on them, as the translation "stool" implies. The Hebrew woman usually crouched on her heels to give birth (as in 1 Sam. 4:19), while another woman knelt between her legs to receive the child onto her waiting lap (as in Gen. 30:3).

The Early Christian Era

There were two basic influences on the cultural attitude of the first-century Christians toward childbirth: that of the Hebrew culture and that of the Greek culture.

The Jews had a high regard for motherhood. Multiple births were considered an event of special honor to a woman, rather than regarded with superstition as in many primitive cultures. As has been noted, in the Pentateuch childbirth is described as a simple process. In Isaiah and Jeremiah, prophets of a leisure-class court society, some illustrations are given that refer to exhausting labors. However, there is no indication that this was the case among the peasants of Palestine in Christ's day. No mention is made of anyone assisting his mother when our Lord himself was born. Indeed, Mary had undertaken a lengthy journey in late pregnancy, as is commonly done among primitives and peasants, who think nothing of giving birth to their babies en route.

Jewish mothers loved their children dearly, and always breastfed their own babies, a function precious to them. Moses' mother was reluctant to let an Egyptian woman wet-nurse her son, and even prostitutes breastfed their own children. Most babies were fed at the breast for two years or more, and later Talmudic regulation forbade a woman to remarry until two years after the birth of her last child, lest the orphan be deprived of her full attention.

Among the Greeks of the pre-Christian era, medicine had reached a high state, which was maintained from the time of Hippocrates until the Roman conquest, when the more barbaric Romans then copied much of the Greek culture. Although the Greeks had no scruples about men attending women in labor (nor did the Jews), most deliveries were conducted by midwives. Physicians were called only in difficult cases. Births must have been relatively simple, since so little mention is made of obstetrics in the medical literature. The Greek woman lived an active, outdoor life and wore loose and free-flowing clothes, especially in pregnancy. The importance of physical preparation for childbirth was recognized and Lycurgus, the ancient lawgiver, instituted exercises for growing girls so that they would have easy labors and produce healthier offspring.

The midwives had high standards of practice and were required to be scrupulously clean, honest, and industrious. As with the Jews, cleanliness was important, and the story of Achilles, who was plunged into the river Styx after his birth by his mother, is well known. He was completely washed except for his heel where his mother was holding him!

But in contrast to the Jews, the Greeks practiced abortion and infanticide freely, and weak-looking newborn babies were destroyed without compunction. The Jews used abortion for therapeutic reasons, such as to protect a mother who had suffered in childbirth from having a similar experience, but they looked aghast at any form of infanticide.

The early church retained the Jewish regard for motherhood and was familiar as well with the Greek teachings of good midwifery. The writings of the earliest church fathers demonstrate their great respect for a woman's creative functions of pregnancy, childbirth, nursing, and motherhood, as the following examples illustrate:

Ignatius (A.D. 30–107) writes:

Children, obey your parents, and have an affection for them, as workers together with God for your birth into the world. . . . Husbands, love your wives, as fellow-servants of God, as your own body, as the partners of your life, and your co-adjutors in the procreation of children.[4]

Clement of Rome (A.D. 30–100) demonstrates the wisdom of God, the great "Creator" and "Designer of the universe," by illustrating his providence in making humankind male and female:

Moreover, the female form, and the cavity of the womb, most suitable for receiving and cherishing and vivifying the germ . . . in which the foetus being placed, is kept and cherished. . . . Who will not, from all these things, acknowledge the operation of reason, and the wisdom of the Creator?[5]

Clement of Alexandria (A.D. 153–217):

Let us . . . understand that the virtue of man and woman is the same. . . . one church, one temperance, one modesty; their food is common, marriage an equal yoke. . . .[6]

As far as respects human nature, the woman does not possess one nature, and the man exhibit another, but the same: so also with righteousness, and every other virtue. . . . Undoubtedly it stands to reason that some difference should exist between each of them, in virtue of which one is male and the other female. Pregnancy, and parturition, accordingly, belong to woman. . . . As then there is sameness, as far as respects the soul, she will attain to the same virtue; but as there is difference as respects the peculiar construction of the body, she is destined for childbearing.[7]

Dark Clouds on the Horizon

Midwifery customs of Roman civilization during the early Christian era were almost identical with those of the earlier Greeks. But Roman civilization became far more dissolute. By the time the early church had come into existence Roman morals were already in a rapid state of decline. Roman rulers set the example, and the masses soon followed suit:

Both Julius Caesar and Augustus led dissolute lives. Caligula kept a brothel in his palace and by taxing the keepers of the *lupanaria* he was able to derive a substantial income from their infamous calling. Nero not only visited the house of the prostitutes and dined in public with a crowd of these creatures, but he also founded, on the shores of the Gulf of Naples, houses of ill-fame, which he filled with the most abandoned women. Commodus was surrounded by no less than three hundred maidens. But perhaps none reached the depths of depravity sounded by the Emperor Claudius Tiberius, whose amours at Capreae cannot be described.

Morally the wives of these Emperors were often little better than their husbands. Agrippina used to leave the palace of the Caesars and go to the brothels of Rome where she would spend the night in debauchery. . . .[8]

The influx of Greek slaves into Rome freed women in the leisure classes from their normal responsibilities, so that they could spend more time at other pursuits including sexual indulgence. There were many more men than women, which increased the temptations to debauchery. But to offset this abnormal sexual activity, induced abortions became so common that some Roman leaders feared the race would die out. There was one full year in a city along the Tiber when not a single birth took place!

Plautus, the Latin playwright, described it [abortion] as a natural step in the life of the Roman woman. Terence, foreseeing the consequence of excess, moaned over its frequency; Juvenal grimly remarked that the Roman wives no longer had any lying-in; Ovid, perhaps facetiously, referred to a league for abortion that was organized by the Roman women.[9]

Rome had become one of those societies in which women consider pregnancy and childbirth a nuisance and an ordeal: furthermore, the

Roman mother refused to breastfeed her own child, turning it over to a wet nurse after the birth. Following weaning, the child was reared by Greek slaves rather than by the mother.

What was the reaction of the infant church to all this? As might be expected, many Christians overreacted—to the extent that they regarded *all* sexual intercourse as sinful, and the "ordeal" of childbirth was considered the inevitable judgment of God upon the woman who had indulged herself. Evidence of this morbid attitude appears by the second century A.D. and continues to develop in the following ones:

Tertullian (A.D. 145–220 or 240):

Therefore when, through the will of God, the husband is deceased, the marriage likewise, by the will of God, deceases. Why should *you* restore what God has put an end to? Why do you, by repeating the servitude of maternity, spurn the liberty which is offered you? . . .[10]

Marrying, let us be overtaken by the last day, like Sodom and Gomorrah; that day when "woe" pronounced over "such as are with child and giving suck" shall be fulfilled, that is, over the married and the incontinent: for from marriage result wombs, and breasts, and infants![11]

Cyprian (A.D. 200–258):

Do you wish to know what ill the virtue of continence avoids, what good it possesses? "I will multiply," says God to the woman, "thy sorrows and thy groanings; and in sorrow shalt thou bring forth children and thy desire shall be to thy husband, and he shall rule over thee." You are free from this sentence. You do not fear the sorrows and the groans of women. You have no fear of child-bearing; nor is your husband lord over you. . . .[12]

Jerome (A.D. 346–420), on a pilgrimage to the Holy Land, was accompanied by a woman named Paula, and one can see the contempt in which motherhood was held by the church in her example:

She resisted the entreaties of all her relatives. In vain her youngest daughter, Rufina, who had recently been affianced, implored her with tears to await her approaching marriage; in vain her little son Toxotius uplifted from the shore his suppliant hands. Paula raised heavenwards her tearless eyes, and, turning her back to the shore, *ignored her motherhood to prove her saintliness.* [Italics added.][13]

What the young church did not realize was that in its reaction to Roman licentiousness and abortions, it was unconsciously absorbing the Roman contempt for marriage, childbearing, and motherhood. *Thus the church became infiltrated with the Roman attitude toward the nuisance of childbearing and motherhood which was in direct contrast to the continuing Jewish concept of the blessedness of marriage and maternity.*

In addition, the gnostic belief that the physical body was evil was accepted by some early Christian writers. Because of this erroneous belief in the sinful nature of the physical body, women, because their very bodies excited the physical desires of men, were thought to be deserving of God's special judgment.

This morbid attitude continued through medieval times. Knowledge of good midwifery almost vanished, and deliveries were frequently attended by untrained, superstitious old women. Physicians were forbidden by the church to be present at the scene of birth, and the midwife had nothing to rely upon except her own "magic." For fifteen hundred years the advances in obstetric knowledge that had been made by the Greeks and Romans were lost to the world.

Because the midwives frequently used ritualistic chants and oblations in aiding a birth, they were often accused of witchcraft. This occasioned such inquiries as:

. . . whether you know anye that doe use charmes, sorcery, enchantments, invocations, circles, witchcrafts, soothsayings or any like crafts or imaginations invented by the Devyle and especially in the tyme of women's travyle.[14]

Of course, from time to time there were women whose midwifery ability was excellent, but they appear briefly in medieval history, and their warnings against abuses were unheeded. The only medical advances of any consequence during this time were among the Arabs and the Jews. The Jewish doctor was never restricted from attending women in labor, nor was he forbidden to destroy the unborn child if the life of the mother was at stake, because the Jews believed that the infant did not become a "soul" until he or she had drawn the first breath. Evidence for this was taken from the account of Adam's creation in Genesis 2:7.

And the Lord God . . . breathed into his nostrils the breath of life; and man became a living soul.

The church forbade any form of abortion under any circumstances, allowing the mother to die as well as the child. The agony of the dying woman, unable to deliver her infant, was considered to be God's judgment upon her for the sin of Eve.

The Renaissance—And Catastrophe!

With the revival of learning the outlook for the woman in labor seemed optimistic. Discoveries were being made in human anatomy and physiology, a greater number of hospitals were being provided, and male physicians were once again reluctantly permitted to attend births.

But it soon became apparent that the parturient woman was in a far more serious plight than in medieval times, for a strange and terrible malady appeared more and more frequently. Puerperal fever (a septic poisoning) attacked women after childbirth, taking them through feverish, racking agony to almost certain death. By 1652 the disease had assumed epidemic proportions, and it raged across Europe unabated for the next two hundred years.

In 1795 Dr. Gordon of Aberdeen, Scotland, announced that he felt certain the disease was of infectious origin, but other doctors ignored him. Oliver Wendell Holmes, the American physician, wrote a treatise in 1843 called "Puerperal Fever as a Private Pestilence," in which he claimed that the disease was contagious and that the doctors themselves were transmitting it. His warning was likewise ignored. It remained for Dr. Philipp Semmelweiss, an Austrian physician, to prove conclusively the direct relationship between the attending physician's lack of personal cleanliness and the resulting puerperal infection of the mother. He was mocked by the medical profession and died before his discovery was really accepted.

Only slightly more than a hundred years ago a physician would frequently go directly from dissecting a corpse to assist a woman in labor, *without even washing his hands in water!* The doctors themselves were infecting the mothers and causing their deaths.

Contrast this practice with the Jewish regard for cleanliness taught by Moses and enforced by Jewish law. This was especially true in regard to disposal of the dead, after which one was required to bathe and wash one's clothes; and was considered "unclean" the rest of the day. Without knowing the principles of sanitation, such observances nevertheless protected the Hebrew mother, and the nation as well, from infections of this origin.

The mortality rate at the lying-in division of the Vienna General

Hospital where Dr. Semmelweiss worked was staggering. But in 1847 he tried an experiment: all physicians under his authority were required to wash their hands in a chloride of lime solution before entering the labor rooms, and the incidence of the fever dropped sharply. Even so, he was labeled the "Pesth fool" (Pesth was his birthplace) by other physicians, and eventually he was forced to leave Vienna. He continued his work at the Pesth hospital, where he could get more cooperation.

In the larger cities of Europe physicians practiced midwifery on cadavers, left the corpses when called to a woman in labor, and transmitted septic poisoning to her because they had not even washed. Then, in the crowded labor wards, after examining one woman internally, they simply wiped the blood and pus from their hands onto their waistcoats, and proceeded to the next patient, thrusting their filthy hands into her birth canal to see how the labor was progressing.

There was always a surplus of motherless children. Vienna's mother and child mortality was enormous. But the world was used to such deaths. There were years when in Paris the Hôtel Dieu lost more than half the women who gave birth there. There were *four years when at the University of Jena not a mother left the hospital alive.* [Italics added.][15]

In 1847 there were so many maternal deaths at the Kiev hospital that the hospital was closed. The director, "heavy with a sense of personal guilt," committed suicide. By 1854 Semmelweiss's theory was well proven in the hospital in Pesth where he delivered the mothers, but it was rejected throughout the rest of Europe.

In the seven years years since the discovery of the cause and the simple prevention of childbed fever had been clearly announced, at least seventy thousand and perhaps a third of a million women had died of childbed fever. As to the babies, there was no counting![16]

With such terrible suffering connected with childbirth for over two hundred years, is it any wonder that Bible translators and scholars began interpreting Genesis 3:16 as meaning "suffering in childbirth"? This pain and death, which women feared and men could not understand, was said to be due to the "hand of God" punishing womankind —the curse of "pain" on Eve!

Yet men could not escape their own sense of guilt over the staggering number of childbirth deaths, and the Puritan concept of the shamefulness of intercourse pervaded Europe. We are not entirely free of this sense of wrong even today. Only a few decades ago the eminent Bible scholar Reverend J. B. Phillips showed the inconsistency of some Christians' thinking about God in relation to sex and other physical matters:

We may, for instance, admire the ascetic ultra-spiritual type which appears to have "a mind above" food, sexual attraction, and material comfort, for example. But if in forming a picture of the Holiness of God we are simply enlarging this spirituality and asceticism to the "nth" degree we are forced to some peculiar conclusions. Thus we may find ourselves readily able to imagine God's interest in babies (for are they not "little bits of Heaven"?) yet unable to imagine His approval, let alone design, of the acts which led to their conception![17]

The common mistaken belief in Western cultures that a woman must be punished for giving a man pleasure in intercourse and that God's whole plan for the reproduction of the human race is a morbid one is strikingly illustrated in Leo Tolstoy's writings. Notice, for example, Prince Andrew's feelings of guilt after his wife Lise dies in childbirth:

Prince Andrew ran to the door; the scream ceased and he heard the wail of an infant. . . . Suddenly he realized the joyful significance of that wail; tears choked him, and leaning his elbows on the window sill he began to cry, sobbing like a child. . . . He went into his wife's room. She was lying dead, in the same position he had seen her in five minutes before. . . . "I love you all, and have done no harm to anyone; and what have you done to me?" said her charming, pathetic, dead face. . . . Prince Andrew felt that something gave way in his soul and that *he was guilty of a sin that he could neither remedy nor forget.* [Italics added.][18]

NOTES

1. E. A. Hoebel, *Man in the Primitive World* (New York: McGraw-Hill, 1958), p. 372. See also Palmer Findley, M.D., *Priests of Lucina, The Story of Obstetrics* (Boston: Little, Brown, 1939).
2. Margaret Mead, *Male and Female* (New York: Morrow, 1949), p. 42. Reprinted by permission.
3. Mead, *Male and Female*, pp. 101, 102, 1069. Reprinted by permission.
4. "Epistle of Ignatius to the Philadelphians," Chap. IV, in *The Ante-Nicene Fathers* (Grand Rapids: Eerdmans, 1951), vol. 1, p. 81.
5. "Recognitions of Clement," Book VIII, Chap. XXXII, in *The Ante-Nicene Fathers,* vol. 8, p. 173, 174.
6. "The Instructor," Book I, Chap. IV, in *The Ante-Nicene Fathers,* vol. 2, p. 211.

7. "The Stromata, or Miscellanies," Book IV, Chap. VIII, in *The Ante-Nicene Fathers,* vol. 2, pp. 419ff.
8. Roy P. Finney, M.D., *The Story of Motherhood* (New York: Liveright, 1937), pp. 42, 43.
9. A. J. Rongy, M.D., *Childbirth: Yesterday and Today* (New York: Emerson, 1937), pp. 162, 163.
10. "To His Wife," Book I, Chap. VII, in *The Ante-Nicene Fathers,* vol. 4, p. 43.
11. "Exhortations to Chastity," Chap. IX, in *The Ante-Nicene Fathers,* vol. 4, p. 55.
12. "The Treatises of Cyprian," Treatise II, in *The Ante-Nicene Fathers,* vol. 5, p. 436.
13. F. W. Farrar, *Lives of the Fathers* (Edinburgh: Black, 1889), vol. 2, pp. 302, 303.
14. Quoted by Rongy in *Childbirth: Yesterday and Today,* p. 86.
15. Morton Thompson, *The Cry and the Covenant* (Garden City, N.Y.: Doubleday, 1949), p. 107.
16. Ibid., p. 108.
17. J. B. Phillips, *Your God Is Too Small* (New York: Macmillan, 1954), p. 38.
18. Leo Tolstoy, *War and Peace* (New York: Simon & Schuster, 1942), pp. 347–354.

18. Theological Considerations

Introduction

That it is possible to give birth without pain has now been demonstrated for over seventy years. This has given occasion for nonbelievers who have experienced the beauty of natural birth to call the Bible false and to scoff at Christians for teaching that childbirth pain is an inevitable result of the "curse of Eve."

It is not the Bible that degrades womanhood in this manner and labels childbearing a curse. Rather, it is this *interpretation* of the Bible that is at fault, just as the interpretation of our forefathers was faulty when they used the Bible to "prove" that the earth was flat. The Bible is not a scientific text, to be abused in this manner, and one neither "proves" nor "disproves" natural childbirth by "using" the Bible.

But if Christianity is relevant to every experience of life, then it is relevant to childbirth. And if the Bible provides broad, underlying principles by which we may examine any philosophy concerning life, then it is imperative for us to examine the philosophy of natural childbirth in the light of these principles. And to do this, we must first discover exactly what the Bible does say about childbirth.

It must be realized at the outset of this survey that it is beyond the purpose of this book to suggest the sources of any text, such as the Genesis account of the Creation and Fall, or to suggest whether the record is to be taken literally, allegorically, or mythologically. The purposes here are three:

1. To determine as closely as possible the accurate meaning of the original Hebrew words.
2. To determine whether or not the English translators have consistently translated these words accurately (the inspiration of the Bible surely cannot be defined as meaning that every translation of it, into any language, is without error).
3. To suggest how inconsistent renderings of certain words have

helped to create and maintain the negative philosophy toward the birth process that is so embedded in our culture.

Since this book is primarily for the lay reader, the word *etsev* is used for either *etsev* or its cognates. This same principle applies as well to all other Hebrew, Greek, or Latin words used.

Also, since frequent mention is made of the Jewish Septuagint, Mishnah, and Talmud, the following brief definitions are given.

1. The *Septuagint* is a translation of the Hebrew Old Testament into Greek by Hebrew scholars during the third and second centuries B.C.

2. Jewish Oral Law, the "tradition of the elders," was at first passed down from generation to generation by word of mouth. When this Oral Law was written down in the third century A.D. it was called the *Mishnah,* and it consists of detailed instructions developed by the rabbis on how to observe the Law of Moses.

3. The *Talmud* is composed of the Mishnah and an interpretation of each of its passages by rabbis. It was written down between the fourth and sixth centuries A.D. Its interpretive approaches are both allegorical and literal.

Etsev and the "Curse of Eve"

It has already been noted in Chapter 7 that *etsev* refers primarily to the emotions. Rabbi Hirsch explains this aspect of the word as follows:

1. *Etsev:* only a *mental* pain and hurt feelings or worry. . . . The root is . . . a modification of . . . "forsaken," . . . leaving something against one's will . . . so that *etsev* is the feeling that we have to give something up that we would have liked to keep, or to have attained: renouncing, forgoing (1 Kings 1:6—"David had never asked his son to give anything up"). . . . Until then Man knew no wrong, and no renunciation. But now for Man nature is no longer at one with his wishes as it was previously, he must wrest everything from her, and only by renunciation, by giving up one thing, one enjoyment, can he attain another.[1]

In our English translations of the Bible *etsev* is frequently given as "labor" or "toil." Although this might not be accurate in the strictest sense, it is so closely related to the concept of "giving of oneself" that it seems to be a legitimate translation. It appears this way in Genesis 5:29, where Lamech says of his son Noah:

This same shall comfort us concerning our work and *toil* (*etsev*) of our hands, because of the ground which the Lord hath cursed.

Etsev is also translated as "toil" in Proverbs 5:10, Proverbs 10:22 (marginal reading), Isaiah 58:3, and elsewhere. Notice how it is used in the Revised Standard Version in Proverbs 14:23 and Psalm 127:2. To be consistent, it should also be translated as "toil" in 1 Chronicles 4:9. Interestingly enough, this verse is the only one in the entire Bible that uses *etsev* in connection with the birth of a child. Furthermore, the mother says that this was her favorite child, because she gave birth to him with *toil* (*etsev*):

And Jabez was more honourable than his brethren: and his mother called his name Jabez [meaning "height"], saying, Because I bare him with *toil* (*etsev*).

After discussing *etsev,* Rabbi Hirsch makes it very plain that in the interpretation of the third chapter of Genesis Judaism and Christianity part company, for it is here that the Christian doctrine of original sin and the consequent need for a Savior begin. He says:

Mankind is in no manner whatsoever placed under a ban for his first disobedience. . . . Still today, every human child comes from the hand of God as pure as Adam did, still today every child is born to mankind as pure as an angel. This is one of the cardinal points of Jewish life and of the essential Jewish nature. . . . Certainly, through this sin, all the descendants of Adam have inherited the task of having to live in a world which no longer smiles benevolently in harmony with them, but that is just because the same sin is constantly being repeated. . . . But that . . . *something else* is required other than the possibility which everyone possesses to *elevate himself* up to faithful fulfillment of duty, against that belief Judaism raises the most vehement protest. For that, no dead, and no resurrected intermediary is necessary. This is taught by the whole of Jewish history.

Adam could well have railed at his wife for the loss of Paradise and he calls her by the loveliest calling of Woman! Man had been allotted renunciation, Woman had been allotted renunication, but the purpose for which Woman had been given renunciation was the higher; *she had become the savior from death, the dispenser of life, in her the immortality of mankind took refuge.* [Italics added.][2]

Clearly, then, the origins of the belief that all womankind is under a curse in childbirth could not have existed in Judaism, as some have claimed. The Jews, in placing woman in the position of "savior from death, the dispenser of life," put her in the place of our Lord Jesus Christ. The origins of the "curse" obviously come later, in the third and fourth centuries, as has already been outlined in the previous chapter.

Rabbi Hirsch's interpretation of the Genesis passage is not new among the Jews, for Josephus, the Jewish historian who lived and wrote in the first century A.D., also points out that since Adam's time, humankind no longer lives in a world which "smiles benevolently in harmony with them":

God said, "Nay, I had decreed for you to live a life of bliss, unmolested by all ill, with no care to fret your souls; all things that contribute to enjoyment and pleasure were, through my providence, to spring up for you spontaneously, without toil or distress of yours. Blessed with these gifts, old age would not soon have overtaken you and your life would have been long. But now thou hast flouted this my purpose by disobeying my commands.[3]

A second-century Christian, Irenaeus, writes prior to the time when the teaching developed that the physical body was evil, that the actual "curse" of Genesis 3 was only upon the ground and the serpent, and that God showed compassion toward the sinners:

For God is neither devoid of power nor of justice, who has afforded help to Man, and restored him to His own liberty. It was for this reason, too, that immediately after Adam had transgressed, as the Scripture relates, He pronounced no curse against Adam personally, but against the ground. . . . But the curse in all its fulness fell upon the serpent, which had beguiled them. . . . For God detested him who had led Man astray, but by degrees and little by little, He showed compassion to him who had been beguiled.[4]

The word *adam* that Irenaeus uses here, is the generic name meaning "Adam and Eve," and was so used by the Jews as well as the Christians:

All the races of men are descended from a single pair, to whom with their posterity God gave the generic name Man (Hebrew *adam*). That God made from one (ancestor) every race of men to settle all over the face of the earth in times and bounds of His appointment, was universal Jewish doctrine.[5]

• The Blessing of Childbirth in the Old and New Testaments

That bearing children was considered a blessing from God in Bible times is abundantly evident. Take the story of Leah, for example, which tells how God blessed her with many children in order to compensate for Rachel's being the favored wife:

And when the Lord saw that Leah was hated, he opened her womb: but Rachel was barren. And Leah conceived, and bare a son, and she called his name Reuben: for she said, Surely the Lord hath looked upon my affliction . . . (Gen. 29:31ff.).

Godly Hannah was also blessed for her faith, not only by the birth of Samuel but with five other sons and daughters as well:

And the Lord visited Hannah, so that she conceived, and bare three sons and two daughters (1 Sam 2:21).

Other passages confirm that childbirth was a blessing, as in Genesis 29:25; Deuteronomy 7:13; 28:11, 12; Ruth 4:13; Psalm 127:3; and many others. That it was considered a judgment of God *not* to bear children can be demonstrated from verses like:

Give them, O Lord: what wilt thou give? give them a miscarrying womb and dry breasts . . . [for] all their wickedness (Hos. 9:14).

The happy comments of Bible mothers is further evidence of the blessedness that they considered motherhood to be. Read the comments of Sarah in Genesis 21:6, 7; Rebecca in Genesis 25:21, 22, who took her worries about her pregnancy to God in prayer; Leah in Genesis 29:31–35 and 30:17–21; Manoah's wife in Judges 13:2, 3, whose spiritual perception was keener than her husband's at this time; Hannah in 1 Samuel 1:10 to 2:1; Elizabeth in Luke 1:24 ff.; and Mary in Luke 1:46 to 2:19.

Even Hagar in Genesis 16:4–13, who was no doubt a pagan before her association with Abraham and Sarah, came to realize God's loving protection over her and her unborn child, so that at the child's birth she named him Ishmael, which means, "God hears."

In John 16:21 Jesus mentions the joy of a new mother at the birth of her child and contrasts it with the sober anxiety that precedes the birth. This contrast between the emotions of sorrow and joy is a familiar one in Scripture, as in Esther 9:22; Nehemiah 8:10; Isaiah 35:10; Jeremiah 31:13, and so forth, and was not new to the disciples to whom Jesus was speaking. In this parallel the same words are used for each: *lupē and chaira* for the mother; *lupē and chaira* for the disciples.

Jesus' understanding of the birth experience of a woman is evidenced further in the use of the word *thlipsis* to describe the labor.

Thlipsis (or the verb forms thlibō, apōthlibō) is sometimes translated symbolically as "oppression," but its literal meaning is to squeeze, compress, or press, as in Luke 8:45 and Mark 3:10, Phillips translation:

... the crowds are all around you and are *pressing (apōthlibō)* you on all sides.

... all those ... kept *pressing (thlibō)* forward to touch him.

The Latin translation of *thlipsis* in John 16:21 as *pressurae* gives conclusive evidence that this is the real meaning of the word. Although some might point out that Jesus was not speaking to his disciples in Greek, it can certainly be assumed that the Greek words John uses are as close a parallel to the original words as he can make them.

It is not strange that Jesus' awareness of a woman's birth experience is recorded, as such things were freely spoken of in the society in which he lived. An example of this is the statement of the woman who called out to him in public one day:

Blessed is the womb that bare thee, and the paps which thou hast sucked! (Luke 11:27).

Jesus did not rebuke her but told her of a far greater truth:

Yes, but a far greater blessing to hear the word of God and obey it (Luke 11:28, PHILLIPS).

The freedom with which such things were acknowledged is pointed out in a description of the social customs of that day:

For the poor inhabitants of Jerusalem's crowded slums ... the newly married couple had to spend their first nuptial night in the same room with the other members of the family. ... In Galilee, this custom did not prevail and the bridal pair were allowed full privacy on the wedding night. The exhibition of delicacy on the part of the Galileans is especially remarkable because in general they were far less modest and refined than the Judeans.[6]

Chul, Yalad, and Related Words

The correct meaning of the words *chul* and *yalad* has already been discussed at length in Chapter 10. It should be noted that *chul* has other apparent meanings when it is not used in reference to childbirth. In addition to this primary meaning of creating or bringing forth, it can also be translated as "patience," as in Psalm 37:7:

Rest in the Lord, and *wait patiently (chul)* for him.

And it can also mean "whirl," which is probably its meaning in Judges 21:21, 23, where it is translated as "dance":

Behold, if the daughters of Shiloh come out to *dance* (*chul*) in dances, then come ye out of the vineyards, and catch you every man his wife. . . . And the children of Benjamin . . . took them wives . . . of them that *danced* (*chul*).

The parallelism of *chul* and *yalad* in reference to birth or creating is found too often to be disregarded. There are examples of it in the Pentateuch, in the Wisdom Literature, and in the Prophets. A few examples will illustrate this:

Knowest thou the time when the wild goats of the rock *bring forth* (*yalad*); Or canst thou mark when the hinds do *calve* (*chul*)? (Job. 39:1).

Art thou the first man that was *born* (*yalad*)? Or wast thou *made* (*chul*) before the hills? (Job 15:9).

Before the mountains were *brought forth* (*yalad*), or ever thou hadst *formed* (*chul*) the earth and the world, even from everlasting to everlasting, thou art God (Ps. 90:2).

Before she was in *labor* (*chul*) she *gave birth* (*yalad*); . . . Shall a land be *born* (*chul*) in one day? Shall a nation be *brought forth* (*yalad*) in one moment? (Isa. 66:7, 8, RSV).

To be consistent, verses like Isaiah 26:18 should be translated in this manner also, where the King James Version says "we have been in *pain* (*chul*)":

We have been with child, we have been in *labor* (*chul*), we have as it were *brought forth* (*yalad*) wind. . . .

The three New Testament Greek words used of childbirth, *tiktō*, *gennaō*, and *ōdinō*, are also interchangeable and do not mean "pain." In the Septuagint, any one of the three is used to translate either *chul* or *yalad*. For example, *yalad* is translated as *ōdinō* in Isaiah 26:17; as *tiktō* in Isaiah 54:1; and as *gennaō* in Isaiah 26:18.

There are six additional biblical words describing childbirth that remain to be discussed—one in the New Testament, and five in the Old Testament.

The New Testament word is *basanidzō*, which describes the efforts of the woman giving birth in the apocalyptic passage of Revelation 12:2. *Basanidzō* does not mean "pained to be delivered," as the passive phrase in the King James Version indicates; it means she was "straining with all her might" to give birth. Reverend J. B. Phillips illustrates this use of *basanidzō* in his translation of Mark 6:48:

He saw them *straining* (*basanidzō*) at the oars.

There is another verse in the New Testament where the King James Version adds the word "pain," although it does not appear in the Greek. This is in Romans 8:22, where the Greek says simply:

The whole creation groans *in labor together* (*sunōdinō*) until now.

The five remaining Old Testament words used in connection with childbirth are *tsir, chaval, qashah, yaphach,* and *tsarah.*

1. *Tsir* is sometimes translated "hinges":

As the door turneth upon his *hinges* (*tsir*) . . . (Prov. 26:14).

Tsir is used of childbirth only once—in 1 Samuel 4:19, where the woman is said to crouch, or bend down, because her *tsir* had come upon her. *Tsir* is translated as "pains" in this verse, but we know this cannot be correct because Eli's daughter-in-law, absorbed with her grief, ignored the birth processes of her body and did not even realize when her child had been born until her attendants brought the fact to her attention.

It is possible that *tsir* refers here to the "hinges," or joints of the body of the woman crouching to give birth, but it is more likely that it refers to the opening of the door of the womb and the vulva. In the Talmud there are references to parts of the body in allegorical form:

In the Talmud the uterus is called the sleeping chamber, the cervix is the porch, the vagina the outer house, the clitoris the key, *the labia the hinges,* and the "seed vessels" the store-room. [Italics added.][7]

Tsir is used twice in Isaiah as a comparison to a woman giving birth. In Isaiah 13:8 it refers to the King of Babylon, and in Isaiah 21:3 to the prophet himself. In these two instances it probably refers to the "hinges" of the body as it assumes a crouching posture similar to "a woman giving birth."

2. *Chaval* is translated "cords, bands, bounds" over fifty times, and when used as a medical term it is said to refer to muscles or nerves in action, as in a birth contraction. It is sometimes translated "pangs,"

but this English word is obsolete today in reference to childbirth, so "birth contraction" would be a more accurate translation. Sometimes *chaval* is translated simply "brought forth," as in Song of Solomon 8:5, which is also a poetic reference to a birth taking place in the out-of-doors:

I raised thee up under the apple tree: there thy mother *brought thee forth* (*chaval*); there she *brought thee forth* (*chaval*) that bare thee.

3. *Qashah* is one of the three words used of childbirth in the Old Testament implying an unhappy experience. *Qashah*, meaning "hard, difficult, fierce," is used of a birth only once and describes Rachel's difficult, abnormal delivery of Benjamin in Genesis 35:16, 17, where it is translated as "hard labor." In the Mishnah, the phrase "hard labor" is used of an animal who has difficulty in giving birth. Out of kindness, the attendant is instructed to destroy the offspring and remove it limb by limb to save the life of the mother animal and to prevent her suffering. The Talmud applies this same principle to a mother who cannot give birth normally.

The two remaining words occur only in the book of Jeremiah in connection with childbirth. It must be remembered that Jeremiah was a prophet among the indolent members of a court society, whose women would be likely to have more tiring labors than the peasant women of the same period. Therefore, these references in Jeremiah cannot be taken to mean that the same conditions applied throughout Old Testament times, or even to women generally in Jeremiah's day. Furthermore, Jeremiah prophesied in a time of national disaster, when fear and apprehension were prevalent, especially at court. It has already been demonstrated how fear creates physical tension, which in turn creates pain. Thus we would expect these women to have more difficulty in their labors.

The two words Jeremiah uses do not mean "pain," but they do refer to conditions that would cause unhappiness and imply suffering. These two words are *yaphach* and *tsarah*.

4. *Yaphach*, meaning "gasping," "out of breath," or "to breathe oneself out," is used of a woman in labor only once in the Bible, in Jeremiah 4:31. This verse describes her condition as one of complete exhaustion, as she labors to deliver her firstborn child. She becomes so weak with exhaustion that she cannot even close her hands around a support any longer to help herself in bearing down.

5. *Tsarah*, used figuratively, is commonly translated "distress," but it can also convey the idea of constriction, narrowness, or "straits," as in the following passages:

. . . the place where we dwell is too *strait* (*tsarah*) for us (2 Kings 6:1).

. . . the place is too *strait* (*tsarah*) for me, give place to me that I may dwell (Isa. 49:20).

The angel of the Lord went further, and stood in a *narrow* (*tsarah*) place. (Num. 22:26.)

For the bed is shorter than that a man can stretch himself on it: and the covering *narrower* (*tsarah*) than that he can wrap himself in it. (Isa. 28:20.)

Tsarah is used in verses that contain a comparison to labor six times in Jeremiah. Three of these times it refers to the woman: (a) 4:31 (see the discussion of *yaphach,* above); (b) 48:41, which also has the element of being surprised, and seems to imply that the woman is afraid; and (c) 49:22, which also implies the presence of fear. Whether *tsarah* refers to the "constriction" of a contraction in these three verses or to an emotional "distress," is not too important, since in each case a distressing situation is implied by the context.

In the three other places where Jeremiah uses *tsarah* there is reference to the approaching confinement of captivity—the nation will be "in a bind." Here again, *tsarah* may have a double meaning and imply distress as well as captivity. In these three passages it is not clear whether the phrase in which *tsarah* appears is a part of the comparison to a "woman in labor" or not. The word is applied to (a) the inhabitants of Zion, 6:24; (b) Damascus, 49:24; and (c) the King of Babylon, 50:43.

The Septuagint and English Translations

It is worthy of note that the simile "as a woman giving birth," which appears fifteen times in our English translations of the Old Testament, appears only nine times in the Septuagint. This simile occurs only once in the Old Testament outside of the prophetical literature, and this is in Psalm 48:6, where it tells of the kings "*laboring* (*chul*) as a woman *giving birth* (*yalad*)." This is a comparison of the effort syndrome in rowing to the effort syndrome of giving birth. The kings are rowing with all their might to escape impending destruction from God, symbolized by the "east wind." The picture is like that of Mark 6:48 (PHILLIPS) where the disciples are "straining at the oars."

The simile "as a woman giving birth" is missing from the Septuagint in Jeremiah 30:6; 48:41; 49:22, 24; and 50:43. Of the nine times it does appear, five times either a phrase is left out or it is interpreted differently from our English translations.

1. In Isaiah 13:8 the phrase "and they shall be afraid" is missing, and the phrase translated into English as "*pangs (tsir)* and *sorrows (chaval)* shall take hold on them" reads:

. . . the aged ones will be thrown into a tumult (*kai taraxthēsontai hoi presbeis*).

2. In Isaiah 21:3 the word translated *pain (chul)* is translated *ekluō,* which means "to give out, become weak, loosen, or become weary." In medicine, when *ekluō* is used in connection with the word for "loins," as it is here, it is a term used for involuntary defecation—a releasing of the contents of the bowel, as a mother releases her child from the birth canal. In this same verse, the Septuagint omits the phrase "*pangs (tsir)* have taken hold on me" (that is, on the prophet himself).

3. In Isaiah 42:14, rather than having the Lord say ". . . now will I cry *(paah)* like a *travailing (yalad)* woman," as the King James Version reads, the Septuagint authors render this verse as:

I have been as *patient (kartereō)* as a woman *giving birth (tiktō).*

The Hebrew word *paah,* then, probably refers in this verse to the groan of effort of the Lord, like the groan of a woman in labor—a groan that is a normal part of the effort syndrome in even the most painless birth. In the Brown, Driver, Briggs *Lexicon,* this phrase is explained as meaning that "the Lord [is] straining himself to deliver Israel."[8]

In Isaiah 26:17, where the woman *crieth out (zaaq)* in labor, this same explanation might apply. In the Septuagint *zaaq* is translated as *ekkradzō* in this verse and means "to call out, cry, or shout." *Kradzō* is even used in classical writings sometimes to describe the noise frogs make!

4. In Jeremiah 4:31 the Septuagint uses *stenagmos (groan)* to translate the Hebrew word *tsarah,* thus relating the word to the effort of labor.

5. The garbled meaning of Micah 4:9, 10, as it is translated into English, is a vivid contrast to its apparent meaning as it appears in the Septuagint. In the Revised Standard Version these verses read:

> Now why do you cry aloud?
> Is there no king in you?
> Has your counselor perished
>   that *pangs* (*chul*) have seized you
>   like a woman in *travail* (*yalad*)?
> *Writhe* (*chul*) and groan, O daughter of Zion
>   like a woman in *travail* (*yalad*);
>   for now you shall go forth from the city . . .
>   you shall go to Babylon.
> There you shall be rescued,
>   there the Lord will redeem you
>   from the hand of your enemies.

The really ironic thing about this translation is that it occurs right in the center of Micah's message of *comfort* to his people, which begins at the opening of the fourth chapter and leads up to the promise of the Messiah in the fifth. In other words, our translators would have us believe that Micah is telling the people that they are going to "writhe" in "pangs" like a woman in labor, because God has graciously promised to rescue them from the enemy.

Translators have inserted concepts of suffering in other passages of comfort and blessing that refer to childbirth, as in Isaiah 54:1–4; 66:7–9; Jeremiah 31:8, and so on. Their doing this reminds one of Job's comment to his friends in Job 16:2: "Miserable comforters are ye all!"

What Micah is saying in 4:9, 10 in comforting Judah is that they should not continue to weep as if there were no hope. He has already given them the glad news that "the mountain of the house of the Lord shall be established" (verse 1). "Is there no king in you?" he asks gently. "Has your counselor perished, that you labor like a woman giving birth?"

Micah's comparison here brings to mind Dr. Dick-Read's picture of the "hard-working woman employing the effort syndrome, which made her appear distressed." Micah encourages Judah to "groan and labor, like a woman giving birth . . . for you will be delivered."

The Septuagint also shows that Micah is here telling the "daughter of Zion" to take courage, as one might encourage a woman nearing delivery:

And now why have you known evils? Was there not a king for you? Or did
your counsel perish that labor as of one who gives birth has taken hold of you?

Be in labor, but be courageous and draw near, daughter of Zion, as one who
gives birth. Because now you will go out of a city and live in the field and you
will go to Babylon. From there He will save you and from there the Lord your
God will redeem you out of the hands of your enemies.

In the remaining four passages in the Septuagint that contain the
simile "as a woman giving birth" (Isaiah 26:17; Jeremiah 6:24; 13:19;
22:23), the words *tiktō, gennaō,* or *odinō* are used where the English
erroneously translates the Hebrew as "travail," "pain," or "pangs."

In order to understand how English renderings can differ so much
from the Septuagint, one must realize that our English and European
translations of the Old Testament are based primarily on the Hebrew
Masoretic text, of which the earliest extant manuscript dates back only
to A.D. 895. The Septuagint, translated from the original Hebrew one
thousand years earlier, obviously had access to documents much closer
to the original. The problem is not in the Hebrew text, however, but in
the cultural interpretations. The importance of the Septuagint, with its
happier renderings of childbirth passages than most of the English
translations, can hardly be overestimated, as it reflects the positive
attitude of an earlier day. And the Septuagint *was the only Old Testament widely used by the early church throughout the Greek-speaking
world until the Latin Vulgate appeared in the fourth and fifth centuries
A.D.*

Many New Testament quotations from the Old Testament were tak-
en by the New Testament writers word for word from the Septuagint.
And although the Septuagint was thoroughly Jewish in origin, it
became so identified with the Christian church that the Jews finally
sponsored another Greek translation of their own by a Jew named
Aquila.

By the time the Latin Vulgate officially replaced the Septuagint in
the church, a change in the attitude of many Christian writers, including Jerome, toward a woman's sexual functions as wife and childbear-
er was already well under way.

However, a negative attitude toward women was still evident at the
time the King James Version was translated in A.D. 1611, so that many
mistranslations of childbirth words occurred. But the really surprising
thing is that it is the translators of some of the newer revisions of the
last half century who have been the chief offenders in this regard. In

their attempts to break away from awkward literal translating and use familiar English words, they have unwittingly "read into" the text the concept of childbirth pain in many places where it is not in the original languages, nor even in the King James Version. This is understandable because of the emphasis on the inevitability of pain in childbirth in our culture and its seeming confirmation by the shocking sufferings in childbirth of many women in the eighteenth and nineteenth centuries.

As a matter of fact, many of us are guilty of careless "reading into" the text our own concepts of childbirth pain. In 1 Thessalonians 5:3, for example, how many people have thought that Paul was comparing the terrifying experience of destruction to the "terrifying" experience of giving birth?

For when they shall say, Peace and safety; then sudden destruction cometh upon them, as travail upon a woman with child; and they shall not escape.

In interpreting a verse like this it is important to determine just what the points of comparison are. In this verse there are two:

1. The *time* of destruction—it comes when it is unexpected, as labor may begin before the mother is prepared. It's "ready or not, here I come!" when a child is ready to be born.

2. The *certainty* of destruction—as certain as that a pregnant woman must someday give birth to a child. She cannot change her mind or put it off to some more convenient time.

The Talmud and Church Interpretations

The Jewish emphasis upon the blessings of marriage and parenthood has already been mentioned. This emphasis is stressed in the Talmud:

An entire section of the Talmud is devoted to "The obligation to marry and to propagate the race." To refuse to do so is tantamount to bloodshed and to expelling the Divine Presence from Israel.[9]

Of the fifty references to Eve listed in the index of the Soncino edition of the Talmud, there is only one passage that mentions any "curse" of Eve. This "curse" is interpreted as being in ten parts, embracing the whole area of a woman's life. The "pain" of childbirth is not mentioned, and the phrase "in *etsev* shalt thou bring forth children" is dismissed with the statement "to be understood in its literal meaning."

The "curse" of Adam is paired with Eve's and is divided into ten parts also. Jewish literature does not single out Eve as bearing a special punishment but mentions her side by side with Adam. In fact, Rabbi Johanan, one of the most prominent of the early rabbis, says that a man's punishment was "twice as great." This is certainly different from the doctrine of the church these last centuries. In another place in the Talmud we read of Eve:

Because she was the mother of all living she was given (to her husband) to live, but not to suffer pain.[10]

Rabbi Jakobovits quotes the Talmud as saying that a woman "is not bound to torment herself on account of her submission to her husband," and that "one need not destroy oneself in order to populate the world."[11]

Among the early Jewish writings outside the Talmud, a reference is found to the "sentence" to which Eve was subjected. In this explanation (c. A.D. 300) of Eve's sentence found in the Tosephta of Rabbi Nathan, the *birth* of a child is not included at all!

As Adam was laid under three sentences, likewise was it with Eve. . . . The first few days of menstruation are painful. So also are the first few moments of sexual intercourse with a man. Also, when a woman becomes pregnant, her face loses its beauty and becomes yellow the first three months.

Since the Talmud does not condemn women to suffering, the objections raised by the church to the use of anesthetics in labor are not paralleled in Jewish thought.

The question about the prohibition of painless birth in view of Gen. III, 16 is never found in the Responsa. As far back as the time of the Renaissance an Italian Rabbi—R. Obadiah Sforno (1475–1550)—did not interpret the Hebrew word "teldi" (thou shalt bring forth) literally. According to him the meaning of the word "teldi" is: "thou shalt bring up," *i.e.,* thou shalt bring up thy children in pain more than any other creature has to endure in bringing up its offspring. Prohibition of analgesics would contradict Jewish ideology, according to which the ways of the *Torah* "are of pleasantness, and all her paths are peace" (Prov. III, 17).[12]

The Jewish attitude toward the Genesis passage gives us insight into other references to childbirth in the Bible. It is a clue to Paul's meaning when he uses the word *teknogonia* ("childbearing") in 1 Timothy 2:15. Although Paul became a Christian, he also calls himself "an Hebrew of the Hebrews" (Phil. 3:5), and evidences of his Hebrew background are seen here. Some have interpreted *teknogonia* as a reference to the "curse of Eve," by which they mean that a woman who lives a godly, Christian life will be protected from pain or death during childbirth and have an easy delivery. Such an interpretation by Christians was sharply questioned even a century ago, when the outcry by the church against any relief of pain in childbirth was at its height:

[One scholar] represents the *teknogonia* as that in which the curse finds its operation (an extravagant statement to begin with, since *death* was plainly set forth as for both man and woman the proper embodiment of the curse), then, that she was to be exempted from this curse in its worst and heaviest effects (of which, however, nothing is said in the original word), and that besides, she should be saved *through*—that is, passing through the curse of her child-bearing trials—saved, notwithstanding the danger and distress connected with these! Surely a most unnatural and forced explanation, and ending in a very lame and impotent conclusion![13]

It is more consistent with the context of this passage to translate *teknogonia* as "motherhood," as the translators of the New English Bible have done. This version, in the margin, also has the most plausible rendering of the rest of the verse: "Yet she will be saved through motherhood—if only *husband and wife* continue in mutual fidelity, love, and holiness, with a sober mind." The Greek has two pronouns, the first singular, the second plural, "she" and "they." Since the previous verses have been talking about husband and wife (Adam and Eve), including the husband in the role of parenting is in harmony with other biblical passages on the subject.

E. J. Goodspeed, in his translation of the New Testament, also translates *teknogonia* as "motherhood." Such a translation is in keeping with the similar injunction to women given by Paul in Titus 2:3 (NEB):

The older women . . . must set a high standard, and school the younger women to be loving wives and mothers, temperate, chaste, and kind, busy at home, respecting the authority of their own husbands.

Protestant theologians are not the only ones who have come to the conclusion that such passages are references to "motherhood" rather than to "childbirth." Pope Pius XII, in an address on natural childbirth in 1956, outlined the official Catholic position. He says in part:

. . . God did not wish to forbid and did not forbid men to seek after and make use of all the riches of creation; to make progress step by step in culture; to make life in this world more bearable and better; to lighten the burden of work and fatigue, pain, sickness and death, in a word to subdue the earth (Genesis, i, 28). . . . God did not wish to forbid—nor did he forbid—mothers to make use of means which render childbirth easier and less painful. One must not seek subterfuges for the words of sacred scripture: They remain true in the sense intended and expressed by the Creator, namely: motherhood will give the mother much suffering to bear.[14]

As has been noted before, the attitude toward motherhood in New Testament and early church days was similar to that of the Jews of the same period. This attitude is little changed today. Rabbi Jakobovits sums up the difference between Jewish and Christian attitudes toward childbirth during some of the intervening centuries by comparing their respective attitudes toward suffering in general:

There is no trace in rabbinic law of the Christian concept in which "Pathos became Ethos; suffering was a sign of grace, not to be evaded but sought." It is true, the moral codes of the Church also modified many of its principles for the sake of mitigating pain. . . . But in general, Christianity is distinctly more panegyrical in its commendation of physical suffering than is Judaism.[15]

Although excesses such as flagellation are no longer countenanced by the church, some Christians still believe that all suffering is the result of sin and that patient bearing of pain is a sign of repentance and humility. But the Reverend J. S. Stewart shows how all suffering cannot be attributed to sin, and that many of the tragedies in life are due to the inexorability of the laws that govern the universe, and yet that it is the very rigidity of these laws upon which life depends:

Take even grim facts like earthquakes and volcanoes. It is hard to discover any trace of beneficence there. But the fact is that the very forces which occasionally produce these devastating outbursts are the same forces which, working continually beneath the earth's surface, make and keep this planet habitable for the sons of men. You cannot have all the assets of life, and refuse its liabilities.[16]

So it is that in the normal process of childbirth there are factors, such as disproportion of the baby's head in relation to the mother's pelvis, or muscular resistance to the birth, which may give rise to pain. But that such pain is the result of Eve's sin is a concept that cannot be considered an adequate Christian explanation.

But what if Genesis 3:16 could be interpreted as meaning that physical pain in childbirth is the judgment for sin; what if the passages in the prophets could be interpreted as meaning that all women in Bible history writhed in pain in childbirth, and that all births everywhere since the beginning of time have been agony—would this "prove" that natural childbirth is not scriptural? Not at all. The basic principles of God's Holy Word, which reveal God as a perfect and loving Creator, also reveal that it is his desire that the sufferings of this present world be alleviated, and that all humankind, through Christ, be brought into physical and spiritual harmony with their Maker. With these principles the philosophy of natural childbirth is in harmony.

NOTES

1. Rabbi Samson Raphael Hirsch, *The Pentateuch* (London: Isaac Levy, 1959), vol. 1, p. 83.
2. Ibid., p. 85.
3. Flavius Josephus, *Jewish Antiquities,* trans. Thackeray, Loeb Classical Library (London: Heinemann, 1889), Book I, p. 83.
4. Irenaeus, "Irenaeus Against Heresies," Book III, Chap. XXIII, in *The Ante-Nicene Fathers* (Grand Rapids, MI: Eerdmans, 1951).
5. George Foot Moore, *Judaism* (Cambridge, MA: Harvard University Press, 1950), vol. 1, p. 445.
6. Louis Finkelstein, *The Pharisees* (Philadelphia: Jewish Publication Society of America, 1946), p. 47.
7. H. J. Zimmels, *Magicians, Theologians and Doctors* (London: Goldston, 1952), p. 16.
8. Brown, Driver, Briggs, *A Hebrew and English Lexicon of the Old Testament* (London: Oxford, 1907).
9. Rabbi Immanuel Jakobovits, *Jewish Medical Ethics* (New York: Philosophical Library, 1959), p. 154.
10. The Talmud, Kheth, I, 364.
11. Jakobovits, *Jewish Medical Ethics,* p. 165.
12. Zimmels, *Magicians, Theologians and Doctors,* p. 7.
13. Patrick Fairbairn, *The Pastoral Epistles* (Edinburgh: T. and T. Clark, 1874).
14. "Text of Address by Pope Pius XII on the Science and Morality of Natural Childbirth," printed in the *New York Times,* January 9, 1956, from the official Vatican translation of Pope Pius' address in French on January 8.
15. Jakobovits, *Jewish Medical Ethics.*
16. J. S. Stewart, *The Strong Name* (Edinburgh: T. and T. Clark, 1941), pp. 137, 138.

19. Contemporary Obstetric Practices

Introduction

It is not surprising, when one realizes the historical background of modern obstetrics, that certain basic misunderstandings persist. One can see how knowledge that the staggering death rate from puerperal fever was caused by filthy conditions led to such an emphasis on sterile, aseptic deliveries that the human relationships became sterile as well. Because of the emphasis on asepsis, the emotional needs of the three human beings involved in the birth are usually overlooked.

Nor is it difficult to see how the terrible suffering and deaths in childbed during the centuries preceding ours have led to overemphasis on the necessity of anesthetic relief in humane attempts to prevent such suffering. Also, a realization of some of the erroneous religious concepts that have influenced our American and European cultures helps us to appreciate why our societies, including the medical profession, have been so slow in accepting a more positive approach to childbirth.

This chapter reveals some of the painful results of the inadequate concepts of childbirth that we have inherited. These facts are not pleasant to relate, and readers must realize that they are accusations against a *philosophy* and the consequent *methods* of modern obstetrics, not accusations against medical personnel or their motives. Doctors too are victims of our negative concepts of childbirth. They have suffered when their patients suffered, and if at times they have seemed indifferent to a woman's pain it is because they felt they had to keep a purely objective and scientific attitude toward their patients to function efficiently as physicians. But humane physicians feel a genuine sympathy for the pain during childbirth that they witness day after day.

Inadequacies

Inadequate Training in Obstetrics for Medical Personnel

The prevalence of medieval and Victorian concepts of childbirth pain among some medical personnel still, in these last two decades of the twentieth century, is a reflection of their inadequate training in philosophy and the humanities. Because of this lack, some of them are unable to comprehend that pain in a typical birth might have a logical, rational explanation. Their concept is that pain during labor and during the delivery is *normal* rather than symptomatic of abnormal conditions. To no other function of the healthy human body is "pain" regarded as a normal accompaniment.

It is not surprising to find this concept of pain in a book written by a doctor in 1929:

The pains accompany the intermittent contractions of the muscle of the uterus as it attempts to expel its contents, and arise from this contraction. . . . The time between them decreases as the labor progresses and their intensity increases. The most severe pain, the agony of childbirth, comes after the child's head has passed from the uterus and while it is propelled through the vagina. The passage is stretched and sometimes torn; the pain is often extremely severe.[1]

It is most surprising to find this concept still expressed in a recent edition of the leading obstetrical textbook for medical students.

Alone among physiologic muscular contractions, those of labor are painful. Therefore, the common designation in many languages for such a contraction is "pain." The cause of the pain is not definitely known, . . .[2]

Inadequate Prenatal Care and Training for Expectant Parents and Inadequate Rapport Between Childbearing Women and Their Doctors

Inadequate Prenatal Care

"Every year in the United States 30,000 infants are needlessly condemned to death, and another 200,000 are born with preventable birth defects. Most cases of mental retardation and other neurological disorders are caused *in utero*. . . . In fact, all of the approximately 11 billion neurons (nerve cells) in the brain are produced before birth."[3]

Malnutrition

The reason for the majority of these tragedies is malnutrition in human pregnancy, malnutrition caused not by poverty, but by women being limited in weight gain during pregnancy and even prescribed diuretics by their physicians to help keep their weight gain down to fifteen to twenty pounds. Not only does this cause problems for the fetus, it is also a health hazard for the mother, especially when the protein intake is inadequate, leading to possible toxemia and even death. Ample medical research has documented these truths for forty years, yet most obstetricians fail to give their clients adequate nutritional counseling.

Harmful Substances

Nor do physicians adequately warn their patients of the dangers of smoking, alcohol, coffee, *all* nonprescription drugs—laxatives, antihistamines, cough medicines, antibiotics, even aspirin. Low birth weight, stillbirths, and slowed growth and development of the child can all be caused by smoking.[4] Marijuana is especially dangerous and is harmful to the brain, lungs, and sexual organs.

Caffeine (found in coffee, tea, cola, and some nonprescription drugs) causes birth defects in animals such as cleft palates, missing digits, and malformed skulls. The U.S. government warns that women should minimize their consumption of these items, particularly during the first three months of pregnancy. Even aspirin can cause problems with blood coagulation or possible chromosome damage. High doses of vitamin C (commonly taken to prevent colds) may interfere with a chemical process in the baby and lead to jaundice. Too much vitamin K can cause a form of mental retardation.

Medications

Not only do physicians often fail to warn their patients of the dangers of harmful substances, but they may actually prescribe them in the form of medications far too freely. Even the nausea drug Bendectin which has been implicated in birth defects[5] is often prescribed in lieu of showing expectant mothers how nausea can be controlled by natural nondrug alternatives.

Ultrasound

Ultrasonography is a noninvasive means of evaluating a pregnancy. Intermittant high-frequency sound waves are produced by an alternating current to a transducer which is placed directly on the skin of the mother's abdomen. Pulse echoes bounce off the contents of her uterus and are recorded on a screen so that a picture of the fetal parts and placenta can be seen.

Some physicians elect to use ultrasound every few weeks throughout the pregnancy, beginning in the earliest weeks. Thus they not only prescribe medications far too freely, but often use ultrasound routinely in normal pregnancies, without warning their patients of the danger to their fetuses. The Department of Health, Education and Welfare states that the use of ultrasound has not yet been proven safe and is known to cause anomalies in animals.[6]

In recent years scientists have . . . reported biological levels of ultrasound, both continuous wave (Doppler) and pulse-echo (sonar). . . . One could argue that the exposure conditions do not mimic those encountered in the clinical situation. For example, one common objection is that the volume of tissue being exposed is relatively greater in a mouse than it is in a human being. In other words, the exposures to the fetal mice represent whole-body exposures. However, I might also point out that when using ultrasound during the first trimester there is a good possibility of whole-body exposure to the human fetus. . . .[7]

The developmental effects of low levels of ultrasound exposure to rodents have included delayed neuromuscular development, delayed neuromotor development, altered emotional behavior, fetal abnormalities, depressed immune response, and spleen enlargement. In rabbits, the effects include changes in the eye. In chicks, the effects included hemorrhaging of bone marrow and blood stasis (when blood stops flowing in the blood vessels).[8] Some researchers believe there may also be chromosome damage.

Amniocentesis

Nor has amniocentesis been proven safe. It is done by inserting a long needle through the abdominal wall of the mother, through the uterine wall into the amniotic sac, and then withdrawing some of the amniotic fluid for examination. It is a painful procedure, often causing severe abdominal cramps after the needle is withdrawn.

Amniocentesis should only be done in high-risk cases to test the fluid for evidence of fetal lung maturity before a cesarean, or when prematurity threatens (to determine whether or not the infant can survive). Sometimes it is done to determine whether or not the fetus is abnormal. Sometimes it is foolishly done simply to determine the sex of the child.

Yet the amniocentesis, or 'tap' as it is often called, will cause one in

150 women to miscarry. Sometimes it punctures the baby, while the major risk is that of puncturing the placenta.[9]

. . . the hazards of amniocentesis include pneumothorax (air in the baby's chest from multiple puncture wounds), gangrene of a fetal limb, hemorrhage, and sudden fetal death.[10]

Fetoscopy

Fetoscopy provides direct visualization of the fetus and placenta for externally visible anomalies.[11] It is performed by making an incision and passing an instrument through the mother's lower abdominal wall, uterus, and amniotic sac. The opening so made also allows for the withdrawal of fetal or placental tissue for examination.

Possible hazards include damage to the fetus from the intensity of the light of the instrument as well as damage that may occur from rupturing the amniotic sac. If prenatal care is to be not only adequate but competent, parents need to know that every "new" device carries some risk, and that they have the option of refusing any tests they feel may not be safe.

Inadequate Training for Childbirth

Not only does inadequate prenatal care often leave expectant women uninformed about proper care of the fetus, it often fails to prepare them adequately for the coming experience of giving birth. After the health examination of the first visit, most women are put through the same routine each time: they are weighed, have their urine tested, their blood pressure taken, and their abdomen palpated (by the hands of the physician or midwife, to determine the size and position of the baby). While these procedures are essential, they should be explained so the woman knows why they are being done. Most doctors ask an expectant mother if she has any questions, but this short interchange is not sufficient to represent the sum total of a woman's training for one of the most important experiences of her life.

One young woman complained to me that the doctor asking if she had any questions didn't help her at all. "My whole mind is one big question," she said. "I don't know enough to ask an intelligent question, and yet there is so much I want to know." This young woman was a college graduate. She showed me her physiology textbook with its description and diagrams of the processes of birth. And yet she said that her mind was "one big question."

Many childbirth classes—especially those run by hospitals—prepare expectant mothers to accept the routine hospital procedures without question: amniotomy, tranquilizers, electronic fetal heart monitoring, pain medication, intravenous fluids, confinement to bed, epidural anesthesia, episiotomy, and, for one out of every four to six women, cesarean section. This is called "education for childbirth"! The dangers, discomforts, and indignities of these procedures may not even be mentioned. Thus while women may be told what to expect in the way of treatment and even taught some "distraction" breathings so they won't feel the "pain," they are not adequately trained to *give birth without artificial aid and with maximum comfort.*

Many "prepared childbirth" classes use the "Lamaze Method," which is erroneously equated with natural childbirth. But there is a vast difference.

Many statements concerning Lamaze techniques are common misconceptions. . . . An excellent example of this is the use of the term "natural childbirth" to describe the Lamaze method. The description of "prepared" childbirth is more appropriate to Lamaze than "natural" (a term that is more often associated with the Read method and its variants, e.g., Bradley method). . . .

In contrast to natural childbirth, most authorities on the psychoprophylactic method (Lamaze) would agree that success has no relation whatever to the use of medication during parturition. . . . Medications are available when needed to enhance the labor experience and to help the laboring woman to remain cooperative and in control. . . . Lamaze techniques do not, for example, preclude the use of fetal monitoring equipment. . . . It is the parents' satisfaction that is ultimately the ideal conclusion. This, and this alone, probably accounts for the present surge of interest in the Lamaze method.[12]

Classes vary not only according to the setting (hospital classes, classes in a doctor's office, classes sponsored by a private group or individual), but also and more importantly, in philosophy (Lamaze, Dick-Read, Bradley, Leboyer, etc.). The greatest variation, however, is in the philosophy of the individual instructor, whose teaching may be true natural childbirth no matter what "name" she is teaching under. The converse is also true, for even a class called "natural childbirth" may not teach relaxed, unmedicated, physiological birth at all. How can a couple discern the difference? There are several helpful clues:

1. Is it implied that childbirth is painful, but that the expectant mother will be taught how to "overcome" or "rise above" the pain? This is not natural childbirth.

2. Are routine procedures explained without an explanation also of the *hazards* of each procedure and without mentioning that the woman has the right of refusal? If so, it is not natural childbirth.

3. Are "distraction" methods taught, breathing patterns that must be "learned," and an explanation that there may often be need for "a little medication" to overcome pain? This is not natural childbirth.

4. Does the class explain the normal physiological processes of birth and how one can cooperate with these processes at each stage so that undue pain is *prevented* from occurring?

5. Does it teach that such pain is symptomatic of something "out of harmony" with the natural process which needs the immediate and continual attention of the birth attendants in order to correct the problem?

6. What percentage of the women who have been trained in these classes have:
   a. received "a little" pain medication;
   b. had their labors induced;
   c. had their labors augmented (speeded up);
   d. had episiotomies;
   e. had an unexpected cesarean due to "dystocia" (failure to progress)?

Not every labor is perfect, even with the best preparation, and we can be grateful for the availability of pain medication and other aids to a labor that is in true difficulty. But if the percentage of women trained are receiving these interventions more than fifteen to twenty percent of the time, the classes do not adequately teach natural birthing.

Inadequate Relief from Pain During Childbirth, in Spite of the Employment of Tranquilizers and Analgesics Beyond the Limits of Safety

It is a common misconception that the natural childbirth patient is a "stoic," while the orthodox obstetric patient is relieved of her pain by means of drugs. Quite the opposite is true. The natural childbirth mother, because she knows how to *prevent* pain by relaxation and relaxed breathing, does not suffer. The untrained orthodox patient, because she is tense, does feel severe pain even under sedation. And maternal fear (which causes her tension) may cause an excessive amount of adrenalin to be present in the baby's system, which increases its need for oxygen and places it at more risk.[13] A recent obstetric text agrees that *tension* in the mother is the source of pain, so that a tranquilizer may be as effective as a pain reliever:

If the woman is made aware that she will never be expected to suffer more than she can stand, and that she will be given a sedative when she feels the need of it, she is less likely to clamor for relief too soon or to lose her nerve. Women who scream during labor do so more from fear than from pain. . . . The woman needs help in coping with apprehension, weariness, tension, and anxiety, therefore tranquilizing drugs are as essential as those with analgesic properties.[14]

Some hospitals routinely give a tranquilizer to every woman admitted in labor, realizing that she is under some "stress." Yet the possible side effects of the most widely used tranquilizers include "drowsiness, confusion, diplopia [double vision], hypotension, changes in libido, nausea, fatigue, depression, dysarthria [abnormal heart rhythm], jaundice, . . . headache, incontinence, changes in salivation, slurred speech, tremor, vertigo, urinary retention, blurred vision. Paradoxical reactions such as acute hyperexcited states, anxiety, hallucinations, increased muscle spasticity, insomnia, rage, sleep disturbances . . .[15] and more. Hardly what a laboring woman needs!

The expectant mother can learn natural means to make these artificial "helps" with their accompanying dangers unnecessary. When there is muscular tension, the pain during labor feels very similar to menstrual cramps when menstruation is delayed. Of course, during labor this pain is distributed over a larger area. In painful menstruation, the pain does not seem to be so much in the tiny uterus itself, as in the tense, aching, congested muscles that surround it. This throbbing pain spreads throughout the lower abdomen, across the lower back, throughout the tissues of the pelvic area, and even down into the thighs. It can become so severe that one can hardly stand or sit up straight. The same thing happens in labor, for the pain of contractions is felt primarily in all the tissues that *surround* the uterus, rather than in the uterus itself. When the muscles of these areas are consciously relaxed, this pain miraculously disappears, and the woman feels only the uterus contracted firmly, which is no more unpleasant than a contracted bicep in her arm.

During my teen years I frequently suffered severe cramps from delayed menstruation. Finally I discovered, by trial and error, that if I went to bed and became warm enough to *relax* all the muscles in the abdominal and pelvic area of my body and fall into a quiet sleep, I would awaken an hour or two later to find the pain gone and the menstrual flow well established. I could then get up and go about my regular duties with no further discomfort. The pain had been caused by muscular tension, which had inhibited menstruation. Years later, when I first read of the relationship of muscle tension to pain in labor, the importance of releasing abdominal and pelvic muscle tension at this time immediately made good sense to me.

Many women trained for natural childbirth have complained that their attendants gave them a tranquilizer on admittance and insisted on a sedative later, so that they lost *conscious muscular control* of their relaxation and found it more difficult to stay "tuned in" to their body and flow with it. Consequently, they reacted to the drugs in the usual irrational, painful way.

In natural childbirth, if sedation is given at all, it is according to individual needs and desires rather than as a matter of routine at a given point in a woman's labor. In a relaxed, confident woman with cooperative attendants, sedation is frequently not needed at all. By contrast, as stated before, most women who go through hospital classes in "prepared" childbirth and/or are trained in "distraction" techniques request at least some mild sedation or medication almost routinely.

Inadequate Consideration for the Laboring Woman's Simple Comfort

Shaving

The removal of the pubic hair brings a sense of shame to some women, a sense of being "denuded" and returned to "little-girl" status. It is not only unnecessary but actually increases infections—the very thing it is supposed to prevent. One large-scale study showed that surgery patients who were shaved had an infection rate of 2.7 percent. Those whose hair was only clipped had an infection rate of 1.7 percent. Those who were neither shaved nor clipped had the lowest infection rate of all, 0.9 percent! Hospital-based infection caused patients an extra 10.2 days of hospitalization.[16]

Enema

One of the most disliked procedures of orthodox obstetrics is the enema. Some doctors are finally becoming aware of this and are omitting the enema unless there is evidence of hard fecal matter in the lower bowel. Early labor often stimulates the bowels to empty, and slight diarrhea frequently accompanies the onset of labor. This is nature's way of preparing the body for giving birth. A medical article states:

The physician who is not present during the administration of the enema is usually unaware of the patient's discomfort and even embarrassment during this procedure. Labor and delivery should be as pleasant and physiologic as possible, yet the patient's admission usually starts with a most displeasing experience. . . . The soapsuds enema has disadvantages in addition to the patient's discomfort. It is irritating to the mucosa. Trauma, including perforation of the rectum, may be caused by the enema tube, and enema fluid may contaminate the small bowel. . . . Side effects caused by general discomfort, mild or marked cramps, and rectal irritation amount to 84.8 percent in the enema group (of the 1,159 patients tested) compared to 1.5 percent for the bisacodyl (suppository) patients.[17]

Vaginal Exams

Vaginal exams are another disliked procedure and should be done as infrequently as possible, with *careful* attention to sterile technique, timed at a moment when the mother is ready (usually not during a contraction, unless a check for full dilatation during a contraction is needed before the pushing stage can begin). Vaginal exams are a prime source of serious infection. In the United States, a woman with ruptured membranes (sac or waters broken) is induced if birth does not begin spontaneously within twenty-four hours, "for fear of infection." Yet if vaginal exams were omitted, most of this risk would be markedly absent.

Many of the organisms leading to infection are probably introduced into the vagina from outside sources, such as the hands of the examiner, and do not arise from the natural flora. . . . Two Melbourne studies made some years apart had shown that there was no risk of infection when women with premature rupture of the membranes were simply hospitalized and put to bed, without any prophylactic antibiotic therapy. In Australia midwives provide most of the obstetric care. They are not allowed to do vaginal examinations. . . . It would be almost impossible in this country [U.S.] to keep a woman with ruptured membranes in a teaching hospital for days without her becoming infected.''[18]

The leading obstetric text in the United States says:

In spite of past reports that vaginal examinations during labor do not contribute to morbidity, clinical experience in certain circumstances strongly suggests the opposite. The likelihood of an injurious effect from repeated vaginal examinations seems most apparent in the case of early rupture of the membranes followed by repeated vaginal examinations casually performed by multiple examiners. . . . A common tendency, especially at large, busy public institutions, has been too little "laying on of hands" to gauge the quality of labor and too much "putting in of hands" to check cervical dilatation.[19]

Confinement to Bed

Confinement to bed is said to be necessary because of some of the routine procedures done. Not only is it unnecessary, it makes labor less efficient. Research by Dr. Caldeyro-Barcia indicates that a woman in both the first and second stages of labor is more comfortable, and her labor more effective, if she is *not* lying down:

The lithotomy position [flat on back, legs in high stirrups] is not natural or convenient for labor. It causes well-known ill effects, such as the compression by the uterus against the spine of the inferior vena cava, aorta, iliac arteries and ureters. This pressure completely disturbs the maternal circulation and the output of urine. Disturbances of the maternal circulation have an unfavorable and distressing effect on the fetus. . . .

The various positions for labor—supine, side-lying, sitting and standing— were studied for their effects on: intensity, frequency, efficiency, and uterine activity. Uterine contractions and fetal heart rates were monitored, recorded and compared while the mothers were in the various positions. Ninety-five percent of women prefer to sit or stand during first stage of labor. . . . The intensity of contractions is greater, and the frequency of contractions is about the same when the woman is standing, than when she is lying on her back. Therefore, the efficiency in dilating the cervix is greater when standing than when supine or in the side-lying position.[20]

Not only is a woman confined to bed in most hospitals, she is frequently required to lie on her back, which is the worst possible position for a woman in labor!

. . . when a pregnant woman near term lies on her back, especially if her blood vessels are vulnerable, the pressure on her great vein may be much greater than can be taken care of by the normal mechanism. In such cases, as long as the mother's blood pressure is abnormal, the fetus gets less of the vital oxygen and food it needs for sustenance and growth. A period of more than a few minutes could seriously affect the baby—especially the baby of a woman already afflicted with high blood pressure. . . . This explains some instances of incomplete development or retardation of the infant before birth. It also clarifies a mysterious syndrome, first reported several years ago and thought to be rare— that is, the case of pregnant women close to term who suffer a rapid decrease in blood pressure, fainting or feeling dizzy, when lying down. Drs. Power and Longo now surmise that this syndrome is more common than was realized.[21]

Lithotomy Position

When it is determined that second stage is underway the woman is usually transferred to a delivery room, where another source of discomfort occurs. The mother is placed on her back on the delivery table, slightly propped up at best, in the lithotomy position with her legs placed in stirrups, high and far apart. In some hospitals a woman's arms may be strapped down alongside her body, as was almost always done until just a few years ago.

The practice of strapping a woman down tightly on her back in an inflexible position is inexcusable. Of course it is necessary when a woman is unconscious under an operative anesthetic, but it has no justification for a conscious, cooperative woman. With her arms pinned stiffly down alongside her body, she can neither bend her elbows outward nor lean forward while bearing down. Her legs are pinned tightly in one rigid position (*higher* than her head!), and her head is left flat on the hard delivery table or, at best, placed on a flat, skimpy pillow.

This customary lithotomy position makes second-stage labor difficult and exhausting, especially for a first baby. Many women have not realized that the severe fatigue and backache that troubled them in the days after their baby was born was due to their having abused their back muscles by arching their backs while pushing—the only way one *can* push when pinned flat on one's back. Imagine trying to lift a weight from the ground by arching your back and throwing your head back! Even a passive delivery in this position may cause backache later, if one is pinned down in this way for any length of time.

The use of this position for delivering a child was first popularized in the seventeenth century by François Mauriceau, a French physician. He found that placing the woman in this position made the birth so much easier—*for the doctor!*

Not only is the lithotomy position uncomfortable, it is also harmful. It prolongs the second stage because it is impossible for a mother to push effectively in this position. Dr. Caldeyro-Barcia states that squatting is the best position for the actual birth as it not only takes advantage of gravity but actually increases the size of the pelvic outlet considerably.[22] Dr. Odent of Paris says that the most comfortable, effective position is the one chosen by the mother herself.

We have also observed that many women during second stage contractions want to flex their knees, especially if they have someone to support their shoulders in a sort of standing squat position. . . . We do not say that there is a best posture for delivery. Some women are delivered on the obstetric chair that we have, others on their knees or side. But the most common scene is of the woman delivering in a standing-squat, supported during pushes. We have observed that the pressure in the pelvis is greater during contractions in this standing-squatting position for delivery, that the pelvis opens much more easily in all dimensions, with the minimum muscular effort and oxygen consumption on the part of the mother. *When the mother is at risk or the baby is at risk, as in twin or breech deliveries for example, the standing-squat position for delivery is imperative.* We know that in a breech delivery what is dangerous is the delay between the delivery of the abdomen and the baby's head. This delay is artificially created or made worse by the dorsal position. When the mother is in a supported squatting position, as soon as the breech is delivered, the whole body comes.[23]

Episiotomy

Perhaps the most intensely disliked procedure is the episiotomy (surgical enlargement at the vulval orifice) and its repair, and the soreness of perineal tissue it causes. New mothers in maternity wards sometimes disrespectfully refer to their painful attempts at walking while this soreness persists as "the hemorrhoid shuffle." The sore area is soaked in sitz baths, heated with lamps, and plastered with salves in attempts to hasten the healing and ease the discomfort. The orthodox physician performs an episiotomy nearly one hundred percent of the time.

There is now ample evidence that the routine episiotomy is not really necessary. A muscle in good condition has a stretch ratio of eight to one, so that when a woman has practiced vaginal contractions during pregnancy, she is able to contract or relax these muscles at will during birth. By relaxing them, she keeps them from offering resistance to the birth of the child. Thus her labor is shortened and her tissues do not tear, although episiotomies may still be necessary in some instances, for example with a very large baby.

Additional advantages of vaginal exercise are: better control of urine incontinence in later pregnancy; quicker healing of stitches following birth if an episiotomy must be performed; restored vaginal resiliency soon after childbirth, so that the pleasure of intercourse is increased for both husband and wife; and a decreased need for surgery on cystoceles (in front) or rectoceles (in back) in which portions of the flabby vaginal wall protrude as masses through the vulva.

Most physicians justify their routine cutting of the perineum of every woman by saying that if they don't, these women will be plagued with cystoceles and rectoceles later on. These arguments have now been amply refuted. Other physicians have pointed out that rectoceles and cystoceles commonly occur in patients who *have* had episiotomies, so this is not an effective prevention. One doctor describes how he preserves the perineum and why he believes it is necessary to do so:

Many women, whether they openly express it or not, have a very real horror of having their perineums cut. Others feel that if while fully conscious and completing the second stage of delivery, they were advanced upon with hypodermic and scissors, it would spoil their moment of triumph. My patients expect me to preserve the perineum intact after delivery, if it is at all possible. . . .
On the question of saving the fetus the "pounding of the head upon the pelvic floor," I am aware of the theory of this "danger" and the measures said to prevent it. . . . I have never seen convincing proof that this is so. . . . The conscientious physician gives his patient what she wants, only if it happens to be good for her. If I believed that I could prevent brain damage in children, or pelvic problems for my patients, I would of course do the episiotomy.[24]

The episiotomy is not without risk. If it is done too early, there may be considerable bleeding from the gaping wound between the time the incision is made and the birth of the baby.[25] If it is done too late, one of the so-called objectives of the operation is defeated[26]—the prevention of the stretching of the perineum (stretching erroneously thought to destroy its muscle tone and normal elasticity).

Another reason the episiotomy is performed on almost all women is to prevent the tearing of the perineum. Yet even with an episiotomy the perineum often tears past the incision on down through the anal sphincter and into the rectum (third- and fourth-degree tears).[27] One carefully controlled research study reported "a 10% incidence of combined third and fourth degree lacerations among patients receiving episiotomies compared to none in 1000 patients who had not received an episiotomy."[28] Another research study "reported a 22 percent incidence of tears in primiparous women who *had* an episiotomy."[29]

The implications of this would be that a woman was *more* likely to tear with an episiotomy than without one (in a carefully controlled birth of the head). But now we are told in the latest edition of *Williams Obstetrics* that tears are not such a traumatic problem and that even a tear down through the rectum (fourth-degree) "is a much less serious accident than it was formerly."[30] We might edit that to read: "a less serious accident than we were formerly *led to believe*." The important factor is the skillful repair, yet in some hospitals "episiotomies and repairs were done primarily by house officers [medical students, interns, or residents] in training"![31] Furthermore, "even when second- and third-degree lacerations were compared with episiotomies, women tended to be more comfortable after having a tear than an episiotomy, and appeared to heal better."[32]

Nor does the routine "speeding up" of the birth with an episiotomy help the baby.

Caldeyro-Barcia has demonstrated that it is prolonged breath-holding and strenuous pushing which may interfere with oxygenation of the fetus, not the length of time in the second stage. In his study women with minimal pushing, and second stages exceeding two hours, produced babies whose Apgar scores were no lower than those of babies delivered after rapid second stages. In the absence of signs of fetal distress it looks as if the episiotomy done to speed up the second stage does not make delivery any safer for the baby.[33]

Nor can it be proven that episiotomy decreases problems with the pelvic floor in later life.[34] It does not lead to "functional normality or increased sexual satisfaction,"[35] as the medical profession claims. The evidence points in quite the opposite direction. Young women frequently complain of pain in intercourse, once it is resumed following the birth of a child when an episiotomy has been performed. This discomfort may persist for months or longer and may permanently affect the sexual relationship even after the pain is gone. Others complain of feeling "violated" by this operation on their sexual apparatus. It has been described in some published material as a "clitorotomy," based upon redefinition of the clitoris as consisting of "the inner lips, hood, glans and shaft, crura, muscles, urethral sponge, perineal sponge and suspensory ligament (fourchette), and hymen. . . . The parts of the clitoris, as newly defined, work together as an organ to produce the sexual response cycle of excitement, plateau, orgasm and resolution."[36]

A young woman vividly expresses the frustration many feel:

> It is now four years since my second child's birth, and I still experience a full day of soreness after each intercourse. If we're not very careful of the angle of penetration, there is an actual tear to the fourchette with each intercourse, albeit a small one. There is definite scar tissue there, which I can feel easily as a "ridge" with my fingers.
>
> And I do feel violated—most definitely. Not only because of a past assault to my person, but because it's an assault that will never go away. I will *never* be physically the same as I would have been had it not been done. Even a rape doesn't cause physical changes in most cases![37]

Technological Interventions

In the twenty years since I first wrote this book on natural childbirth, tremendous advances have taken place. At that time I was cautioned against using the word "natural," yet now the term is widely accepted. No longer are most women heavily sedated in labor and anesthetized routinely for the birth. Husbands are not only admitted into hospital labor rooms, but are often accepted in delivery rooms as well. Breastfeeding is permitted on the delivery table. A period for bonding is often provided and mothers are discharged early if desired. Prenatal classes are common.

However, it seems that for every battle overcome, another "novel" intervention has arisen to take its place. In the last ten years we have seen interventive methods proliferate in obstetrics: routine amniotomy, induction of labor, intravenous glucose during labor, external or internal fetal monitors, epidural anesthesia, manual removal of the placenta, and an alarming increase in the percentage of cesarean sections. While there are thousands of physicians and health professionals who believe in and promote natural childbirth, they still face an uphill battle. The following recent statement in an obstetric newsletter makes this evident:

Consumerism has given rise to the "natural childbirth movement," the home birth organizations, the Lamaze and Bradley advocates, and many other lay organizations whose allegations and claims are totally lacking in scientific verification or support. . . . Extensive media exposure . . . has panicked some hospitals into providing some poorly thought out gimmicks . . . i.e., the practice of "bonding," of putting the baby to breast on the delivery table, the "ABC Room," the birthing chair and other cult rituals. . . . If we are to avoid being done in by the malpractice problem we must reassert our control over the patient and insist that we exclusively make the decisions relative to patient care, putting an end to the non-physician interference in this process. . . ."[38]

It seems incredible that any physician should make such a statement. The author apparently has not read the extensive research that has been conducted and published in medical journals that supports each of the practices about which he complains.

Only brief mention is possible here of some of the more common obstetric interferences, but resources for further study are listed in the appendix. Among these interferences are amniotomy, routine induction of labor and augmentation of labors that are "too slow," routine fetal monitoring, and cesarean section.

Amniotomy

Amniotomy is the artificial rupturing of the "sac of waters," if it is still intact when a woman arrives at the hospital in labor. This may even be done without informing the mother, who may think she is just being cervically examined. (This happened to me.) It is estimated that in about two-thirds of women with uncomplicated, unmedicated labors, the amniotic sac, if it is not broken artificially, will not rupture until the end of the first stage of labor or later.[39]

The use of amniotomy has become so routine that intact membranes during second stage labor may be perceived as abnormal rather than as normal physiologic progress in labor. Many experienced labor attendants have seldom seen a woman push her baby down the birth canal with the ovular membranes still intact.[40]

Amniotomy may shorten the length of labor slightly (one purpose for which it is performed), but there is no evidence that a shorter labor is necessarily beneficial to baby or mother, and the reverse is more likely true.[41]

When the membranes have been ruptured, the protection of the fluid, which is particularly important during contractions, is lost. This protection of the amniotic fluid is mostly accepted on the head and the umbilical cord. After rupture, the fetal head will suffer the effects of uneven pressure accepted during uterine contractions. Also, the umbilical cord will be compressed, and in many cases, occluded during contractions. . . .

Once the membranes are ruptured, . . . the absence of the pressure of the forewaters [causes] the parietal bones [to] protrude with a marked misalignment, causing deformation of the head and deceleration in fetal heart rate. . . . In this situation [of uneven head compression] if you study the EEG of the fetus you will see abnormal changes in the EEG, indicating that the brain is not in a normal position.[42]

Induction and/or Augmentation of Labor

A few years ago routine induction of labor was considered a great advance. Births could now be "scheduled" at a time convenient for the obstetrician and for the parents. The medical profession itself soon began warning of the dangers inherent in indiscriminate "birth by appointment," but that has not stopped the practice.

There is still widespread use not only of induction of a labor but also of artificial stimulation of a labor that is "abnormally slow" or shows "lack of progress in cervical dilatation." By whose standards is the labor "too slow"? When at *least* thirty percent of labors or more are classified as dysfunctional and in need of artificial stimulation (most frequently by synthetic oxytocin given intravenously), perhaps a second look needs to be taken at what constitutes a "normal" length of labor.

Dr. Caldeyro-Barcia concluded (after a collaborative study in twelve Latin American medical centers) that in oxytocic-induced labors, even with all proper precautions—such as the lowest effective dosage given and proper monitoring of mothers—almost seventy-five percent of the mother's uterine contractions were shown through fetal heart monitor tracings to result in a reduction of oxygen to the baby's brain.[43]

Women who have experienced an induced labor have much more difficulty relaxing during contractions and usually state that their labors were "painful." But unless the procedure is very carefully done, there are far more serious consequences for the mothers as well as the babies. *Williams Obstetrics* warns:

The mother should *never be left alone* while the infusion is running. The uterine contractions must be *observed continually* and the flow shut off immediately if they exceed 1 minute in duration or if the fetal heart tones show any significant alterations. . . . The frequency, intensity, and duration of contractions, and uterine tone between contractions must not exceed those of normal spontaneous labor. Oxytocin is a powerful drug, and it *has killed or maimed mothers through rupture of the uterus and even more babies* through hypoxia from markedly hypertonic uterine contractions.[44]

The italics are mine, for how many women are "never left alone" and "observed continually" by medical personnel while labor is being augmented by "pitocin drip" or something similar? The presence of the husband alone and the use of the fetal monitor is not adequate for ensuring safety. Furthermore, augmented labor causes more cases of uterine rupture than do previous cesarean sections!

The Golan study concerned 93 cases of uterine rupture during a five-year period. Of these, 61 occurred in normal uteri while 32 were found in patients who had undergone a previous section. There were nine maternal deaths, and *all* occurred in the group of mothers who had *not* had previous cesarean surgery. The fetal mortality was also much worse for the women without previous cesareans. The fetal mortality for the previous cesarean group was 22%, while it was more than triple, or 74%, in the unscarred group. The ruptured uteri in the normal, unscarred group were, for the most part, associated with oxytocin administered during labor.[45]

Intravenous Glucose Drip

Even more common than artificial stimulation of labor is the intravenous glucose drip, often given to every woman in labor. In a recent symposium on obstetric anesthesia, it was stated that maternal intravenous glucose administered during labor may cause hypoglycemia in the newborn. This increases the risk of central nervous system abnormalities which may only become apparent as the child grows older. "Within approximately 10 minutes of a maternal bolus infusion of glucose, a rise in fetal blood glucose occurs which will usually persist for at least an hour."[46]

For a woman who is sugar-responsive and tends to become hyperactive, a glucose infusion would make it much more difficult to relax. Or if a woman is mildly hypoglycemic or has diabetic tendencies, a glucose drip could dangerously upset her blood sugar balance. The same would be true of her baby. The dangers outweigh the benefits. There are simpler ways to restore a mother's fluid and blood sugar, such as giving her orange juice to drink. Dr. Harlan Ellis insists that the woman in labor should have "all the fluids she wants."[47]

Routine Fetal Monitoring

This has become the "norm" in many hospitals, even though the risk of internal fetal monitoring has quickly become apparent:

The risk of contamination of amniotic fluid during internal fetal monitoring may be as high as 50%. . . . In a series of 30 pregnancies, intrauterine fetal monitoring produced contamination of amniotic fluid in 15 women and puerperal fever in 11. Since the monitoring equipment was sterile, the fluid was probably contaminated by introduction of flora from the cervix.[48]

One might question whether the monitoring equipment was in fact sterile. Why blame the poor cervix? Couldn't the contamination have crept up the wires from the machine that's been sitting on a table at bedside for days, weeks, months, and years? And hasn't it been handled by scores of nurses (without sterile gloves), not to mention the technicians coming around to check it for accuracy (if they bother, that is)?

The disadvantages of routine monitoring greatly outweigh the advantages. Although a woman may still move around on the bed, her freedom of movement away from the bed is greatly limited. If she is wearing an external monitor, the pressure of the transducer against her contracting uterus makes it difficult to relax. The abdominal muscles cannot release tension and rise above the contracting uterus, so that each contraction "hurts." The nerve endings in the abdominal muscles are pinched between the uterus and the transducer.

The theory is that monitoring saves many babies' lives and prevents such problems as brain damage due to oxygen deprivation during birth. Yet "an analysis of literature in the field showed little evidence that the monitoring prevented death or long-term disability. . . . The possibility of preventing brain damage, through fetal monitoring and cesarean section, is 'purely speculative.' "[49]

Not only is there a question that it helps prevent damage—evidence shows that it *causes* damage. The FDA has warned of the dangers of fetal monitoring because it depends upon constant low frequencies of ultrasound, and ultrasound has never been proven safe. Unlike ultrasonographic exams during pregnancy where the transmitter is moved around, during labor it is directed *continuously* to the *same spot* on the baby.

And the monitoring poses risks to the mother as well.

One mother is sacrificed for every eight babies saved by electronic monitoring, and gravidas [expecting mothers] should be told, prior to the procedure, to fulfill informed consent requirements. . . . Dr. Munsick, professor of obstetrics and gynecology, University School of Medicine, Indianapolis, arrived at the 1:8 ratio by extrapolating statistics on increased neonatal survival attributed to fetal monitoring, increased cesarean section rate associated with monitoring, and increased maternal mortality associated with cesarean section. . . .

His remarks followed a presentation by Dr. John G. McFee on a controlled, prospective study showing that electronic monitoring did not improve perinatal outcome in high risk pregnancy but did result in a threefold increase in cesarean section.[50]

Cesarean Section

The greatest danger in the routine use of the fetal monitors is that it has led to a rapid increase in the number of cesarean operations being performed, often due to a misreading of the data. With the introduction of fetal monitoring in the mid-sixties, the cesarean rate more than tripled in thirteen years (from five percent in 1965 to fifteen percent in 1978) and it is still rising.[51] In some hospitals it is as high as thirty percent, so that one out of every three or four women who enter the hospital door in labor is operated on. The most frequent reason given is *dystocia,* "failure to progress," which accounts for about thirty percent of the increase in cesareans. It is now the tenth most common surgical procedure in the United States.

Maternal mortality, although rare, is about four times higher following a cesarean compared to a vaginal delivery. About half of this increase is due to the complications leading to the cesarean or maternal disease, and about half to the risks of the surgery itself. The risk of maternal death in a repeat cesarean is about twice the risk in a vaginal delivery, and the risk is *not* declining. . . . Maternal morbidity is also much greater after cesarean, most of it infectious. Since a major contributor to maternal mortality is the use of general anesthesia, we recommended that all parents should have the choice of regional anesthesia, except for the few times where it is medically contraindicated.[52]

There is a growing acceptance of the validity of planned vaginal births after a cesarean, supported by the National Institutes of Health Cesarean Birth Report: "Data from national and international sources suggest that labor and vaginal delivery, after a previous low segment cesarean birth, is of low risk to mother and fetus in properly selected cases."[53] And on February 24, 1982, the American College of Obstetricians and Gynecologists announced a significant policy change that could have a major impact on the soaring cesarean rate. Speaking for the College, Dr. Cefalo, Chairman of the Committee on Obstetrics, stated:

After reviewing detailed studies carried out since since 1951 on over 28,000 vaginal deliveries following prior cesareans, the College's Committee on Obstetrics has determined that under proper conditions, many women who have had a cesarean birth may safely be considered for vaginal delivery.[54]

Morbidity and Mortality

There are far more serious consequences of orthodox obstetric methods than pain and discomfort for the mothers—illness, damage, and even death of either mother or child or both may occur. The United States makes a poor showing for safety to mother and child among nations of similar standards of living and similar culture. While the infant death rate has fallen about fifty percent in the last twenty years, as much credit—and no doubt more—can be given to the natural-childbirth movement and improved knowledge of proper nutrition during pregnancy as to medical advances. An increasing number of women are choosing to give birth without medications or interventions, in or out of hospitals. Some credit must be given, of course, to improved technology, especially in saving the lives of premature infants, but this is only part of the story.

Even so, the United States still makes a very poor showing, compared to other nations, in its infant mortality statistics. We are now *seventeenth* down the list, the lowest ever, even though our infant mortality rate continues to decline. A glance at the U.N. statistics reveals the grim truth.[55] Surely we can do better! Many of the countries achieving better rates than ours are doing so largely without the technology we employ. Perhaps this is part of the reason their rates are better.

Morbidity in infants continues to be a problem, often unnecessarily, due to the analgesics and epidural anesthetics commonly used for laboring women:

Experts now estimate that only 1 in 5 American newborn infants is born in optimal conditions; 1 out of every 3 newborn infants admitted to U.S. intensive care nurseries come from mothers who were diagnosed as completely normal when labor began.

Infant Mortality for Selected Countries**

Country	1979	1980
Sweden	7.3	6.7*
Finland	7.7	7.4*
Japan	8.0	
Switzerland	8.5	
Denmark	8.7	
Norway	8.8	
France	10.0	
Canada	10.9	
Belgium	11.2	
Australia	11.4	11.0*
Hong Kong	12.3	
Ireland	12.4*	
New Zealand	12.6	
Spain	12.7*	11.1*
England and Wales	12.8	12.2*
German Democratic Republic	12.9	12.1*
United States	13.0	12.5*
Singapore	13.2	11.7*
German Federal Republic	13.5	
Austria	14.7	13.9*
Italy	15.3*	14.3*
Israel	15.9	14.1*
Czechoslovakia	17.7	16.6*
Greece	18.7*	

** Data from United Nations, mortality rates based on deaths per 1,000 live births.
* Provisional data; figures from France exclude live-born infants dying before registration of birth.

One out of every 35 children born in the U.S. today will be diagnosed as retarded. In 75% of these cases there is no known familial, sociologic or physical predisposing factor.

One out of every 10 U.S. children is learning disabled, and 1 in 20 is hyperactive.

In one large Boston study 80% of the children demonstrating significant brain dysfunction were not premature but were within the normal range of gestational age and weight.[56]

While heavy sedation and general anesthesia are no longer widely employed for laboring mothers, the use of tranquilizers when a woman enters in labor, some form of analgesic sedation later, and an epidural for the birth are still common practices. There is some risk in all of these.

The respiratory center of the infant is highly vulnerable to sedative and anesthetic drugs, and since these agents, if given systemically, *regularly traverse the placenta* they may jeopardize reparation after birth. . . . The sensitivity of the fetus to the effects of almost all forms of maternal anesthesia poses one of the most difficult problems in obstetrics.[57]

Obstetric anesthesia is the greatest risk, although it is now used primarily for cesarean rather than vaginal births:

Gastric emptying is likely to be delayed appreciably during labor, *especially after analgesics for pain relief.* . . . Vomiting with aspiration of gastric contents is, hence, a frequent threat and a major cause of morbidity and mortality in obstetric anesthesia.[58]

The data from thirty-five studies on damage to infants, conducted by Dr. Yvonne Brackbill, was submitted to the U.S. Senate Subcommittee on Health and Scientific Research on April 17, 1978:

Almost all investigators have found statistically significant adverse effects of obstetric medication on infant behavior—namely, on the ability to see and hear, the development of motor skills, language ability, intelligence and so on. The direction of these effects is, without exception, toward behavioral degradation and interference with normal function.[59]

The deleterious effects are not limited to analgesics taken by mouth, but also result from local infiltration anesthetics in a pudendal or paracervical block. For a pudendal block, a very long needle is inserted deeply through one side of the vaginal wall, through the sacrospinal ligament and on into the pudendal nerve (which supplies sensations to the whole genital area. A paracervical block is performed by passing a needle through the vagina and inserting it into the areas on each side of the cervix in the upper vagina. Anesthetic agents are passed through the needles into the pudendal or paracervical nerves.

Complications of the pudendal block anesthesia include "serious systemic toxicity characterized by stimulation of the cerebral cortex leading to convulsion and depression of the medulla to cause respiratory depression. . . . Deaths and severe permanent impairment in some survivors have been recorded."[60] Complications of the paracervical block include fetal *tachycardia* (too rapid heartbeat) or *bradycardia* (too slow heartbeat). It can also induce *cyanosis* (lack of oxygen making baby "blue") in the newborn and cause possible breathing difficulties.[61]

Another unfortunate result of the use of analgesic agents is the depression of the woman afterwards, commonly called the "third-day blues," often accompanied by difficulty in bonding with the new baby. Eugene Marais, the South American naturalist, reported that throughout his study of a herd of sixty half-wild Kaffir deer over a period of fifteen years, he saw no case in which a mother refused her young under normal conditions. But when, as an experiment, he gave anesthesia to six animals, rendering them unconscious during the birth of their offspring, *each of the six refused to accept her own fawn* and had to be coaxed to do so![62]

There can be frustrations for a new mother caused by, say, a painful labor, worry over an apparent inability to breastfeed, or by separation from and worry about her other children at home. But none of these even begins to explain the thousands of times this unhappiness occurs following a labor the mother did not consider too unpleasant and a birth she did not feel. Nor does it explain the thousands of times this depression occurs, sometimes with increasing severity, following the birth of a second, or third, or fourth child. The mother's unhappiness seems to have no obvious reason.

There is a hormonal change in the mother that can cause a mild, temporary spell of the "blues," though this is often absent in the natural-childbirth mother, particularly if she is breastfeeding. The estrogen-progesterone level that has risen gradually during the pregnancy drops sharply on about the third day after childbirth and can make her feel restless, a condition similar to premenstrual tension. But if the "blues" continue, it is well to look for more serious causes. One of these may be a change in thyroid activity,[63] which should be carefully checked by a physician if the depression lasts for more than a few days.

The most important factor contributing to a continuing depression following childbirth is a subconscious feeling of being robbed, a sense of loss. For nine months of pregnancy and several hours of labor, a woman has been gradually brought to a peak of emotional and physical expectation. An adequate emotional and physical climax at the moment of birth provides a most essential catharsis for this pent-up emotion. This climax, of which one mother said, "What an exhilarating sensation!'' and another, "It was the most tre*men*dous orgasm!'' and which still another described as "a sensation of glowing warmth and comfort that is hard to describe!'' is a most important part of childbearing. As the birth is completed, the sudden release, the change in physical sensations, is so dramatic, so profound, that one reacts to the sudden change and the sight of the baby by laughing, or crying, or both at the same time.

This climax is essential. A mother who has missed it and had a passive, frigid birth due to analgesics and local injections, is emotionally still in a state of expectancy. She looks at her child, but experiences no euphoria, no sense of exhilaration. It is with difficulty that she identifies herself with the child at first, although this happens in time. She touches the baby gingerly, unbelievingly.

For the natural childbirth mother, identification with her child is not broken at birth. She looks with awe at this infant in her arms who was harbored so long within her body and recalls with keen pleasure the pleasant sensation of the warm, little body moving from her own. Her baby seems an extension of her own being, with no break between the bonding before birth and the bonding after birth. The process has come full circle. She feels no sense of loss, and this identification with her child continues as he or she grows. She laughs when the child laughs, glows with pride over each little achievement—holding up the head, the first tooth, the first word, the first step, and when he or she cries because of bumps and bruises, she weeps as if she herself had been hurt.

Conclusion

The joy inherent in a natural birth is a philosophy that represents a universal truth. But the *application* of that philosophy must be on an individual basis. No two women are alike. No two labors are alike, even for the same mother. The happy outcome may depend on the cooperation of the husband and other family members, as well as the wholehearted encouragement and support of the medical team involved. Many women like myself have had happy natural birth experiences without receiving any encouragement—not to mention receiving open skepticism—from the doctors who attended us. But we must continue to work toward a greater understanding among birth attendants, in order that every woman may give birth in dignity and freedom, even in "high-risk" circumstances where intervention may be a necessity.

We are most grateful to those outstanding physicians and other medical personnel who have the courage to provide leadership in the desperately needed reforms in our obstetrical systems. We are confident that increasing numbers of them will also assume such leadership as they become aware of the many benefits of natural childbirth to mother and baby and will help train women everywhere for such wholesome birth experiences. We fully believe that obstetricians will become determined to keep the Hippocratic oath more fully in their practice of obstetrics in the years ahead:

I will prescribe regimen for the good of my patients according to my ability and my judgment and never do harm to anyone. To please no one will I prescribe a deadly drug, nor give advice which may cause his death. . . . If I keep this oath faithfully, may I enjoy my life and practice my art, respected by all men and in all times; but if I swerve from it or violate it, may the reverse be my lot.

NOTES

1. Howard W. Haggard, M.D., *Devils, Drugs, and Doctors: The Story of the Science of Healing from Medicine Man to Doctor* (New York: Harper, 1929), pp. 119, 120.
2. *Williams Obstetrics,* ed. Jack A. Pritchard and Paul C. Macdonald, 15th ed. (New York: Appleton-Century Crofts, 1976), p. 300.
3. Tom Brewer, M.D., "Society for the Protection of the Unborn through Nutrition" (SPUN). Undated pamphlet. 17 North Wabash Ave., Suite 603, Chicago, IL 60602.
4. "Young Women Who Smoke Should be Warned of Risks to Fetus," review in the International Medical News Service of an article by Dr. Wm. Hollingshead, M.D. in *Ob. Gyn. News,* Vol. 14, No. 20.
5. "Bendectin and Birth Defects," *ICEA News,* 19:4:80.
6. "Diagnostic Ultrasound Equipment," *Federal Register,* Department of Health, Education and Welfare, Food and Drug Administration, February 13, 1979.
7. M. E. Stratmeyer, "Research in Ultrasound Bioeffects: A Public Health View," *Birth and the Family Journal,* reprint, 1980. Reprinted by permission.
8. Ibid.
9. Margot Edwards and Penny Simkin, "Tests for Fetal Well-Being," *Obstetric Tests and Technology* (Seattle, WA: Pennypress, 1980).
10. Robert Mendelsohn, M.D. "The Hazards of Amniocentesis and Ultrasound," *The People's Doctor* (Chicago: A Medical Newsletter for Consumers) 3:11.
11. *Williams Obstetrics, op.cit.* P. 278.
12. Judith Anderson, R.N., ASPO-certified instructor, "A Clarification of the Lamaze Method," *Journal of Obstetrical, Gynecological and Neonatal Nursing,* March/April 1977. Reprinted by permission.
13. Report on Neonatal Respiratory Therapy by Bill Kingsepp, Certified Respiratory Therapy Technician, in *California Association of Midwives (CAM) Newsletter,* Spring 1982.

14. Margaret F. Miles, *Textbook for Midwives, with Modern Concepts of Obstetric and Neonatal Care*, 9th ed. (New York: Churchill Livingstone, 1981), pp. 258, 259. Reprinted by permission.
15. "Valium (diazepam)," *Perinatal Press*, 1:2, 1977.
16. Ronald Kotulak, "Shaving Surgery Patients Seen As Infection Peril," *Chicago Tribune*, January 1978.
17. Isadore B. Fogel, M.D., "The Enema—Is It Necessary?" *American Journal of Obstetrics and Gynecology*, vol. 84, no. 1, September 15, 1962, pp. 825, 830. Reprinted by permission.
18. Doris Falk, "Return to 'Aseptic' Exam During Labor is Advised," *Ob. Gyn News*, vol. 13, no. 22.
19. *Williams Obstetrics*, pp. 325, 321. Reprinted by permission.
20. Roberto Caldeyro-Barcia, M.D., "The Influence of Maternal Position During the Second Stage of Labor," *Highlights of the Tenth Biennial Convention of the International Childbirth Education Association*, (Seattle, WA: Pennypress, 1978), pp. 32, 33. Reprinted by permission.
21. Louise L. Henriksen, "University Scientists Urge Adoption of New Childbirth Method to Protect Unborn Infant," *Scope*, Loma Linda University, April 16, 1970.
22. Roberto Caldeyro-Barcia, M.D., "Supine Called Worst Position During Labor and Delivery," *Ob. Gyn. News*, June 1, 1975.
23. Michel Odent, M.D., "The Evolution of Obstetrics at Pithiviers," *Birth and Family Journal*, vol. 8, no. 1, Spring 1981, p. 13. Reprinted by permission.
24. Morris Gold, M.D., personal communication.
25. *Williams Obstetrics*, p. 346.
26. Ibid, p. 347.
27. Ibid, p. 347.
28. Carol Brendsel, Gail Peterson, and Lewis Mehl, M.D., "The Role of Episiotomy in Pelvic Symptomatology," *Episiotomy: Physical and Emotional Aspects*, ed. Sheila Kitzinger (London: The National Childbirth Trust, 1981), p. 38.
29. M. J. House, MRCOG, "To Do or Not to Do Episiotomy?" *Episiotomy*, p. 6.
30. *Williams Obstetrics*, p. 347.
31. Ibid.
32. Sheila Kitzinger, "Emotional Aspects of Episiotomy and Postnatal Sexual Adjustment," *Episiotomy*, p. 45.
33. Roberto Caldeyro-Barcia, M.D., "The Influence of Maternal Bearing-Down Efforts During the Second Stage on Fetal Well-Being," *Birth and the Family Journal*, vol. 6, 1979, pp. 17–21. Reprinted by permission.
34. Brendsel, Peterson, and Mehl, "The Role of Episiotomy in Pelvic Symptomatology," *Episiotomy*, p. 38.
35. House, "To Do or Not to Do Episiotomy?" *Episiotomy*, p. 10.
36. *How to Stay Out of the Gynecologist's Office* (Los Angeles: Federation of Feminist Women's Health Centers, 1981), pp. 78, 4.
37. Personal communication. Printed by permission.
38. Marsh Steward, Jr., M.D., "Consumerism and the Malpractice Problem," *CAOG Newsletter*, 3:3, 1981, reported in *Napsac News*, 7:1, Spring 1982.
39. R. Caldeyro-Barcia, R. Schwarcz et al., "Adverse Perinatal Effects of Early Amniotomy During Labor," *Modern Perinatal Medicine*, ed. Louis Gluck (Chicago: Year Book Medical Publishers, 1974), p. 433. See also "Amniotomy," *ICEA Review*, vol. 3, no. 2, Summer 1979.

40. *ICEA Review*, vol. 3, no. 2, p. 1.
41. *Williams Obstetrics*, p. 331.
42. Roberto Caldeyro-Barcia, M.D., "Some Consequences of Obstetrical Interference," *Birth and the Family Journal*, reprint, 1977. Reprinted by permission.
43. Suzanne Arms, *Immaculate Deception* (New York: Houghton Mifflin, 1975), p. 58.
44. *Williams Obstetrics*, p. 551. Italics mine. Reprinted by permission.
45. J. Morrison, M.D., review of an article by A. Golan et al. in *Obstet. Gynecol.* 56 (5):549, November 1980. Reported in *Napsac News*, Fall, 1981.
46. Reported in *International Medical News Service*, from *Ob. Gyn News*, vol. 13, no. 15.
47. Helen Wessel and Harlan F. Ellis, M.D., eds., *Childbirth Without Fear*, 4th ed. (New York: Harper & Row, 1972), p. 200.
48. *International Medical News Service*, *Ob. Gyn. News*, vol. 13, no. 15.
49. *Los Angeles Times*, December 3, 1978.
50. "One Mother Dies for 8 Newborns Saved with Electronic Monitoring," *International Medical News Service*, from *Ob. Gyn. News*, vol. 13, no. 24.
51. Elizabeth Shearer, "NIH Consensus Development Task Force on Cesarean Childbirth: The Process and the Result," *Birth and Family Journal*, vol. 8, no. 1, Spring 1981, pp. 26, 27.
52. Ibid, p. 27. Reprinted by permission.
53. Donna Heath, "Freedom of Choice for Cesarean Parents—Vaginal Birth After Cesarean," quoting from the NIH Task Force, *ICEA Bookmarks*, Supplement, May 1981, p. 3.
54. Diony Young, "Policy Reversal for Vaginal Delivery After Cesarean," *ICEA News*, 21:2, May 1982.
55. Data from United Nations, reported in *Pediatrics*, vol. 68, no. 6, December 1981.
56. Doris B. Haire, "Obstetric Medication—Better for Whom?" *Highlights of the Tenth Biennial Convention of the ICEA*, pp. 52, 53. Reprinted by permission.
57. *Williams Obstetrics*, p. 351. Italics mine. Reprinted by permission.
58. Ibid, p. 355. Italics mine.
59. Haire, "Obstetric Medication," p. 55.
60. Ibid., p. 361.
61. Ibid., p. 363.
62. Eugene Marais, *The Soul of the White Ant* (New York: Dodd, Mead, 1937).
63. Virginia L. Larsen, M.D., *Prediction and Improvement of Postpartum Adjustment* (Fort Steilacoom, WA: Division of Research, 1968).

20. Family-Centered Birthing

Education for Childbirth

The importance of adequate education for childbirth cannot be overestimated. Expectant young couples, in today's intelligent societies, are eager for such education and respond to it with enthusiasm. But facts concerning the physical processes of sexual reproduction are not enough. Far more important is the instilling of the right attitudes toward both mating and childbirth as God-given privileges and blessings.

Ideally, the instilling of right attitudes should begin in the home when the child is small. The child is affected, through actions if not through words, by the attitudes prevalent in the family in which he or she grows up. Too often the home fails to provide either the factual information or the positive attitudes the child needs. Thus sex education is left to the schools and childbirth education is left to the hospitals.

Churches are finally beginning to become aware of their responsibilities to families in this important aspect of their lives. Many churches are now providing sex education for their young people along with attempts to instill in them Christian attitudes toward it. Courses for young married couples in marriage and the family are also beginning to appear in the churches. Education for childbirth can hardly be omitted in such courses. And it is here that the presentation of childbirth as God's wonderful plan for the completion of the Christian home belongs. God's plan assures a welding of the bond between husband and wife as co-creators of a "family."

The great need for more adequate teaching materials in the churches on the practical aspects of family life (including natural family planning, natural childbirth, breastfeeding and related subjects) led me to found Apple Tree Family Ministries in 1978. For information on

ATFM materials for both individuals and groups, readers are referred to Appendix A.

The Husband's Role

One of the greatest changes in the past thirty years in conventional obstetrics has been the attitude toward the husband's role in birth. In my revision of this book only ten years ago it was still necessary to truthfully say:

There is one caricature in contemporary publications that is familiar to all of us. This is the caricature of the helpless, jittery male pacing the waiting-room floor or reading a magazine upside down, as he waits for his wife to give birth to their child beyond the doors which read NO ADMITTANCE.

Medical personnel and hospital administrators are aghast at the thought of bringing this helpless, jittery creature into the sacrosanct "halls of birth." . . . Many hospitals are letting down their barriers and permitting husbands in the labor rooms. But the same old rule still applies to too many delivery rooms. The wife is wheeled in, and the door is shut in the husband's face. . . . Is the wife to be subjected to such horrors in the hands of the medical attendants that it is better for the husband not to know about it? . . . The argument that the husband will "contaminate" the sterile room is invalid. Soap and water are cheap, aren't they? And there are plenty of sterile caps and gowns around. . . . Sometimes the nurses are embarrassed by the presence of the husbands and don't quite know what to do with them. . . . Some hospitals provide "amphitheaters" where the husband may observe the birth from beyond a glass. What a revolting thought! A husband does not want to be present as a "spectator," as if the birth were a "spectacle." . . . His place during the birth is not beyond a cold glass, but by his wife's side, supporting her when she pushes, whispering words of encouragement in her ear, and letting her see the love in his eyes.[1]

Most hospitals today have childbirth classes for both husbands and wives. It is common for the husband to be with his wife in the labor room throughout the labor and it is not uncommon for him to be present with her in the delivery room. This tremendous change is partly due to the outspoken efforts of Dr. Robert Bradley of Denver, Colorado, who has insisted through all these years that the husband's place during labor and birth is with his wife. He has been variously maligned as "a nut," "a crank," and various other uncomplimentary epithets. Yet today few of his former accusers would admit to having ever been opposed to the husband's presence. How times change!

One frequent objection to the husband's presence was the effect it would have on him if something went wrong at the birth. Dr. Bradley answers that objection admirably:

What if there were unforeseen complications? . . . Complications are exceedingly rare to begin with (96.4 percent of vaginal deliveries are spontaneous births). However, when they occur, completely honest explanations are made to the parents at the time, and their assistance elicited. . . . A forceps bruise on a baby will be far better accepted by a husband who, by his presence, clearly saw the lack of progress necessitating the forceps, than a bewildered, doubtful husband who, by his absence, imagines all sorts of mismanagement. . . .
What if the baby were deformed? For this exceedingly rare occurrence we have no way of "keeping it from" the parents. . . . In the absence of anesthetic depression of the mother we feel there is no contra-indication to complete honesty to both parents at birth.
In our opinion it would be a crime to deprive thousands of the joy of seeing their normal babies at birth in order to postpone the inevitable stress of the exceedingly few with abnormal infants.[2]

Many intelligent young husbands today are not only attending child-birth classes with their wives and staying with them throughout the labor and birth—many of them are also actively participating in the process. The caresses of lovemaking are far safer than artificial stimulation for encouraging labor. The loving husband, his arms supporting his wife, breathing encouragement in her ear, stroking her breasts, her body, kissing her, is a one hundred percent change from the births of yesterday where the strapped, unconscious woman had the baby dragged from her body by professionals. Several years ago some physicians began letting a husband "cut the cord," a token act reaffirming his importance in the whole process.

Today many husbands are "catching" their own babies, bonding with their newborns at the moment of birth. A husband participates at the birth of his child not just as an observer, but as a helper—a very special helper because of his loving touch. His gentle stroking of the perineum is a pleasurable sensation for his wife which helps her relax the perineum and release the baby into his hands. Attendants may stand by, alert to making suggestions if necessary, but doing so unobtrusively. The husband need do nothing to "hurry" the descent of his baby except for this loving, intimate touch.

A husband can learn to do the perineal massage with his wife. His hands should be well scrubbed and the nails smooth and clean. Light lubrication such as olive oil may be helpful. Then gently, lovingly, he can stroke his wife's vagina under her guidance, stretching the perineum slightly as he does so, in preparation for coitus. If a couple is accustomed to this intimacy, it will not be difficult for the husband to use stroking and stretching of the perineum in late pregnancy, in preparation for the birth. Then at the time of birth, it will be a familiar touch, in which husband and wife are in tune with each other.

Elizabeth Davis, a practicing midwife, describes how a birth attendant can do this massaging or assist the husband with it during the second stage of labor:

Start out slowly and be sensitive to response. Unless a woman really loves the massaging, do it only *between* contractions early on so you don't interfere with her efforts to feel through her contraction sensations and establish a flow. Once the baby's head is down and the woman is really pushing, you can massage more frequently. Always concentrate on the areas closest and immediately surrounding the descending head and just work your way down.

For working on the internal muscle bands, the best strokes are either smooth, full-range ones following the sweep of the entire band, or else direct, deep, ball-of-the-fingers pressure penetrations on the tightest areas. Both are good; the first thins out and stretches, the second breaks up and un-knots the tension. Often on one side the musculature is tighter, and deep pressure should be concentrated there. You need not focus on the perineum while the head is still high, unless the muscles are drawing closed or remaining rigid during a push. Then it's good to do a sensitive, sensual massage of the outlet. . . . Work gently around the area and ask the woman how it feels, taking your cues from her response. . . . It's very important while doing massage to communicate to the woman all you are seeing and feeling. So strong is the desire in most women not to tear, that the response to a comment like "You're a little tight right here, now really try to let go," can be rather miraculous. . . . I often feel that massage is only 40–50 percent of preventing tearing, and that the main factor is the mother's cooperation and subtle attunement to her own sensations, as well as her intuitive understanding of verbal cues. . . .

The father should also be encouraged to massage the woman (especially if he's planning to assist with delivery). He needs to be tuned in to the power and force and feeling of the contractions. Touching the baby's head internally will convince him and ground him in the reality that birth is imminent. Many a father gets really nervous at this first feel, first contact with the baby, and you may need to steady him with an arm around the shoulders and some very clear instructions on what to do. Put your fingers close to his, showing the pace and movement of the strokes. Excited fathers tend to overdo at first. You should ask the woman how it's feeling and with some positive feedback, he'll probably loosen up and start to enjoy it. Check from time to time to see how well tense areas have responded to his touch, and give more guidance if necessary.[3]

One wife described her husband's perineal touch at this time as "sheer ecstasy," though he was barely touching her with his finger tips. When a wife is in a vertical position, looking into her husband's eyes and experiencing his touch, giving the baby into his hands will be an unforgettable experience for them both.

This is not advocating the foolishness of a couple "going it alone." Adequate prenatal care is essential. Careful study and preparation on the part of the couple is essential. Quality medical attention readily available during the birth is essential. But within the safety of these boundaries, may the children of tomorrow know the blessing of bonding with their fathers as well as their mothers at the moment of birth.

Bonding

The term *bonding* has become widely used to describe the imprinting of a newborn (animal or human) to the first person seen, heard, and felt in the first few moments and hours after birth as well as the bonding of the caretaker to the newborn. Animal studies have shown its importance, and the term has become popularized through the well-known work of Drs. M. H. Klaus and J. H. Kennell.[4] The importance of allowing this bonding to take place between the newborn and his or her parents in the crucial moments after birth is no longer a matter of controversy.

What is less recognized is that bonding needs to begin at *conception*, and that the unborn child is profoundly affected psychologically not only by the mother, but also by the father, although less directly, either negatively or positively. The late Dr. Frank Lake, well-known British psychiatrist and Christian, stated in the foreword of his latest book:

For most of my psychiatric life I have been working in a half-light, oblivious of the earliest and severest forms of human pain. We have always known, whether taught by St. Augustine, Søren Kierkegaard or Sigmund Freud, that infants suffered abysmally, and that human beings crawling out of their abysses into life have damaged perceptions, distorted goals and a lifetime bondage of primal fears. What we had not known, and even now are somewhat terrified to know as clearly and rigorously as in fact we do, is the contribution to this soul-destroying pain and heart-breaking suffering that comes from the distress of the foetus in the womb when the mother herself is distressed. *The focus for psychopathology is now, for us, the first trimester of intra-uterine life.* These first three months after conception hold more ups and downs, more ecstasies and devastations than we ever imagined. . . .

Those who have benefited from a counselling course based on a theory of origins stemming back to birth and the first year of life may well be disturbed by the rumour that we now regard these as not going back early enough. My psychiatric colleagues and I "stuck our necks out" twenty-three years ago in affirming birth and the early months as powerfully relevant occasions of stress. . . . Now, by taking birth and maternal bonding seriously, we have had to push further back still . . . and recognize that life in the womb is a potent source of psychopathology.[5]

For this reason, Dr. Lake says that it is imperative that a young couple, even before they intend to have a baby, plan *"to give priority to the provision of a peaceful and harmonious environment for the mother."* The italics are his. He goes on to say:

A young couple could decide, on learning that a baby is on the way, to devote half an hour a day to being quiet or singing to it in celebration of the person who was coming to awareness within, to assure him or her, with equal delight, of a joyful welcome. There is firm evidence that music heard *in utero,* associated with a restful, peaceful mother, continues to be recognized and to have the same effect after birth, reproducing in the baby the mother's state of calm.[6]

It is recognized that the child in the womb can remember as soon as the cortex of the brain is developed enough to record an impression, at about the sixth month.[7] The infant hears and recognizes his parents' voices, their joy and their anger. He can see, and if his mother is standing in a bright light, his world is a rosy glow, such as one sees when holding fingers up before a light. He can remember strains of music and may show definite preferences for some music over others. But Dr. Lake goes on to show that memory occurs even before the development of the brain. "It seems that there may be structures in the protein molecule of the single cell which . . . subserve learning and memory in the zygote stage before and after implantation."[8]

The mother/father/infant bond is more crucial than we realized! The expectant mother who does not receive the love and affection she craves may be transmitting her own sense of rejection to their unborn baby. Bonding is a continuity, from conception through pregnancy, through the labor and birth, on into the arms of the mother and father.

Both parents need to participate in the birth. Both need to handle and fondle their baby skin to skin, fondling him from head to toe, the mother holding him or her close to bare arms and breast, the father holding him against his own face and neck and arms and bare chest. This establishes a mutual closeness and sense of security from the very beginning.[9]

Pediatricians have long been aware of the symptoms of mental illness in small babies separated from their parents:

Infants under 6 months of age who have been in an institution for some time present a well-defined picture. The outstanding features are listlessness, emaciation and pallor, relative immobility, quietness, unresponsiveness to stimuli like a smile or a coo, indifferent appetite, failure to gain weight properly despite the ingestion of diets which, in the home, are entirely adequate, frequent stools, poor sleep, an appearance of unhappiness, proneness to febrile episodes, absence of sucking habits.[10]

No one can measure the emotional trauma inflicted upon a tiny baby whose needs are not met. One associate professor in the nursing care of children says there are infants in nearly every central hospital nursery for the newborn who show some evidence of maternal deprivation. She says that in the average hospital nursery, each infant cries an average of 113.2 minutes a day—almost two hours.[11] By contrast, Niles Newton says that in one hospital she visited where each baby was with its mother, "there was almost a church-like hush as each mother nursed, or rocked, or slept with or near her baby."[12]

Those of us who have mothered several children know that this kind of coddling of a tiny infant does not lead to spoiled, demanding babies. On the contrary, they become contented, happy, and quickly responsive to affection. When this loving attention is given right from birth, we have not had the exhausting task of caring for a fussy baby who has developed the habit of long and frequent crying spells during the first few days in a central hospital nursery. When this has occurred, it has taken days, and sometimes weeks, to break the frustrated crying habit and restore contentment to the baby.

Not only does the child need the mother, but the mother needs her child. Reva Rubin, associate professor of maternity nursing at the University of Pittsburgh, has demonstrated how the narcissistic introspection of the pregnant mother carries over to include her newborn, if the child is taken away from her and kept in a central nursery:

[There is] the compulsive need to ascertain that the baby is whole and intact. . . . The mother sees the minutest blemish with anguish: milia, petechiae, lanugo, dry skin, et cetera. There is an intolerance for anything short of perfection. . . . Her desperate need for both bodily intactness and perfection in her infant serve mother and infant richly and poignantly in a specifically maternal way. . . .

During the first week, each of the normal functions is checked on by the mother. If he never cries, she is relieved to learn that he can cry. If he never opens his eyes when she sees him, she worries and fusses until he does open his eyes. If he never has a wet diaper or a soiled diaper, she is silent until she finds that he can wet, he can move his bowels. How much she worries about his capacity to function physically can be realized by her expression of relief in laughter or tears when she finds that this, too, is all right.[13]

This hidden anxiety is spared the mother who bonds with her infant from birth on. The father present through the labor and birth also bonds with his baby in this precious time after the baby's arrival. Others who may have been invited to be present at the birth—grandparents, siblings of the baby—also bond to the infant.

Researchers first explored maternal-infant bonding after noting the high rate of child abuse among children who had spent their first weeks in premature care nurseries. The baby's chances of being a victim of child abuse at some point later in his life, are dramatically reduced when bonding is early.[14]

It has been stated that "newborns can learn better on the first day of their life than they ever will be able to again."[15] The newborn can tell if a sound comes from the right or from the left and turn his eyes in that direction. He knows his mother's voice and turns his face toward that sound shortly after birth. If the father spoke often in his presence during the pregnancy, he will also recognize the father's voice. He can explore his surroundings and make eye contact with his parents.

For this reason, silver nitrate should not be put into the baby's eyes unless it is known that the mother has gonorrhea. It has been used to prevent gonorrhea-caused blindness in the newborn, but it is now known that there is time to treat the baby's eyes if the infection develops. "Apparently the baby does not instantly go blind from the gonorrhea. Within the first day or two after birth the baby's eyes will ooze and become irritated, and if this happens it can be treated."[16] Since less than five percent of mothers giving birth have gonorrhea, if silver nitrate is routinely given ninety-five percent of the babies have their eyes needless treated with a caustic substance that causes their eyes to become puffy and swollen and appears to cause temporary blindness.

And this at a time when the baby's alertness and ability to take in his new surroundings is at its most acute stage! Some states still require that silver nitrate be put in the baby's eyes. If this is true in your state, work to get state laws changed, at least so that alternatives such as tetracycline or erythromycin can be used. Even if one of these alternatives is available, the parents must *request* it, or the silver nitrite will be used on the baby. For attendants who insist that it doesn't hurt the baby, you might ask if they would be willing to prove it doesn't hurt by having a drop put in each of their own eyes.

Professionals in large hospitals are beginning to recognize the importance of the first few hours and days of life. No longer are babies always whisked away to a central nursery immediately after birth. Many hospitals even "allow" the parents an hour or two with the baby after birth, in token recognition of the importance of bonding. But there are other alternative settings in which bonding may take place more freely and completely.

Birth Settings

There are three major alternatives to the usual birth setting of hospital labor/delivery room. These are alternative birth rooms in the hospital, birth centers outside the hospital, and the home.

The ABC Room

Some hospitals have arranged for one of their labor rooms to be made into an "alternative birth center," commonly called "the ABC room," for couples wanting natural childbirth, laboring and birthing in the same bed, husband present throughout, and ample time for bonding. The advantages of the ABC room are many. In addition to the above freedoms, if the bed is double, the husband can lie down and rest during the labor if desired. There are comfortable chairs, including a rocking chair for the mother, so that she can be up as much as she likes. There is a private bathroom, and the decor is comfortable and homelike. After giving birth the couple may stay together with their baby for bonding for a couple of hours and then go home if all is well. Other family members can sometimes come to the birthing, if the couple so desires—their other children, the grandparents, occasionally an invited friend. The purpose of the ABC room is to make the birth as "homelike" as possible, while still within the "safety" of the hospital, in case medical complications arise that require the use of the standard facilities such as those for a cesarean section.

There are problems with the ABC room, however. The biggest problem is that a number of the hospitals that have yielded to pressure and allowed one make so many restrictions for its use that very few couples can get permission for it. Another problem also related to the hostility of some of the medical profession toward the ABC room, is that it sometimes is not a true one. Curtains on the window, a double bed, and a rocking chair do not in themselves ensure an uncomplicated, comfortable, companionable birth, if all the hospital paraphernalia for intervention procedures are still present or brought in to be applied at any time regardless of the desires of the parents. In short, the ABC room can be a ploy, a guide for forcing the usual standard measures upon the unsuspecting couple.

We need to guard against "improvements" that begin to hospitalize alternative birthing rooms so that they are unlike the home. One of the great advantages of the birthing room is that the mother can give birth *in bed,* with no anxiety about her baby falling to the floor because of the "bottomless" delivery table. But now, expensive "break-away" single beds are being installed in hospital birthing rooms. Although the woman stays in the bed, the bottom of the bed is pulled right out from under her and stirrups are moved into place!

Another big seller these days is the "birthing chair." The mother sits in it with her bottom over the U-shaped opening and her feet in special footrests. Since it's all one piece, she's sitting up in the normal position. But then—an attendant lowers the whole chair back into a near-reclining position. Since it's motorized, she can be lowered anytime the attendants want, whether she wants it or not. And of course the advantage of the upright position is lost and she's right back where we started—with the standard delivery table, stirrups and all.

Another problem is that the demand by intelligent, trained young couples for the birthing room is greater than the number available. Couples are told they may use it "if no one else is using it at the time." Few hospitals have more than one, so that arrival at the hospital may find the room already occupied by someone else. Some of our more cooperative hospitals in that case allow a natural childbirth mother to labor and give birth in a standard labor room, though it is less convenient and comfortable and there are also more restrictions.

But *why can't every labor room have the same comforts as an ABC room,* even those rooms in which special equipment must be kept for the high-risk mother in labor? Does she not deserve the same freedom and courtesy and comfort as other mothers, even if she or her baby is at "high risk"—or should we say, *especially* if she is at high risk?

Birth Centers

The last ten years have seen a phenomenal rise in the number of out-of-hospital birth centers all over the United States. They have developed as an alternative to the hospital setting, where intervention is routine and inevitable, and to the home setting, where medical assistance often is not available.

Birth centers, which used to be called "maternity homes," are not a new concept, but they practically disappeared during the decades when the trend was toward hospitalization of all patients for births. Only a few centers continued to operate in areas serving the rural poor. Now the trend has changed. Ruth Watson Lubic, General Director of the Maternity Center Association of New York City, reports:

But the centers which attracted the questioning and alienated middle class began to develop in 1973. By the end of 1975, three were operating, the demonstration model Childbearing Center of the Maternity Center Association in New York, the Southwest Maternity Center in Albuquerque and Birthplace Lucinia in Eugenia, Oregon. In spite of initial vigorous opposition from organized obstetrics and neonatalogy, six years later, in 1981, there were an estimated 125–150 out-of-hospital centers operating in at least 27 states. About one third of the centers are operated by or utilize nurse-midwives as the primary providers of care expertise. Others are sponsored by physicians and/or lay midwives.[17]

There is growing acceptance of the concept among obstetricians and gynecologists, since it is obviously impossible to stop the trend, and since it does provide some bridgehead against the rapidly growing home birth movement. But, again, birth centers are not completely without some problems that both those who run the centers and parents who wish to use them need to be alert to:

Although many freestanding birth centers (and I am most familiar with those operated by nurse-midwives) continue to pay scrupulous attention to screening and risk management, there are recent disconcerting reports of physician-operated centers where operating rooms are being added so that cesarean sections may be done on site![18]

In a 1980 statistical study an attempt was made at a scientific evaluation of out-of-hospital birth centers. A collaborative study in eleven birth centers was set up with several strict criteria. The centers were stratified by size. "This gave a sample of labours over the time each centre had been in operation—total, 1938. All women, whether delivered in the centres or transferred to hospital, are included in the sample and analyses."[19] Among the findings were the following:

Nearly 60% of the labours were conducted without analgesia, anaesthesia, sedatives, hypnotics, or tranquilisers. 89% of deliveries were spontaneous, 4% were assisted by forceps and 1% by vacuum extraction, and 5% ended in cesarean section at a back-up hospital. . . . The neonatal death rate for birth centre infants including transfers is 4.6/1000 live births, and excluding transfers 3.0/1000 live births. 15% of the birth centre families were transferred to hospital after the onset of labour owing to a change in their risk status.[20]

This excellent record of 4.6 infant deaths per 1000 live births cannot be fairly compared to the United States infant mortality record of 12.5 infant deaths per 1000 live births during that same year (1980). For one thing, women selected for the birth center were "low risk," and there is no comparable hospital study with data controlled for statistical purposes. But one of the main reasons for the birth centers' fine record is that they provide homelike care.

In the Home

The majority of births in the United States now take place in hospitals, because home births are not considered safe. Yet when mothers have been carefully selected for home births, any in whom a possible complication is suspected being referred to a hospital, statistics compiled according to adequate standards show that home births can be safe.

For example, between 1931 and 1951 when the Maternity Center of New York City was still conducting home births, they had

. . . a neonatal death rate of 14 per 1,000 births or 15 per 1,000 live births. In this group there was a high incidence of poor nutrition, poor home conditions, low income, unmarried mothers, and high parity. In spite of this [the] neonatal death rate is much lower than the rate for the whole Clinic area.[21]

This fine record is all the more remarkable when it is realized that most of these births occurred before or in the early days of the development of antibiotics! And it is almost as low a record as the 1980 overall U.S. infant mortality rate of 12.5, in spite of all the medical advances, new drugs, cesareans, intensive care newborn units, and so on!

Although what we now call the "methods of natural childbirth" were not yet known in the United States and there was no "education" or training for childbirth, the methods used in these home births were undoubtedly very similar to those of natural childbirth. Women learned from their mothers and sisters about birth. Birth was a common occurrence in the lower-class communities, and people were familiar with what to expect. Ether was made available at these home births by the attendants from the Maternity Center, but the mothers seldom wanted it. In fact, during the last nine years of this twenty-year period, it wasn't used at all, even though it was available if mothers asked for it!

The usual procedure for a home birth is to have the mother supply all the essentials for herself and the baby. This includes a rubber or plastic sheet (a clean old shower curtain or plastic table cloth would do), old linens which may be discarded after the birth (placed over the plastic sheeting), newspapers, and disposable bed pads (giant disposable diapers work fine). Clean linens, blankets and clothes for both mother and baby will be needed following the birth.

It is also helpful to have on hand a small bottle of alcohol, a bottle of an antiseptic solution, a sauce pan in which to boil instruments (like a good size dutch oven), a tea kettle, infant ear syringe (with rubber tip and nozzle) for suctioning baby's nose and throat if necessary, scissors, and a flashlight. Two large boxes of sterile 4″ by 4″ gauze pads and hospital-sized sanitary napkins and belt will be needed. The couple may also want to have a loaded camera and tape recorder ready.

The attending physician or midwife brings his or her own clinic bag and medicine kit. Apparatus for treating complications is thus either right at hand or readily available. Back-up plans for transport to the hospital should be made in advance in case this becomes necessary.

The biggest single worry in a home birth is postpartum hemorrhage, which may occur suddenly and profusely. Yet the Maternity Center Association of New York City during the same twenty-year period mentioned earlier, delivering 4988 women at home, lost not a single mother due to postpartum hemorrhage, although it did occur in 4.3 percent of the births.

The Chicago Maternity Center, which also delivered thousands of babies in the poorest of homes, lost *not a single mother* from any cause during a sequence of 12,106 births. During that same period of time the national average was one maternal death for every 500 babies born. During a three-year period in the 1950s, 9,000 consecutive home births were conducted by the Center without a single maternal death.

Part of the success of these home birth programs was due to the use of well-qualified nurse-midwives. Delores Henne, a certified nurse-midwife, describes her experiences in delivering babies at home:

From February to June I did home deliveries in the cosmopolitan city of New York, chiefly among Puerto Rican mothers of whom many spoke only Spanish. Home deliveries are unique. The children have the advantage of seeing the baby shortly after delivery, and what a thrill it is to see their interest and enthusiasm in their new baby brother or sister. The father is given the opportunity to stay and to encourage his wife during labor and delivery. And mother has the advantage of rooming-in, having the baby with her in the same room. [22]

Following her training in New York, Delores Henne went to Africa as a missionary, where she spent several years delivering babies. I met Delores at about the time I was first writing this book, in the early 1960s. When I asked for her counsel and advice, her humble answer made such an impression that I have never forgotten it.

In spite of her vast obstetric experience under all kinds of conditions, she replied, "I really don't know how much I can help you. You see, I've never had a baby." She was affirming *me,* a mother, as knowing more about birth than she knew, with all her training and experience!

During the last decade there has been an increasing trend in the United States toward giving birth at home. Young couples of the more traditional middle and upper classes of society as well as those in the counterculture movement are rebelling against being robbed of the right to have their children born in the dignity and peace of their own homes. It is a movement whose time has come, one that cannot be stopped.

The main medical argument against home birth is that it is not safe. (Though if the full truth were known, the hostility of at least some of the professional community may be because it is an economic and political issue. Physicians, hospital, pharmaceutical and medical equipment companies all lose money when women choose to stay home and give birth to their babies with only midwives in attendance.) The question of safety is a valid one, however, and a number of statistical studies as well as the records of personnel who have been doing home births demonstrate the safety of home birth.[23]

There has never been, however, any data to support the contention that one hundred percent *hospitalization* is safe!

Let us set the record straight once and for all: *Hospitals have never been proven to be the safest place for most mothers to give birth.* Since the founding of NAPSAC in 1975, we have searched for the data, if it exists, that supports 100% hospitalization for birth. . . . We have formally asked the ACOG, the AMA, the AAP and any other professional organization who supports 100% hospitalization to share, with us, their data. . . . To date, they have failed to produce even one legitimate study in support of their contention.[24]

. . . The ACOG did write a news release in January of 1978[25] and subsequently published their own adaptation of the news release in their own newsletter. The news release, which is frequently quoted as if it were a valid statistical study, is actually a fraud when cited in the context of planned home births. It claims in bold headlines that "Out-of-hospital births pose a 2–5 times greater risk to a baby's life than hospital births." This was based on raw vital statistics from 11 state health departments. The vital statistics do not concern planned home births, but concern "out-of-hospital" births. These include spontaneous abortions after 20–28 weeks of gestation (all stillbirths) and accidental births in taxis, on the street, etc. They also include involuntary home births of impoverished mothers, often ill and malnourished, who should be in the hospital, and want to be in the hospital, but who were refused prenatal care and entry into the hospital because they had neither money nor insurance. These statistics also include home births without competent attendance, prenatal care or backup because no attendants were available and accessory care denied by a hostile medical establishment. These data also include homicides by unwed mothers who did not want their babies and left them to die of exposure and neglect.[26]

This infamous 1978 news release has been thoroughly rebutted. The out-of-hospital births it included obviously cannot be compared to planned home births attended by qualified personnel, with adequate back-up plans for emergency. In regard to safety, David Stewart says:

A truly informed discussion concerning home birth does not debate whether or not it is safer because home birth has already been proven to be the safest and best place for many mothers and babies. The question is not whether it is "safer," because this has already been answered. The answer is, "Yes. For many it is safer. For some it is not." Truly scientific discussions go beyond that and address the question of "for whom is it safer to give birth at home, and for whom would it be safer to give birth in a hospital?"[27]

One carefully controlled study has been done in North Carolina. The results, reported in 1980 in the Journal of the American Medical Association,[28] clearly distinguish between planned home births attended by midwives, which resulted in 3.0 neonatal deaths per 1000 live births, and planned home births without attendants ("do-it-yourself" births with only the husband or a friend), which resulted in ten times as many neonatal deaths: 30 per 1000 live births. But for *un*planned home births, such as those listed above (spontaneous abortion, homicide, accident, etc.) there were 120 neonatal deaths per 1000 live births! "Planning, prenatal screening, and attendant-training were important in differentiating the risk of neonatal mortality in this uncontrolled, observational study."[29]

During this same period, the hospital neonatal death rate was 12 per 1000, slightly less than the overall national average. Thus the burden of proof for the safety of hospital births over home births rests with the medical profession.

General statistical studies comparing the safety of home versus hospital are not much help to a couple wanting a home birth. What they need to know is the quality of service provided by those who attend home births in their own community and how good their safety records are.

Birth Attendants

Until recently, almost all women were traditionally delivered by other women. By physical and emotional endowment women are particularly well suited for this task. But the traditional midwife, while she gave the mother warm understanding and encouragement, too often lacked sufficient medical knowledge to protect both mother and child.

This is no longer true in the United States. Professionally, the certified nurse-midwife has quality training in obstetrics that greatly exceeds in number of hours the obstetrical training given the aspiring general practitioner. Her midwifery training is graduate training, after nursing education. She is highly skilled in all aspects of normal prenatal, obstetric, and postnatal care. She is skilled in recognizing a problem early and referring her patient to a physician for further care.

The statement has been made that "the need for a female birth attendant is worldwide and as natural as the fact that small children need the loving care of a mother."[30] David Stewart quotes the late Dr. Nicholson Eastman, a great American obstetrician, who observes:

"Who manages the first stage of labor in the great majority of hospitals? Is it not the nurse? If this be true, should not the nurse receive special training for that function? In our small rural hospitals, without house staff, who performed the deliveries? Most of them, it is true, are performed by doctors, mostly general practitioners. However, I have evidence (which I cannot, however, document or prove) that in such hospitals as many as 20% of the deliveries are performed not by doctors, nor by midwives, nor by graduated nurses, but by practical nurses or aides. Doctors, of course, ultimately sign the birth certifications, so that our national statistics indicate that all hospital births are attended by doctors. But in respect to the small rural hospitals, I am certain that these statistics are misleading.''

Eastman points to a situation that in my opinion presently exists all over the world, and that situation could be summed up as follows: If a well-trained professional midwife takes care of a woman in labor, then she gives this care personally; if a doctor takes care of delivery, he unloads a big part of his task on the shoulders of untrained female aides.[31]

Noninterventive obstetrics is "midwifery" by definition. We are blessed that there are an increasing number of physicians and obstetricians in this country with the humility to respect the normal physiological process and to "stand by," ready to assist only if needed. A number of these physicians employ certified nurse-midwives or well-trained lay midwives as birth assistants to work with them in their practice. This frees the obstetrician to handle critical cases, cesarean births, and so forth, and to provide back-up care for birth center and home births. There will always be a need for the doctor and his or her specialized skills for particular, special needs.

There are now well-qualified birth assistants delivering babies in all fifty states. Some of these are nurse-midwives, some are lay midwives, some are birth assistants working out of a doctor's office. It is a growing trend that means greater comfort and safety for mothers and babies and greater freedom and involvement for husbands and other family members in the celebration of the birth of a baby.

For the young woman looking for an area of service one can think of few more needed and rewarding areas in which to serve than midwifery. This is also a service in which older women who have raised a family could also contribute a great deal, having learned patience and understanding during the years of coping with the tantrums and trials of the two-year-olds and the teens. In earlier cultures, a woman must have reared a family before she was considered eligible to enter the honorable calling of midwifery. But whether young or middle-aged, today's woman can look for opportunities to develop her skill and train as a midwife. She can then approach her responsibilities with the same sense of dedication as the old granny midwives in Georgia, who claimed that they had "always been called by the Lord, like preachers are."[32]

These older women in the black community were carefully trained as midwives by the Public Health Service in Georgia and worked under its supervision. Their records of safety were excellent. They took their calling as a spiritual service to God, and the example of their personal self-sacrifice and devotion to duty remain a challenge to anyone working in obstetrics. One aged woman at the time of her retirement said, "I been passing faithful and never quit till the Lord knowed I can't hardly get along, and He lifted all the burden He laid on me." Another one said:

I caught a lots of babies when their mothers birthed them. . . . Over forty years I been a granny midwife and no mother ever died with me. But I don't take credit to myself. I always had the Lord and one or the other Doc Powells to call on in trouble. . . .

Now I'm old and bent over and sometimes when I get called in the nighttime, I says, "Lord, I'm old and tired. Give me my long rest, and let me come up there to stay." . . . But the Lord He says, "You ain't so old as you will be. I got work yet for you to do down there and I'll give you strength. Go long now, and do your job!"[33]

NOTES

1. Helen Wessel, *Natural Childbirth and the Family*, (New York: Harper & Row, 1973), p. 235.
2. Robert A. Bradley, M.D., "Fathers' Presence in Delivery Rooms," *Psychosomatics*, vol. 3, no. 6, November/December. 1962, p. 5. Reprinted by permission.
3. Elizabeth Davis, *A Guide to Midwifery, Hearts and Hands* (John Muir Pub., P.O. Box 613, Santa Fe, NM 87501, 1981), pp. 102, 103. Reprinted by permission.
4. M. H. Klaus and J. H. Kennell, *Maternal-Infant Bonding: The Impact of Early Separation or Loss on Family Development* (St. Louis; MO: Mosby, 1976).
5. Frank Lake, M.D., *Tight Corners in Pastoral Counselling* (London: Darton, Longman and Todd, 1981), pp. vii, viii. Reprinted by permission.
6. Ibid., p. 39. Reprinted by permission.
7. Thomas Verney, M.D., with John Kelley, *The Secret Life of the Unborn Child* (New York: Simon & Schuster, 1981).
8. Lake, *Tight Corners in Pastoral Counselling*, p. xv. Reprinted by permission.
9. Ashley Montagu, *Touching: The Human Significance of the Skin* (New York: Columbia University Press, 1971).

10. Florence G. Blake, R.N., *The Child, His Parents and the Nurse* (Philadelphia: Lippincott, 1954), p. 6, quoting Harry Bakwin, "Emotional Deprivation in Infants," *Journal of Pediatrics*, vol. 35, 1949, p. 512. Reprinted by permission.
11. Ibid, p. 10.
12. Niles Newton, Ph. D., "The Medical Case for Routine Rooming-In," *Child and Family*, January 1962. Reprinted by permission.
13. Reva Rubin, R.N., C.N.M., "Basic Maternal Behavior," *Nursing Outlook*, November 1961, pp. 684–686. Reprinted by permission.
14. Ralph W. Gause, M.D., "Dr. Ralph Gause Discusses Maternal-Newborn Bonding," American Baby Magazine, May 1979. Reprinted by permission.
15. T. G. R. Bower, *A Primer of Infant Development* (San Francisco: Freeman, 1977).
16. Nancy Whittaker and Judy Strasser, "The Silver Nitrate Challenge, *Mothering Magazine*, Reprint 19-3 (Albuquerque, NM: Mothering Publications, 1981).
17. Ruth Watson Lubic, M.A., Ed. D., "The Rise of the Birth Center Alternative," *The Nation's Health*, reprint, January 1982. Reprinted by permission.
18. Ibid. Reprinted by permission.
19. Anita Bennets and Ruth Watson Lubic, "The First National Collaborative Study of Birth Centers," *Cooperative Birth Center Network News* (Perkiomenville, PA, February/May 1982), p. 12, from *The Lancet*, February 13, 1982.
20. Ibid., p. 13. Reprinted by permission.
21. Marion D. Laird, M.D., "Report of Maternity Center Clinic," *American Journal of Obstetrics and Gynecology*, vol. 69, no. 1, p. 184. Reprinted by permission.
22. Delores Henne, R.N., C.N.M., in a letter for a column "We the Women," *The Baptist Herald*, (Forest Park, IL: North American Baptist General Conference), January 24, 1957, p. 16. Reprinted by permission.
23. Lewis Mehl, M.D., Gail Peterson, M. Whitt et al., "Outcome of Elective Home Births; A series of 1,146 Cases," *Journal of Reproductive Medicine*, vol. 19, 1977. pp. 281–291. G. White, "A Comparison of Home and Hospital Delivery Based upon 25 Year Experience of Both," *Journal of Reproductive Medicine*, vol. 19, 1977, pp. 291, 292. See also D. Stewart and L. Stewart, *Twenty-first Century Obstetrics Now*, 1977, pp. 27–32 and *Safe Alternatives in Childbirth*, 1976, pp. 73–100 (Chapel Hill, NC: NAPSAC).
24. David Stewart, Ph. D., *The Five Standards for Safe Childbearing* (Chapel Hill, NC: NAPSAC, 1981), p. 204. Reprinted by permission.
25. Ibid, pp. 221, 222, from "Health Department Data Shows Dangers of Home Birth," ACOG News Release, ACOG Headquarters, Chicago, January 4, 1978.
26. Stewart, *The Five Standards*, pp. 201, 202. Reprinted by permission.
27. Ibid, p. 220.
28. Claude A. Burnett, III, M.D. et al. "Home Delivery and Neonatal Mortality in North Carolina," *Journal of the American Medical Association*, vol. 244, no. 24, December 19, 1980, pp. 2741–2745.
29. Ibid.
30. Stewart, *The Five Standards*, p. 156. Reprinted by permission.
31. Ibid, p. 156. Reprinted by permission.
32. Marie Campbell, *Folks Do Get Born* (New York: Rinehart, 1946), p. 109. This book is a delightful report of the personalities of the black midwives who worked under the direction of the Public Health nurses in Georgia.
33. Ibid.

21. Natural Childbirth

A Humanitarian Philosophy

One of the main tenets of natural childbirth is that every pregnant and parturient woman must be cared for on an individual basis, according to her individual physical and emotional needs and desires.

A woman longs to remain a *person* throughout her childbearing experience. When a young wife, pregnant for the first time, enters a doctor's office, does the doctor attempt to get to know her or does he or she dispense with her feelings and immediately conduct a thorough physical examination? Is the doctor aware that she may not yet be emotionally prepared for such an invasion of her spirit? These young women often leave the office blushing and subdued.

When, therefore, the young married woman enters the consulting room believing, hoping or fearing that she is going to have a baby, the physician's first investigations should be to confirm that she is pregnant. This may be ascertained by clinical signs, without an internal or vaginal examination. Such an examination can be a severe shock to many young women and, apart from the discomfort it may cause, it is an experience that frequently produces a lack of confidence in the attendants. If at thirteen weeks the uterus is not in the correct place and position, a vaginal investigation should be carefully performed for sound clinical reasons.[1]

Such thoughtful consideration for preserving the integrity of her innermost needs as a person helps a young woman to confide in her doctor. She becomes more responsive to guidance toward a rewarding birth experience. She realizes that the physician does not regard her simply as a reproductive machine, to be prodded and examined, doped and delivered when her time comes.

Thorough training in the principles of natural childbirth and how to achieve it is the right of every pregnant woman. But because each woman is an individual, not all will respond favorably to such teaching. The doctor who is aware of the emotional needs of the patient will courteously comply with her wishes to be "knocked out" to the extent that it is considered safe to do so. Dr. Dick-Read was the first to write:

. . . a serious word of warning—no one who uses these methods [natural childbirth] must expect invariable success. There are women who will never learn control, who will never concentrate upon doing their antenatal work well, and whose upbringing has given them a psychological background upon which fear thrives. Analgesics and anesthetics are the correct treatment for such. Whatever happens, no woman should ever be allowed to persist in pain.[2]

Such women are in the minority, however. There are also a few women who have physical abnormalities that necessitate anesthetics. But the majority of young women respond eagerly to adequate childbirth training and are profoundly grateful afterward for the guidance they receive. In their happy natural birth experiences they come face to face for the first time with the real meaning of being *woman,* and they find it good.

Doctors may not understand this intuitive need for fulfillment in the childbearing experience that a young woman feels. What they do not understand, they do not approve. When they do not approve, they are unwilling to help her to achieve her goal. When they are unwilling to help her, they are failing in their responsibilities as physicians. Fortunately, situations like this are on the decline.

The Miracle of Birth

The First Stage of Labor

Civilization has imposed one handicap upon us that primitive women did not have to contend with. Most women today have to puzzle over whether labor has or has not begun, in order to know whether to go or not to go to the hospital. In the majority of women the beginning of true labor is signaled by contractions that occur at regular intervals. But for some this is not an infallible sign of true labor. A woman may have contractions occurring every three and a half minutes. She is told to report to the hospital. She packs her bag and goes. Several hours later she is dismissed, the regular contractions having ceased. She is told that she was in "false" labor.

Then again, a woman thinks she is in labor. She calls the doctor, who asks, "Are the contractions regular?" She replies that they are not. She is told to call again as soon as they become regular. An hour later the parents and doctor rush to the hospital, and the baby appears shortly. Her contractions never did become regular.

How is it possible to know whether labor is "true" or "false"? A safer criterion is especially necessary for the mother who has learned to relax, as some contractions may pass unnoticed, and she will think they are not "regular."

Because this may be a problem, certain sensations that are true indications of labor should be recognized. The surest way to tell if the contractions are real or "practice" ones is by noticing whether or not there is this mild feeling of tightening *down in the area of the pubic bone and lower spine*. This is a sign that the uterine muscles are pushing *down*. A false contraction will often be much larger, expanding the abdomen up and out, rather than giving the sensation of tightening *low* in the abdomen. This sensation disappears when one relaxes, so *do not go to bed to relax if you think that you are really in labor*.

Another way to discern false labor is to change activity. If you are resting when contractions start, try activity, and vice versa. The contractions will often stop or become erratic with the change in activity.

But when a woman knows she is in labor, she should wait to completely relax until she has notified her attendants that she is in labor. If she's going to the hospital, she should wait until admitted to completely relax.

One strange thing occurred that puzzled me. From time to time, the nurse would put her hand on my abdomen and say, "Are you having a contraction?" And in all truth I would answer, "I don't think so, I don't feel anything." "Well, you are," she would answer, "only you must be so relaxed that you don't feel it."[3]

Medical attendants in the labor wards should realize how much pain they can actually indirectly *cause* by their constant concern over the strength and regularity of labor contractions. "Be sure to tell the nurses when your *pains* get too bad," the doctor says kindly. Or, "Oh, that's a *good* one," the nurse remarks, her hand on a rising abdomen. She stands expectantly, watch in hand, waiting for the next one. Unconsciously the woman begins to tense in anticipation of the "next one" along with her, embarrassed at keeping her waiting when she is so patient. All this preoccupation with contractions contributes to pain. As one obstetrician aptly said, "If we paid this much attention to the processes of digestion, we'd all have nervous indigestion!" Another eminent doctor reminds us of this:

Our organs actually work much better when we leave them to their automatic functioning and do not think about them. That this is so is clearly shown in the case of the hypochondriac, who suffers from all kinds of functional disorders simply because his mind occupies itself with his body. These disorders attract the attention of his mind, and thus he is caught in a vicious circle.[4]

Whether in the hospital, at a birth center, or at home, once labor begins one can more or less ignore the contractions during most of the first stage of labor. Light activity and movement is helpful in keeping labor progressing. A variety of positions may be used for comfort during contractions: leaning over the back of a chair while relaxing the abdomen; resting in a rocking chair or recliner, knees supported, head dropping forward, abdomen relaxed, breathing deeply and slowly. If the contractions begin to cause discomfort it may help to lie on one side or the other, bending one's head forward and drawing up the knees ("curling up in a ball"). Extend the upper knee slightly above the lower leg and rest that knee and thigh on a good-sized pillow. The pillow should support the weight of the thigh and knee so completely that the muscles all through the thigh and across the abdomen and lower back can be totally limp. Keep the back rounded.

It is impossible to remain in one position for a long period of time. For those who seem unable to get comfortable in the lateral position and prefer to lie in the recliner-chair position, the back and knees must be elevated and supported to prevent pressure tension on the abdominal muscles. Sometimes the labor-room bed is too narrow for lying in the lateral position. In this case, a mother can lie on her side, her legs straight, with a large pillow between her knees. This will hold them apart, keep the weight of the upper leg from resting on the lower one, and help her keep the pelvic floor relaxed.

The woman may get up whenever she feels rested and walk or rock in a chair. (The only exception is if the water has broken, and the baby's head is not yet firmly engaged in the pelvic basin. In this case, the mother should remain in bed to help prevent a loop of the cord from slipping out of the cervix before the oncoming head. Once the head is firmly engaged this is no longer a problem.)

As transition approaches, squatting or kneeling—or the recliner-chair position—may be more comfortable than lying on one's side, and these positions can be used on through the birth. (Yes, baby can be delivered while lying on one's side.) In any of these positions, however, the mother should be fully supported by others so that she may keep her balance easily and keep her abdomen and perineum relaxed.

The Transition Period

There are certain emotional signs of the progress of labor that a woman shows. These make it possible for attendants to tell how her labor is advancing without frequent vaginal examinations, which always interfere with relaxation. By observing these phenomena, both mother and attendants can tell when the transition period is near. Dr. Virginia Larsen writes:

The inexperience of the hospital team with trained parents may make them under-evaluate the shortened labors and the woman's self-awareness of labor progress; consequently the obstetrician is apt to be called too late. Many nurses are not aware of the emotional pattern of labor and miss the importance of the signs of the transition period from the first to the second stage. As the emotional guideposts in labor become more appreciated, the labor room nurse, and the intern will find these a valuable adjunct to the vaginal exams that otherwise tend to be overdone and discomforting.[5]

These emotional guideposts have been outlined as follows: the mother appears mildly euphoric and frequently likes to carry on conversation between contractions until the cervix is dilated to about four centimeters; at three to four centimeters she becomes more serious about her labor; as transition approaches, the mother may find difficulty in relaxing, experience some backache, and feel chilled to the point where her legs will tremble. When this happens, the attendants should wrap her warmly in blankets, give her a hot water bottle, and have her change to the recliner-chair position on the bed.

Transition contractions usually last a full minute or more, and they may come so close together that they seem almost continuous. This is the point in labor when an uninstructed woman may go all to pieces emotionally and remain out of control for the rest of the time. *No woman should ever be left alone after labor has begun,* especially not at *this stage.*

During transition (eight to ten centimeters until complete dilation) there is often a feeling of confusion between the need to *relax,* as for first-stage contractions, and the need to *push,* as for second-stage contractions. The mother should be reminded not to bear down until the doctor gives permission, since pushing too soon can damage the cervix. It helps to be raised to a sitting position during transition, with the knees raised and supported by pillows so the legs can remain limp.

The strength of transition contractions may alarm a woman having her first baby. If she has had a relaxed, comfortable first stage, the sensation of the strong contractions will be similar to that of tensing her biceps firmly in the upper arm. She should be reminded that transition is very short and that she will soon be more comfortable.

If pain occurs in the labor of a well-prepared, relaxed woman, this is most often the time when it may occur and become a problem. She may have severe backache from the pressure of the descending baby against her backbone. Since the baby must pass down through the bony rim of the pelvis, she may have discomfort in the pelvic area due to the baby's size or position and/or to the size and shape of her pelvis. Although the pelvis may be adequate for a vaginal birth, if its shape is slightly irregular or contracted, the pressure of the baby's bony skull pressing the mother's flesh against the bony rim of her pelvis can give rise to pain. (The pressure "anesthetizes" the baby's head from feeling the pain, unless this period is greatly prolonged.)

When a woman complains of pain, it should *always* be taken seriously. The first step is to try and determine the cause, in order to take measures to alleviate it enough for her to be able to cope with it adequately, medication being a last resort. Simply changing positions, squatting, kneeling, or "squat-standing" may help. An experienced labor companion can make a great difference by suggesting to the husband ways in which to help his wife through this trying period. It may be, if these things are not adequate, that experienced medical attention is necessary.

As the transition stage ends, the bearing-down reflex begins. This reflex may not begin immediately after the cervix is completely dilated; the uterine muscles need time to shorten, since the baby is now farther down. If pushing causes any discomfort, the mother should be told to wait and not push until it does not hurt. If her body is ready, bearing down will feel good.

The Birth of the Baby

The second stage of labor is the really exciting period. At last one can *do* something to help bring this baby into the world! As one mother wrote, "Tell them that if they can get out of the labor room" without having been given any medication, "whatever they do, don't take any in the delivery room . . . or they'll cheat themselves of the most fascinating, thrilling series of sensations they've ever experienced!"[6]

Frequently a young mother needs to be reminded not to "squeeze up" the muscles of her pelvic floor as she feels the baby's head coming down, but to keep them slack. Often she will hesitate to relax this birth outlet and bear down properly because of embarrassment over this part of her body. Turning her attention to her baby as soon as possible helps to relieve her self-consciousness and relax the outlet by taking her mind off herself. If the muscles of the outlet remain tense, she will have pain.

A common mistake that is made is instructing the woman to bear down "as if moving the bowels." This increases her embarrassment and confusion and causes her to tighten the vagina in order to open the anus, which hinders rather than helps her efforts. Pushing this way also causes her to push with her abdominal muscles rather than from the diaphragm.

As mentioned earlier, there are a variety of positions for birthing, but the important factor is that the mother be upright, so that gravity can be used to full advantage.

As the baby's head descends and the initial stretching of the vulva begins, the mother may appear alarmed. Although this "pins and needles" sensation is only mildly uncomfortable, it brings all our negative cultural misconceptions about childbirth to mind. The common belief that the approaching moment of birth *will* be painful causes the mother to hesitate with doubt at this crucial point.

It is a wise attendant who can reassure her with confidence that the birth outlet will be insensitive in a moment, and that she will feel only the bulging of the baby's head. She will be grateful for this after the birth is over, if she is not robbed of the wonderful orgasm of birth by the administering of an anesthetic, or pudendal block, or hypnotic analgesia, against her wishes.

One cannot feel either the incision for an episiotomy, or minor laceration during the birth, once the baby's head has cut off circulation of the blood to the perineum. What one does feel is the thrilling expansion of the vagina to its maximum capacity.

Mrs. Dick-Read describes a properly conducted delivery as follows:

As the head is about to be born, the attendant will place a hand firmly on the area between the anus and the birth canal (perineum) supporting the head towards the mother as it emerges. . . . She will feel no pain as the head is born (contrary to popular belief) because nature provides a perfect numbing, for a few minutes, of the area surrounding the outlet. During the crowning and birth the mother can think of herself as "a rose unfolding" bringing her baby forth gently and beautifully as it should be.

Irrespective of whether the attendant is present or not, the oncoming *head should never be held back forcibly* but should be allowed to be born slowly and gently. Nor should the baby be pulled straight out from the mother. The natural rotation of the head should be allowed to take place without interference, and the baby allowed to come gently of its own accord, supported *upwards* towards the mother's abdomen.

. . . there is no immediate need to cut the cord which attaches the baby to its placenta. . . . [Wait until] pulsation has ceased.[7]

The description Dr. Dick-Read gives of his delivery of a child is vastly different from orthodox deliveries in America:

. . . the mother will be holding the hands of the child before the body is born. The head emerges and with the next contraction the shoulders are freed. The child is then rotated and lies upward facing his mother. That rotation gives relief and takes the tension from the points where it has been greatest on the perineum. It is then we see an astonishing transfiguration of a hard-working woman employing the effort syndrome, which made her appear distressed, to a mother who suddenly becomes happy and smiling and sits up and waits for the baby to be fully born. Women in these circumstances will complain because the doctor is not yet able to tell them whether it is a boy or a girl. They will ask him to hurry, and I have to say to them, "I will hurry when you give me a contraction to hurry with."

. . . These children are all handed to the mother immediately after the cord is cut. Every woman takes her child in her arms and holds it to her breast, not necessarily to suckle it. This stimulates a reflex contraction of the uterus which is definitely of physiological value. I think women were meant to take their babies when born. They will say what a funny looking thing it is. "Is that the right colour, doctor?" "It really is like my husband!"[8]

The Delivery of the Placenta

Mrs. Dick-Read describes the proper delivery of an afterbirth, which every mother should know and understand:

The close contact between mother and child and the suckling of the child at the breast will cause the uterus to contract strongly, thus preventing excessive bleeding. There need be no hurry and there will be little maternal loss (bleeding) provided there is no pummelling or squeezing of the uterus.

Any violent form of extrusion of the placenta is a violation of the purely natural function and has no place in a normal delivery. One should never attempt to hurry the birth of the placenta by impatient pulling on the cord. A sharp cough will usually jog the placenta and bring it forth if it is ready to come. . . . Injections to hurry the placenta and to prevent bleeding should only be given if there are clinical indications. There is very little loss of maternal blood after a carefully managed labour. . . . Once the placenta is delivered and the mother is refreshed there is no reason why she may not walk immediately if she wishes to do so.[9]

If a slight abrasion occurred during the birth, doctors who understand natural childbirth take the stitches immediately, while the perineum is still insensitive. It is only later, after the delivery of the afterbirth, that they are tied. This tying, if not carefully done, can cause more discomfort than the stitches, since feeling has by then returned to the perineum. On the rare occasions when an episiotomy is necessary in a natural birth, some doctors use one or two percent Novocain for the stitches if feeling has returned to the perineum.

The birth is not completed until the afterbirth has come. None of us can fully appreciate the miracle that has taken place within this simple structure. Dr. Dick-Read often uses this occasion to point his patient to God's part in the creation of a child:

Years ago it was unheard of that a woman should wish to see the afterbirth. Today nearly every woman who watches her baby born asks me to show her the placenta. This I do, and point out the bag in which the infant, now lying peacefully in her arms, developed and became a perfect little human being. . . . "Madam, when man can make one of these, he will have reached the foot-stool of the Creator; as I hold this discarded mass in my hand, I am humbled by the limitations of Science."[10]

Having given birth without an anesthetic, it is astonishing how exuberant and energetic the mother feels right afterward. Mild activity, as well as rest, helps all body functions return to normal. Breastfeeding the baby a few moments from time to time aids the uterus in contracting. One can feel it knot into a hard ball as the baby takes the nipple. If he will not take the nipple into his mouth, help him to nuzzle it with his nose or cheek. This will have the same stimulating effect on the uterus.

Breastfeeding the Baby

The tiny baby needs much more than warmth and food. He also needs the kind of affection that the reassuring kinesthetic warmth of his mother's body gives him. Ashley Montagu suggests that a child's nine months in the womb may represent only half of the gestation period, the last half being completed after birth, when he or she still needs the closeness of the mother's body.

Food is not simply nourishment; it is also an expression of love and friendship. Guests come to pay us a visit. We are glad to see them, and slip into the kitchen a bit later to prepare refreshments for them. Obese persons may stuff their bodies with food because they are starved for human affection and understanding. Our toddler falls and hurts himself. We comfort him with a snack, or with a few moments at the breast, as well as a hug and kiss. In this same way we comfort him when he is tiny:

The baby is put to the breast whenever he indicates discomfort. This feeding act helps to warm and soothe him. He may stay at the breast for a half hour or an hour at a time. The comfort he receives there encourages him to fuss for frequent repetition. The hours of sucking each day vigorously stimulate lactation. Milk in large quantities appears rapidly, often within 24 hours after birth.

The baby and mother stay near each other through the first few months. Each night they sleep within touching distance, and in the daytime the baby is carried everywhere his mother goes. Feeding continues on demand day and night. The baby seldom cries for he is constantly within reach of the soothing comfort of his mother's breast, the warmness of her body, and the gentle touch of her skin.[11]

Thus breastfeeding gives the infant the security of love that he needs. Theoretically bottle-feeding can do this too, *if* the person feeding the baby stops and holds him close each time he takes the bottle, at least until he is several months old. We may have every intention of doing this, but we may not always follow through. It is too easy, after the first few weeks, to pop a bottle in baby's mouth, prop it on a pillow, and rush off to other pressing tasks.

One of my own toddlers at eighteen months occasionally showed this need for affection with his food. He had weaned himself from the breast a few months earlier, but still wanted to be held each time he took the bottle. (How I wish I had known then that he could have been a nursing toddler and never have needed a bottle for his sucking instincts! But back in the early sixties I had already nursed him longer than anyone else I knew had nursed.) No matter how hungry he was, or how much he enjoyed his bottle, occasionally he refused it. He would pull me away from the sink, where I was washing dishes, or tug at my arm as I sat by the typewriter. He wanted more than food; he wanted *me*, his mother. So I would lay aside the task at hand, and rock him as he drank his milk. And then, his need for food and affection satisfied, he would play contentedly near me the rest of the morning as I went about my work.

Breastfeeding is as important for the mother as for the baby. It demands of her that she stop and relax frequently, which helps her to regain her strength more quickly. As she rocks and feeds her baby, or lies on the bed with him, she can doze, or read, or just enjoy admiring him. Breastfeeding is the most fun *after* the first three or four months, as the baby becomes more responsive. He stops drinking to smile at his mother, as if to say thank you. He pats the breast playfully with his little hands. He teases—now he will take the nipple in his mouth, now he will not, until she scolds him laughingly, "You naughty baby, get busy now!" This give-and-take relationship provides the mother with the security of love, too, that the child gives.

An additional advantage to breastfeeding for the mother, which few American women realize, is that it gives her a physical, as well as spiritual, sense of satisfaction and well-being. This is clearly explained in Niles Newton's article "The Sexual Implications of Breastfeeding":

There is just as much physical basis for believing a woman should get pleasure from breastfeeding as there is a physical basis for believing a woman should get pleasure from intercourse. Her nipples are extremely sensitive tissue which become erect when stimulated.

Nipple stimulation, or psychic stimulation such as the baby's hunger cry, causes the discharge of a pituitary hormone which has the . . . effect of causing the uterus to contract rhythmically for as long as twenty minutes. . . .

Undoubtedly, many frigid breastfeeders exist. However, the existence of frigid breastfeeders does not indicate that this condition is inevitable, any more than the existence of frigid males indicates that sexual frigidity is inevitable. Naturally, intercourse can involve more intense feelings; but breastfeeding gives more frequent sensations. . . . As the infant grows older the frequency of breastfeeding recedes. However, at the same time the child's sucking strength increases and the amount of milk discharged increases—thus increasing the physical pleasure possibilities of each nursing. . . .

Successful breastfeeding, as practiced by a large proportion of peoples all over the world, is entirely different from the unsuccessful frigid breastfeeding attempt by the modern urban American mother. Successful breastfeeding is a simple and easy procedure. The hungry baby is merely lifted to the bared breast, and he and his mother join for a while in the lactation embrace. Doubt, worry, fear, and embarrassment are absent; and thus the mother is free to enjoy the physical sensations of the act. The mutual pleasure of the act is so satisfying that breastfeeding often continues into the second or third year, or even longer.

It is indeed curious that the suggestion that women can and should get pleasure from sucking shocks many more than the suggestion that women can and should get pleasure from intercourse.[12]

Picture for a moment some of the Renaissance paintings that capture the elusive beauty in the faces of mother and child, as they share the physical and spiritual pleasures of the "lactation embrace." Can we imagine feeling the same moving response to a painting in which a mother is feeding her child with a bottle?

The great majority of mothers who have had a natural birth prefer to breastfeed their babies. Perhaps the common painful frigid birth experience forced on the American woman has inhibited her ability to breastfeed successfully and makes these attempts frigid also.

Breastfeeding is becoming much more widespread among the younger mothers in the United States. However, without personal encouragement from a friend or helper, many of these do not continue for more than a few days or weeks. Mothers who live in areas where breastfeeding is not popular or who cannot find local help will find real encouragement from the La Leche League International (see Appendix A).

The Birth Climax

Because the birth climax is so important and yet so poorly understood, discussion of it has been left until now. The one thing that puzzles doctors most about natural childbirth is the enthusiasm of mothers who have experienced it to repeat it again and again and to pass on what we have learned to other women. One young mother, now a missionary in Japan, said to me, "People think that by 'painless' we mean that we don't *feel* anything. That's not true! We feel a great deal, but what we feel doesn't hurt."

Some doctors, realizing that we do "feel" something, have defined these pleasurable sensations as a sublimation of pain! People who feel pain as pleasure are masochistic or sadistic. They are not normal. Clearly, this explanation is inadequate. The simple truth is that when a woman says, "It was such a thrill!" or, "I wouldn't have missed it for

anything!'' she is not just referring to the emotional excitement of
being present when her child appears but is also referring to a physical
climax of her whole being that words simply can't describe.

The emotional excitement that accompanies the physical stimulation
of the birth demands relief through expression. This results in a ''crying out'' similar to the involuntary gasp or cry as intercourse approaches the height of its climax. Too often this ''crying out'' is misin-
terpreted by attendants as a sign of pain!

An excellent example of this phenomenon is found in an early Rus-
sian novel, written by a woman, Lidiia Nikoloevna. The heroine, Veri-
nea, is speaking:

"I want my child to come into this world in joy. I have waited for it a long
time. . . . I will not cry out, I wish it to have an easy birth." And she uttered
a single cry, a loud strong one. It did not seem to be a cry of pain, but one of
joy. And then her body was pierced by an indescribably sweet, light sensation
and she heard the marvellously lusty voice of the newborn child.

This ''sweet, light sensation,'' which is similar to the release from
the emotional impact at the height of orgasm in intercourse, is demonstrated in the dazed and happy expressions of a woman whose baby
was born in a car on the way to the hospital:

"Better get a doctor," she said calmly. "The baby's here already." At this
instant I heard it cry. It seemed incredible. . . . Dotty, *at peace,* lay against the
seat. . . . The attendant and I helped Dotty, who seemed *dazed and happy,* into
a wheelchair. (Italics added.)[13]

The euphoric emotion that follows the birth climax subsides slowly,
just as does a woman's excitement following the climax of intercourse,
and the new mother should have companionship for a while after her
child has been born naturally. She will relax and rest contentedly after
this first happy wave of emotion has had time to subside.

This euphoria of newly delivered mothers is rarely witnessed by
American doctors who try to apply the principles of natural childbirth,
because most of them *insist on dulling the final climax, or birth orgasm,* as the baby emerges, by using a pudendal or saddle block, an
inhalant anesthetic, or hypnotic analgesia and amnesia to deaden sensation in the pelvic area.

Fortunately, some doctors are now recognizing the similarity of a
natural birth experience to a sexual experience. Dr. N. Kalichman, a

graduate of McGill Medical School with postgraduate training at the Allen Memorial Institute of Psychiatry in Montreal, writes:

An analogy drawn between childbirth and sexual intercourse sheds a new light on this idea. In labor, the descending baby can be considered the equivalent of the penis in intercourse. In both situations, the to and fro movements of the penis or baby accompany increasing intensity of stimuli received from the genitalia. A possible explanation now arises as to the mysterious dozing that occurs between contractions during the second stage, and of the amnesia experienced during a great part of the labor. These two phenomena are characteristic also for the period close to the climax of intercourse. A possible explanation for both situations in psychological terms presents itself. The ego withdraws from the too-intense stimulation into a semi-consciousness. . . . To continue the analogy, as the climax is reached in both situations, the woman utters involuntary sounds and performs involuntary pelvic movements. With the expulsion of the child, as in reaching the climax of the orgasm, the woman suddenly relaxes, and there appears a calm ecstatic look on her face. The analogy applies as well to the post-delivery state. The woman's remarks are now directed to both the child and physician and are usually tender and loving and are reminiscent of remarks following intercourse. . . . As in intercourse, the ideal may not be attained, and the expression of some of these various natural phenomena may be inhibited.[14]

The following delightfully uninhibited account of the birth of a child verifies Dr. Kalichman's observations. The mother who wrote it was twenty-four years old when her child was born. It was her first child, weighed nine pounds, twelve ounces, and was twenty-one inches long. She titled her account, completed when her baby was ten days old, ''I Want a Thousand Babies'':

Doctor said. . . . ''When you feel a contraction coming, pull.'' Doubtfully I tried pulling, and it seemed pleasant, but only that. Then, on the next contraction I started to pull, and was suddenly swept away with primitive strength. Everything went blank and lightninglike streaks flashed, it seemed. It was ecstatic, wonderful, thrilling! I . . . heard myself moaning—in triumph, not in pain! There was no pain whatsoever, only a primitive and sexual elation. From my grimace, the nurse thought I was in pain and started to put the mask over my face. How annoying! In the middle of a push, I gasped, ''Go away! It doesn't hurt.''

I felt as if I had enough strength to pull the world apart—everything was bright, illuminated. In between contractions, I shouted deliriously, *''This is wonderful!* My husband only wants two babies, but I want a thousand.'' . . . And then another contraction started. The doctor said, ''I know it feels good to shout, but don't do it; that wastes your strength.'' So again, as I pulled, the dark, magic whirlwind caught me, and she said, ''You're doing beautifully; couldn't have done it better if you'd had a dozen babies!''

. . . After about two more thrilling pushes and a breath of oxygen, I heard the doctor say, ''Hang on to this one and push the baby out.'' With the most spiraling, fascinating thrill of all, I felt the baby slither out. I wanted to shout with joy. Doctor held baby in her arms, baby cried, and I saw a perfect child attached to the cord. Doctor said reverently, ''You have a little girl.'' . . . I wanted to stop and rest and drink in the thrill of having the baby. It was about five minutes before I wanted to push again. And then the last, slightly weaker, slightly less thrilling, but wonderful push, and out the placenta slipped.

. . . Bill walked with me to the elevator and I felt so good that I said, ''It's silly to wheel me; I can walk. Bill, I feel as if I could do a day's washing right now.'' But after talking to him ten minutes in the maternity ward, I felt a little tired. He left—I started this letter, and then just rested.[15]

Does it seem a strange paradox that the birth of a child, which can cause such an agony of pain to a mother under certain conditions, can be a source of physical pleasure to her under other circumstances? Life is full of paradoxes. Love and hate are not so far apart as they seem, nor are tears and laughter. Sex itself carries the potentials of great pleasure or great tragedy; it can be uplifting or degrading, depending on the circumstances.

Some people may be shocked at the thought that the birth of a child can bring its mother physical pleasure. But what is their concept of the character of God? Is he a tyrant, who denies us pleasure, as some of our forefathers believed? Is he not rather a loving God, who delights in bringing pleasures to his children?

Conclusion

Adequate prenatal education is essential for a successful childbirth experience. Because of this, some members of the medical profession are now calling natural childbirth ''psychophysical'' or ''psychosomatic'' obstetrics. By this they mean that attention must be given to the ''mind,'' *psychē,* as well as to the ''body,'' *sōma,* of a pregnant woman. This is all right as far as it goes, but it leaves out the most essential component of a natural childbirth experience, which is *pneuma,* ''spirit.''

What the birth of this particular child means to me, the mother, is not just a matter of the mind, nor of the body, but is essentially a matter of the spirit. It is the spiritual significance of a birth that gives it dignity and beauty, for creativity is a spiritual function. Dr. Paul Tournier, in *The Meaning of Persons,* makes this distinction clear:

The body and the mind are only the means of expression of the spirit, which coordinates and directs them both at once. The body and the mind which we study appear simply as mechanisms . . . the instruments by means of which the spiritual reality which is the person expresses itself.

. . . Dom Weisberger . . . expresses it thus: "To defend the person it is not enough to confine oneself to the specific nature of man as a composite mind-body, a reasoning animal. To defend the person is to defend man as being somebody . . . unique, incommunicable, irreplaceable, willed and loved by God. . . ."[16]

Two of us stand looking at a sunset. Our bodies are in the same place. Our mental perception is of the same scenery. But the *impression* that this sunset gives to each of us is individual, unique, a thing of the spirit. Though we have had the same mind-body experience, the spiritual significance will be different for each of us. If we each paint a picture of the sunset, these pictures will be different. They will reflect the spiritual perception and creativity of our own, unique personalities.

So it is with natural childbirth. Its principles have a universal application, for all women desire fulfillment in their childbearing experiences. But what this particular childbirth experience *means* to one is not just a matter of mind-body. It is a unique, personal, spiritual experience of creativity. Each woman is unique. Each child in a family is unique, different from his or her brothers and sisters. Giving birth to this particular child has a unique spiritual meaning to the mother, whether the child is her first or her tenth. It is this spiritual aspect that makes natural childbirth so rewarding.

"She talks," I heard some say today,
"As though none else had ever had a baby!"
How right they are!
No one else has ever borne this child, my husband's child.
It is our own unique gift to the universe,
The living symbol of our faith in the dignity of life,
In the destiny of man,
And in the reality of an eternal, living God.
And God, Who made me for this hour,
Will not desert me now!

Women are most grateful for being taught how to give birth in a way in which it is to them a beautiful, personal miracle. One young woman wrote, after the natural birth of her first child:

Mrs. Wessel, I want you to know how grateful I am to you for all your helpful advice. . . . It has been such a blessing to me that I want to share my experience with others, too. So I have definitely made up my mind to try to help any expectant mother in our future pastorates to see that it can be a wonderful and blessed experience. The natural way which the Lord intended it to be. I shall always be indebted to you and deeply appreciate it—more than you will ever know.

My file is full of such letters I've received through the years. They all reflect a similar sentiment, so beautifully expressed by the letter first quoted in this book in 1963 describing the birth of a first child, a seven-and-a-half-pound girl:

I am an RN and first saw "Natural Childbirth" as a student nurse ten years ago. After observing deliveries of all types, I had a chance to observe "Natural Childbirth," so asked to stay overtime and watch this mother's delivery. I was completely "sold." Could it be possible that labor, which to me before was accompanied by moaning, groaning and screaming, could be an experience that was capable of such powerful, exultant yet humble emotions? This patient was fully alert, was calm and confident throughout the whole first stage.

I shall never forget the look on the woman's face as her baby was held up, still attached to the cord, to the mother who lost her first baby because of medication that made the baby so sluggish it died. The mother had a look of profound joy and her eyes filled with shining tears and her face looked as if a miracle had just happened to her. I remember as I stood there, that I had tears in my eyes too as did the other nurses, and I decided then and there, that if I ever got pregnant, I wanted to remember my baby's birth as this woman would, as an experience that was a beautiful miracle, not one of fright and pain from the contractions or a complete blank of the birth of the baby in second stage.

My experience with "Natural Childbirth" was just as I hoped it would be, and I must admit tears flowed down my cheeks when I first saw my baby, I was so happy. There were 8 or 9 student nurses in the delivery room when I delivered, and like ten years ago when I first saw "Natural Childbirth" and was "sold" on it, these students came to me later on in the maternity ward to say they were just thrilled with my delivery and the sight of joy on my face. They went to class after my delivery and told the rest of the class about it. They also said every student in the delivery room who watched the delivery wants to try it when they get pregnant, so as a nurse and as a mother, I want to say "Thank you" to the Institute for making my dream a reality.[17]

Should we not all stand humbled in awe at such evidence of God's love in our world, which has made such happiness possible? We can say with the Psalmist:

> Praise the Lord for his goodness,
> And for his wonderful works to the children of men!
> For he satisfies the longing soul,
> And fills the hungry soul with goodness. . . .
> He turns the wilderness into a standing water,
> And dry ground into watersprings. . . .
> He lifts the poor high above affliction,
> And makes his families like flocks.
> The righteous shall see it, and rejoice:
> And all iniquity shall stop its mouth.
> Whoever is wise will observe these things,
> And shall understand the loving kindness of the Lord.
> —Psalm 107:8–43

NOTES

1. Grantly Dick-Read, M.D., *Childbirth Without Fear*, 4th rev. ed. (New York: Harper & Row, 1972), p. 40.
2. Grantly Dick-Read, M.D., "The Birth of a Child," *Child-Family Digest*, June 1953. Reprinted by permission.
3. "Letter from 'Natural Childbirth' Mother to Instructor," *Child-Family Digest*, February 1952, pp. 49–51. Reprinted by permission.
4. Paul Tournier, M.D., *The Meaning of Persons* (New York: Harper, 1957), pp. 106, 107.
5. Virginia Lawrence Larsen, M.D., "Comments" on the article "An Evaluation of Childbirth Training in Seattle," *Child-Family Digest*, May 1955, p. 79.
6. "I Want a Thousand Babies," *Child-Family Digest*, January 1952, pp. 94–99. Reprinted by permission.
7. Mrs. Grantly Dick-Read and Prunella Briance, *What Every Woman Should Know About Childbirth* (Grantly Dick-Read Childbirth Training Centre, 1960), p. 5. Reprinted by permission.
8. Grantly Dick-Read, M.D., "The Discomforts of Childbirth," the substance of a lecture delivered before St. Mary's Hospital Medical Society in October 1948, printed in the *British Medical Journal*, April 16, 1949, vol. 1, p. 651.
9. Mrs. Dick-Read, *What Every Woman Should Know About Childbirth*, p. 6. Reprinted by permission.
10. Dick-Read, *Childbirth Without Fear*, p. 230.

11. Michael Newton, M.D., and Niles Newton, Ph.D., "The Normal Course of Lactation," *Child and Family*, October 1962, pp. 6–12. Reprinted by permission.
12. Niles Newton, "The Sexual Implications of Breastfeeding," *Child-Family Digest*, November 1952, pp. 16–18. Reprinted by permission.
13. Marvin R. Weisbord, "Our Baby Wouldn't Wait to Be Born," *Reader's Digest*, June 1962, p. 138, condensed from "Our Baby Was Born at 30 M.P.H.," *Parents' Magazine*, March 1962.
14. N. Kalichman, M.D., "On Some Psychological Aspects of the Management of Labor," *The Psychiatric Quarterly*, vol. 25, no. 4, 1951, pp. 655–671. Reprinted by permission.
15. "I Want a Thousand Babies," p. 97. Reprinted by permission.
16. Tournier, *The Meaning of Persons*, p. 169.
17. First printed in *Preparation for Parenthood News*, Mary Jane Hungerford, Ph.D., editor, by The American Institute of Family Relations, Los Angeles, Calif. Reprinted by permission.

22. Breastfeeding

A Mother's Breasts

Soon after a child is conceived the mother's breasts begin their preparation for his or her arrival, for one of the earliest signs of pregnancy is a slight swelling and perhaps tenderness of the breasts. Obviously, breasts and babies were "made for each other"!

What an awesome experience it is to nurture a new life, in the womb and at the breast, in the continuity of love and sustenance that God planned for everyone born into his world. But baby is not the first to be blessed by the mother's breasts. Until now, they had been solely the possessions of the husband, his comfort and joy. Against their softness he rested his head, and upon them he pressed his loving kisses. And his doing so was right and beautiful, for the Bible says (Prov. 5:18b, 19, NIV):

> May you rejoice in the wife of your youth.
> A loving doe, a graceful deer—
> may her breasts satisfy you always,
> may you ever be captivated by her love.

The husband who is sensitive to his wife may know almost as soon as she that their love-child is on the way, for she may draw back a bit when he touches her breasts or say "ouch!" when he bumps them accidentally. Can he release his "sole" right to them and share their delights with another? In the providence of God, he need not adjust overnight; he has nine months to enlarge his heart and to make room for his child at his own wife's bosom. For it is *his* child. He can open his arms for "one more" in his encircling embrace.

The breast tenderness of the early days soon passes, but the fullness remains. Many women enjoy their "filled-out" bosom during pregnancy, especially if they felt underendowed before. The husband too can take pleasure at the sight of his wife's firm, full breasts and at the rounding of her profile by the form of his child within her body. And once the breast tenderness passes, he can once again enjoy his wife's breasts, at her invitation and for her pleasure. His caresses during love-making help stimulate the breasts to function. She can guide him by her preferences and show him what is most helpful.

During later pregnancy gentle breast massage is helpful. The expectant mother can first use moist heat on the breasts to stimulate circulation and help herself relax by directing the shower onto the nipples or by placing warm, wet washcloths over the breasts while in the tub. Soap or anything drying should not be used on the nipples. While still in the bath or shower, she can massage gently, encircling the breasts with her thumb and fingers pressed against the chest wall, and gradually moving her hands outwards. After the bath, she can rub with a terry cloth towel and then grasp the nipple, pulling it out, and turning it up and down. It can then be lubricated with a skin cream or vegetable oil.

If the nipple is flat or inverted (barely projecting out, or shrinking back into the breast when the areola is depressed), La Leche League suggests using the "Hoffman technique."[1] The woman draws an imaginary cross on the nipple, places a thumb on each side of the nipple along one line of the cross, presses in firmly and at the same time pulls the thumbs *away* from each other. (The thumbs should be directly at the base of the nipple, not at the edge of the areola.) The stretch should be repeated five times once a day, first along one of the lines of the cross, then along the other. This stretches out the nipple and loosens the tightness at the base, making the nipple move up and outward. Plastic breast shields that encourage the flat or inverted nipples to protrude are also very helpful when worn in late pregnancy. (These are not to be confused with the nipple shields sometimes recommended for use during feeding after the baby arrives.) Another help is to have the husband draw out the nipples by sucking during lovemaking, if both find this pleasurable.

During pregnancy, both parents can delight in the reality of the baby for whom these preparations are being made. Touching the mother's stomach they can stroke him, feeling the roundness of his little bottom, the line of his back—perhaps the soles of his feet when he stretches against the boundaries of his nest. Baby loves to hear them talk or pray or sing to him. "Little one, we are so happy to have you as our own. We are getting ready for the day when we can hold you in our arms and cradle you at your mother's bosom. Be at peace, child. Keep on growing in beauty and strength in your warm haven. You are covered within the safety of your mother's love, your father's love, and we are all surrounded by the protection and wisdom of your heavenly Father.''

Breastfeeding the Newborn

When the happy day arrives, parents and child are not strangers to one another, and the parents are already the familiar safe boundary within which the child can explore new freedoms. The new baby has a message for the parents too.

I am your baby. I have just come from inner space where I was warm and held in a close, tight nest. I heard the rhythm of your heartbeat and felt the patting sensation that your breathing gave me. I was continuously tube fed; therefore I was never in pain from hunger. I would occasionally drink the warm amniotic fluid that surrounded me. Maybe you noticed it when I had the hiccups. The thumbsucking that relatives object to—why, I have done that for months! I heard your voices and even Dad's when he came close to talk to me. I did not sleep all the time. You may have been aware of that fact when I had my exercise sessions.

Please re-create for me the familiar surroundings of inner space. Allow me time to make the transition to outer space and to fulfill your expectations of what a baby is.

Feed me—I have never been hungry, or full.
Pat and stroke me. I'm used to this "touching."
Talk to me. Let me continue to hear your voice.
Hold me close. I was swaddled in the uterus and heard your heartbeat.
Look into my eyes. Let me study you and become acquainted with you.[2]

Baby is meant to go from his mother's body into his mother's arms at her bosom.* This is essential not only for the continuity of his emotional security, but also to take advantage of his inborn instinct to seek the breast.

The sucking reflex of a full-term healthy newborn is usually at a peak about twenty to thirty minutes after he is born, provided he is not drowsy from drugs or anesthesia used during labor and delivery. If this prime time to begin nursing is missed, the baby's sucking reflex may be less acute for about a day and a half.[3]

---

*Baby is "he," to distinguish from the mother, "she."

Baby may not take the breast in the first few moments, but even the touch of his cheek against it will cause his mother's uterus to contract, helping to expel the afterbirth, for there is an acute physiological interaction in addition to the social interaction between mother and baby. They are finely attuned to each other through the long months of close association in the womb.

The father's presence sheltering his wife and child enhances the happy balance of their relationship and he is an integral part of this crucial early bonding period. He too is being bonded to his baby. And it gives him the opportunity to see, for the first time, *someone else* intimately at his wife's breasts, which until now had been for his pleasure alone. His presence transmits in a profound, unspoken way the right of the baby to be there. He gladly makes way for his child and, rather than feeling left out, is aware that he is himself an important element in the happy nursing relationship between his wife and his child.

When the infant is placed in his mother's arms and at her breast for the first time, appreciate that this is also *a new experience for the baby*. It is possible that the new baby will immediately take the nipple and nurse vigorously, even right after birth. It is also possible that he will make very little response, and the mother may feel a little worried or disappointed. But remember that the baby has just come from intrauterine life. He has never nursed before. He is comforted by the warmth and smell and rhythmic breathing of his mother, yet alert to all the newness around him—a bigger world, air rather than water, light rather than semidarkness, voices taking on a different timbre than in the womb. From the security of his mother's arms he may first look around, search for her eyes with his eyes and look into his daddy's face, full of wonder. How blessed he is if in these first few moments in a "new" universe, his visual, auditory, and tactile impressions take place within the security of his mother's and his father's arms.

Soon enough he will seek the "fountain of joy," that source from which he will not only be sustained but from which he will find his primary source of comfort and security for months to come. The baby will quickly learn to breastfeed well, especially when he remains continually with his mother from birth on.

Breastfeeding is a baby's reassurance of security, in which he feels again the rhythm of the mother's breathing and heartbeat. This experience at her breast continues the love and acceptance he experienced in the womb, but in greater psychological depth, mother and baby giving and receiving warmth and love from each other as the baby's hunger is satisfied.

The physical benefits to the baby are immeasurable. Scientists are continually discovering new intrinsic values of breast milk. The milk not only contains immunoglobulin antibodies, which act against viruses and bacteria, but it is also easily digested and has the proper amounts of lactose, protein, calcium, and other minerals, the proper biochemical balance for the human infant. It is now known to contain substances such as *taurine,* an essential element for brain growth. The human baby does not metabolize taurine well from sources other than the mother's milk. Because of these and other important elements, breastfed babies are ill less often and have fewer allergies.

Breastfeeding is on the increase, for knowledgeable young parents are increasingly rejecting artificial feeding by bottle for their babies. These young people are looking at life honestly and making choices objectively, rather than blindly following professional or traditional advice without question. They are discovering the positive values of nature, of clean air and water, and of natural foods; they are concerned for less wastefulness, better care of the environment, and more love for humanity. As the incidence of breastfeeding has increased there have been unexpected dividends for parents as well as for baby.

When the mother feeds her baby at her breasts, she also experiences both psychological and physical benefits, for these are closely inter-woven. Dr. Deborah Tanzer in *Why Natural Childbirth?* writes:

There are exceptionally close ties between reproductive and psychological functioning. We take for granted the influences of moods and feelings on courtship behavior and on sexual activity, as well as vice versa. . . . The in-teractions of body and mind in the woman's reproductive cycle are not at all surprising for there are events that start them, specific places in the body where they begin, pathways they follow and places where they end.

The most obvious major pathway is the body's nervous system. . . . The involuntary nervous system . . . is intimately concerned with psychological activity, including emotions. It also provides the main direct supply to the organs of the female reproductive system, especially the uterus. . . .

One neurohormone, oxytocin, is involved in mating behavior, birth and lactation or nursing. In orgasm, for example, oxytocin is thought to be related to contractions of the uterus. In labor and delivery, it helps stimulate uterine contractions. In breast feeding, it brings about "letdown"—release of the

262 / NATURAL CHILDBIRTH AND THE CHRISTIAN FAMILY

mother's milk. Particular smells, sights and sounds can send oxytocin out along internal pathways to stimulate specific responses.[4]

When the baby touches the breast, or cries in anticipation of feeding, oxytocin is released from the mother's pituitary gland, which stimulates the uterus to contract pleasurably (as in female orgasm), although in the first few days after birth this can be uncomfortable. This in turn stimulates the anterior lobe of the pituitary gland to release *prolactin,* a woman's built-in "tranquilizer." Many women have admitted a "baby-blues" period during the early weeks, when all the changes of daily life seem just too much. But there are women, honest and aware of themselves, who say, "Yes, a cloud of discouragement did descend. But I nursed my baby, and it went away!"

The disappearance of this depressed feeling is not just the result of cuddling the baby close and enjoying him, it is also due to this release of prolactin into the mother's bloodstream. Thus the best cure for a "nervous" mother is nature's built-in tranquilizer, released automatically into her system as her baby suckles at the breast.

The person who was breastfed herself by a mother who was comfortable and natural about it may have no psychological barrier to overcome. But the new mother attempting to breastfeed without this support will need to discover how to deal with the negative attitudes of others, for any anxiety will affect her ability to breastfeed successfully during the months after birth and may cause her to wean her baby early. Negative statements may come from well-meaning friends and relatives who have had poor experiences in breastfeeding or who are actually offended by the thought and cannot resist letting the mother know how they feel. Some have the concept that breastfeeding is "dirty," and that the nursing mother should never be seen. I remember nursing one of my babies in the front room of the home of relatives one time. The only persons at home were my cousin, her teenage daughter, and my husband, across the room reading. My cousin's husband was gone. My cousin said, "Would you mind going into the bedroom? I don't want my daughter to see you nursing when your husband is in the room!"

It helps to remember that reactions like this only mirror the dissatisfaction some women feel with themselves, those who may think of their breasts as nonfunctional sex objects created only for the admiration of the opposite sex. In *Modern Motherhood,* Dr. Liley suggests:

Breastfeeding is actually such an intimate part of our human life cycle that our reaction to the question reflects our approach to life. The proportion of women who breastfeed their babies is not so much a measure of our economics or sophistication as it is of our confidence and joy in motherhood.[5]

The encouragement and support of the husband helps offset the negativism of many of these people. His approval and his reassuring attitude that breastfeeding is the best feeding provide a shield for his wife and baby against the well-meaning disapproval of others. He will be rewarded in this. He will share the joy that comes to his wife as she gains confidence in her role as an adequate mother. He will see her womanly beauty unfold as she nurses their baby and will also discover that nature is maturing her capacity as a sex partner. And, of course, nature's tranquilizer, prolactin, released in her body as she nurses, makes her not only a calmer mother but also a more pleasant companion to live with.

A man whose baby is breastfed can hold the baby and help care for him as much as he wants to, without the infant ever confusing him with the mother. He can wash diapers or help with meals or any other chores without ever been thought of as "effeminate," for femininity does not reside in what tasks are performed, but in what bodily functions can be fulfilled. The daddy need not keep his distance from the baby to prove his manliness.

The Early Weeks

Most of the problems encountered in breastfeeding occur in the early days and weeks, so that it is important to make a good start. This is easiest when mother and baby are continually near each other from the moment of birth on.

It is extremely important that the new baby not be imprinted with the feel of the rubber nipple. He should not be given *any* bottles until his sucking reflex is well established (preferably not until after several weeks of breastfeeding, if at all). The baby who bottle-sucks has a much weaker sucking reflex by four days of age and sucks less vigorously when put to breast.[6]

A baby quickly develops his own oral habits, so that it is important for these to be set in the right direction from the start. A mother may have breastfed other babies, but not *this* baby. Each baby has his own unique oral mannerisms and some habits, such as thumb sucking or tongue sucking, may already be well established.

In Chapter 15 there is a summary of initial instructions for breast-feeding. Here are a few more helpful suggestions:

1. Stroke the baby's mouth or cheek with the nipple. The baby will turn *toward* the side stroked, open his mouth, and put his tongue down. Make certain that his tongue is *down* before inserting the nipple. A baby who has been tongue-sucking before birth must be trained to suck with his tongue down *under* the nipple, or he will not be getting milk and the mother will soon have very sore nipples. In the tongue-thrusting position, the baby dimples his cheeks and is on the breast with the tongue thrusting above the nipple. When the baby is nursing well the nipple is fully grasped in his mouth above the tongue, and one can feel and hear his productive pumping action. His jaw is thrust upward, milk is expressed, and the baby swallows. The action of his jaws around the areolar area above the nipple not only draws the milk but also stimulates the mother's milk supply.

2. A new mother may not recognize the feeling of her milk letting down, but if she is relaxed, she *will* simply "let" the milk down. The baby cannot suck out the milk until the mother relaxes enough to release it. If she is inhibited, upset, or tense, she can use the abdominal (sleep) breathing she used for relaxing during pregnancy and labor. As she releases muscle tension and breathes more deeply and quietly, the milk will be able to come down. It may take two or three minutes for the milk to be released in any quantity, especially in the early days, but the baby will be getting the needed colostrum. After the first few weeks of breastfeeding most women (though not all) can recognize the milk "letdown" as a tingly, full feeling in the breasts, even before the baby is put to the breast, or in the breast on which the baby is not nursing. The breasts may leak when letdown occurs while baby is not at the breast, so it is wise to wear clean, absorbent pads—a large handkerchief will do—inside the brassiere. If letdown is felt while baby is not at the breast, cross both arms across the breasts and press firmly. This helps stop the leaking.

3. A newborn enjoys being held close and enjoys sucking. He should be nursed frequently, even every couple of hours, in the early days. Remember that nursing is not just for food, but also to satisfy baby's sucking needs and show him love. Baby may nurse a bit, then rest a bit, then nurse some more. If he seems satisfied, remove him from the breast, but be sure to let him back again frequently. Shorter,

frequent nursings also help prevent the mother's nipples from becoming sore.

4. A baby literally creates suction as he nurses. To remove baby from the breast, break the suction by depressing the breast away from one corner of his mouth. If he does not release the nipple, gently insert a finger between his *gums*, where the vacuum is being created. It is not enough just to slip a finger into the corner of his mouth. Never pull the nipple out of his mouth until he has released it.

5. Alternate the breasts each feeding. Begin feeding on the breast that was second at the previous feeding, so that each breast receives the same amount of stimulation and the baby doesn't favor one side more than the other. It is helpful to use a safety pin on the bra strap as a reminder of the breast last nursed.

Another important reason for changing sides is that the fat content increases in the milk that is formed after the "let-down" reflex. Protein content is also increased in this "hindmilk," so the end of the feeding provides baby with richer milk.

6. It is wise to vary the positions used for nursing, sometimes lying down, sometimes sitting up, sometimes in a rocking chair. The "football" hold may be helpful if the nipples are becoming sore, or if nursing two babies at once. Hold baby under the arm, his head cradled in your hand so that he can grasp the nipple on the same side as your arm.

7. Leave the nipples exposed to the air for a few minutes after each nursing. The milk acts as an antiseptic agent on the skin of the nipples, so no washing is needed.[7] The baby's saliva is also a healing agent.

If the nipples become tender, limit nursing to ten minutes on each side, being sure to continue frequent feedings. Applying ice to the nipples just before nursing can help make the first few minutes of baby's sucking less uncomforatble. Also, the initial tenderness tends to disappear after the milk is flowing well. It is wise to take extra vitamin C with lots of fluids. The doctor may prescribe a mild pain reliever or ointment for the nipples. Pure hydrous lanolin applied to the nipples after nursing may be helpful (for those not sensitive to wool). It may also be helpful to take supplemental zinc.

Whenever there is a tender or bleeding nipple, try to discover what is causing the problem. Check the position of the baby's tongue, making sure it is under the nipple. Make sure he gets the whole nipple in his mouth and is not just sucking on the tip. And be sure to break the suction of baby's gums before taking him off the breast.

A mother can continue to nurse even with nipples that are cracked and bleeding. The slight amount of blood won't hurt the baby, and the bleeding will soon stop. If the soreness is extreme, the milk can be hand-expressed each time and fed to the baby with an eyedropper or a spoon temporarily. (Again, get the spoon on *top* of his tongue so that it goes down his throat, or the "thrusting" action of his tongue will make it seem as though he is spitting it out.)

8. Milk supply is produced in response to stimulation. The more frequently the baby nurses, the more stimulation there will be. Even if medication has been inadvertently given by the attendants to "dry up" the breasts, the stimulation of the baby's sucking will gradually overcome it. Mothers should know that taking birth control pills hinders milk production. Getting enough rest, drinking ten to twelve glasses of fluid a day—including some milk or a milk substitute (cheese, yogurt, etc.), and eating a balanced diet will assure enough milk.

Sometimes a mother may think she doesn't have enough milk because the baby seems hungry and wants to nurse all the time. This is normal nursing behavior for a new baby and is no reflection on an adequate supply. If a hungry baby were *not* getting milk, he would pull away from the breast and cry. In this case, wait a few moments, and then put him on again. The milk will be there.

9. If the baby is with the mother continually from birth, engorgement is not as likely to be a problem. If engorgement does occur, use moist heat to increase circulation. (Do not use ice packs!) Breastfeed still more frequently to draw off the excess milk, and follow the techniques for relaxing to allow the "let-down" to occur.

Massage the breasts gently as described for late pregnancy. It may be helpful to have the husband massage the breasts and/or stimulate the nipples. His touch will help stimulate the "let-down" reflex.

Express the colostrum or milk as described in Chapter 15 if the breasts become overfull, but only during the few days of engorgement. Once this has subsided, expressing "extra" milk will only cause more to be produced. Using a breast pump for early engorgement is ineffective and painful. (Later on a breast pump will be all right, if it is necessary to express milk for the baby.) Be careful not to wear a brassiere that is too tight.

10. Engorgement can make one more susceptible to breast infections, so it is important to keep the breasts soft, making sure that there are no "hard" places on the breasts. If one is found with the fingers,

massage it gently as baby nurses so that the duct will empty. If a "plugged" duct is emptied early, infection, with its flu-like symptoms of achiness and fever, can usually be prevented.

If a breast infection does occur, keep on breastfeeding and treat it as you would engorgement. Go to bed if possible, keeping baby in bed too, for frequent nursing, and rest as much as possible. Nursing during a breast infection is not harmful to the baby and plays a big part in preventing abcess in the breast. Sleep without a bra and make sure that no clothing constricts the breasts. If the doctor prescribes antibiotics for a more serious infection, be sure to take the full treatment and not stop when feeling better, or the infection may flare up again. If the infection recurs or does not seem to improve, contact the La Leche League leader in your area, and also ask for their materials on breast infections and what to do about them.

As the Months Pass
The experience of breastfeeding changes considerably as the baby grows and as mother and baby continually adapt to each other. If mother or baby is ill, it may affect the milk supply. If they must be separated (which is only very rarely necessary), the mother can keep expressing her milk and then breastfeed more frequently again when reunited with her baby until the supply is back up to normal. If hospitalization is required, mother and baby should be allowed to remain together if at all possible. The simple fact is *they need each other*.

A boy baby is often circumcised on the day the mother's milk begins to replace colostrum, although the biblical guide for circumcision is that the child is not to be circumcised before the eighth day.[8] There is a good medical reason for this latter timing. The substance in the blood necessary for coagulation (prothrombin) decreases in all infants during the first days of life, and the lack of this substance is most pronounced on the second to fifth day (the days during which most circumcisions are performed!). The prothrombin rises again spontaneously between the seventh and the tenth day so that there is less bleeding and more rapid healing if the circumcision is not performed until that time. Also, by that time the mother's milk is well established.

The baby is tired following the experience of circumcision and may not nurse well. If the procedure is done on the third day, the mother may also be feeling low due to the hormonal changes in her body after the birth. At such a time, the mother breastfeeding her first baby may become pessimistic about ever breastfeeding properly, particularly if she and baby were not bonded from birth and are not allowed rooming-in. Or, she may worry about the baby and feel rejected if she has ample milk and he won't breastfeed after his surgery.

Even if the baby is born in the hospital, circumcision can be post-poned until the proper time. Baby and mother can go home and the baby can be returned to the hospital as an out-patient if circumcision is to be performed. However, the New Testament indicates that circumci-sion is not mandatory,[9] and an increasing number of both professionals and parents are questioning its validity when it is not performed for religious purposes.[10] It is perhaps the most unnecessary routine surgery in the United States.

The two most frequently mentioned problems for uncircumcised boys are the inability of the foreskin to retract over the head of the penis and the problem of cleanliness. In regard to the first, if the foreskin is not tampered with it will eventually retract when the child is from three to five years old, as a normal part of his maturing.[11] And cleanliness is no problem, for once it retracts easily, a boy can be taught to draw it back when bathing as naturally as he is taught to wash behind his ears. A natural secretion, *smegma,* is secreted under the foreskin as a boy grows older, in which bacteria may be deposited and cause infection if it is not regularly cleansed. And a husband should always be sure the smegma is washed away before intercourse. But to routinely circumcise millions of boy babies because these factors may occasionally be a problem makes no more sense than routine episioto-my for childbirth.

There are other occasions in addition to illness or circumcision in which nursing may not seem to go well. At about one week of age, at about six weeks, and again around three months of age many babies have a growth spurt and suddenly demand more milk than is being produced. The reactions of the mother (and the suggestions of others) too often are to give a supplement, to start baby food, and to think that breast milk alone is not enough for the baby to thrive on.

When this growth spurt occurs, the mother can take off a day or two to relax, feed, and just enjoy the baby. The work can wait. Daddy can help. The phone and doorbell can go unanswered. There is no reason to panic. A baby does not need a large amount of food immediately and is in no danger of starving. He can be nursed every couple of hours, while he and his mother rest together, or rock together, and she takes time to talk and sing to him and play with him. As she rests more, spends more time with him and allows him to feed more often, the supply will soon adjust to the new demand.

Among my own most precious memories are those of breastfeeding my last three children. I had looked forward to breastfeeding our first baby, as related in the Preface, but was told I could not. I had had tuberculosis as a child and supposed that perhaps that was the reason. When preparing for my first natural birth (fourth child) I asked my doctor if it might be possible for me to breastfeed, in spite of my childhood illness.

"If you can carry a baby," he said, "there's no reason you can't feed it." His reply shocked me, for I realized I had been cheated of something I had wanted and longed to do, because I had not pursued the question with my first three babies! The same is true for any mother: if she can bear a child, she can nurture it at the breast. If there are problems, she can learn how they can be overcome. As time goes on, she will discover that the interaction between herself and her nursing baby is among the most blessed of life's experiences, for both baby and mother.

My first attempt at breastfeeding was not without problems. It was difficult to get the baby to take the breast. She was born six weeks prematurely and had little sucking reflex. She would take the breast and then fall asleep after only a few moments. I had been told never to nurse more than twenty minutes at a time, and I of course was trying to follow all the "rules." After twenty minutes, every four hours, baby was back in her bed where she slept most of the time until her next feeding. When taken to the doctor at three weeks, she had barely gained three ounces and still weighed less than five pounds!

"Well, Peanut," the doctor said as he checked her over, "you're healthy enough, but why aren't you gaining?" He suggested giving her canned baby food meat in addition to the nursing. Although I did that (fortunately, it seems to have done no harm), I also decided to lie down with my baby every time she nursed, for a full hour, to be sure she had enough. We did this every two to three hours. This way she could nurse a little, doze, nurse, doze, without becoming overtired, while I restfully gave her my full attention. If it was difficult to keep her awake to nurse enough, I would get up and change her or do something to rouse her enough to feed well. She began to gain, and within a few months took no longer to nurse than any other baby.

Try to wake the baby if he falls asleep before nursing from the second breast. Baby nurses only to a comfortable feeling, even if he is not full. Change his diapers, give him a bath, rub his feet lovingly, or loosen his clothing to help him wake up and be alert enough to nurse for a while on the second breast. If he is sleeping soundly and *won't* wake up, let him sleep. Perhaps he has received enough milk for that feeding.

Something else I didn't know was that a breastfed baby needs to nurse more often than a bottle baby, including nighttimes. It is no great achievement to have the baby sleep through the night. In fact, it is normal for him to nurse two or more times during the night. If baby sleeps in bed with his parents, it is a simple matter to roll over and "put him on." The baby even learns to "latch on" to his mother's nipple without her waking! There is no need for her to ever get out of bed, unless he needs changing.

If the parents feel reluctant about baby being in the bed with them all the time, at least he should be nearby in the same room during the early weeks. As the months pass, he can gradually be adjusted to his own bed, perhaps in another room with siblings. Throughout history in most cultures, most babies have slept in bed with their parents.[12]

Transitions

"Solid" foods need not be offered until the baby is at least six to nine months old, or even twelve months for some babies. Breast milk provides all the nutrition he needs. When solids are introduced, breastfeed on both sides before offering them, for the first few months.

As time goes on and baby is over a year old, solids may be substituted for a few nursings, such as at mealtimes. But for the first few months solids should be thought of as supplemental to nursing; baby is beginning to need more than just milk, but he still needs the milk too. Solids do not replace mother's milk, only add to it. Mother's own milk is still baby's most healthful food.

The time to introduce solids is when the baby shows signs of needing them, such as very frequent nursing for more than several days, chewing on everything in reach, grabbing food out of the parents' hands, and so on. The food on mama's or daddy's plate becomes a great attraction!

Breastfeeding is not one hundred percent assurance that the mother will not ovulate and conceive while still nursing. The prolactin released while breastfeeding is thought to inhibit ovulation, so that no egg is discharged from the ovary to be fertilized, but the fact that the mother is not menstruating does not mean that she may not begin ovulating, though the majority of women will menstruate before the first ovulation. Sheila Kippley's book *Breastfeeding and Natural Child Spacing* (see Appendix B) is an excellent resource for those concerned about conceiving while breastfeeding.

The return of menstruation is no reason to discontinue breastfeeding, for the milk will continue to be produced as long as the baby wants it. He can even be breastfed through another pregnancy, although the milk will gradually disappear and be replaced by modest amounts of colostrum. He may not like that taste and decide to wean, but since toddler nursing is more for comfort than for food, he may want to continue even after another child is born. This is called *tandem nursing,* in which both the newborn and the toddler nurse. A mother can have an ample supply for both, since it is the sucking stimulation that increases the supply. If the older child has not weaned before the new baby arrives, tandem nursing helps his acceptance of the new baby. He does not have to "make way" for the new brother or sister, until ready to wean on his own.

Toddler nursing is quite different from newborn nursing. The newborn needs to be breastfed frequently, day and night, so that at first it seems that this is *all* a mother is doing! The older baby, on the other hand, receives most of his nutrition from other foods and nurses only to "touch base" with mama, as when he is hurt, at naptime, at bedtime, on waking up in the morning. It is also greatly enjoyed by most mothers, and the interaction between a nursing mother and her small child becomes a precious memory to both.

Most babies, if allowed to wean when ready, will continue nursing beyond one year of age, and some for as long as three or four years, the feedings becoming gradually shorter and less frequent. Children eventually wean themselves, if it has not been forced on them earlier. Weaning should be very gradual, both for the mother's sake and for the child's.

Toddler nursing is once again becoming accepted in our own culture, as it has been in most cultures throughout the world. It was common in biblical days, for we read (1 Sam. 1:24, 2:18, 19, NIV) that the child Samuel was breastfed until he was old enough to wear special garments and run errands for Eli the priest. He would have had to have been at least three years old before weaning occurred, and may even have been six or seven, which would not have been unusual.

After he was weaned, she took the boy with her, young as he was, . . . and brought him to the house of the Lord at Shiloh. . . . Samuel was ministering before the Lord—a boy wearing a linen ephod. Each year his mother made him a little robe and took it with her when she went up with her husband to offer the annual sacrifice.

NOTES

1. *The Womanly Art of Breastfeeding,* 3rd ed. (Franklin Park, IL: La Leche League International, Inc., 1981), p. 30.
2. Ilene S. Rice, *A Breastfeeding Guide* (St. Joseph's Hospital, St. Paul, MN), p. 1. Reprinted by permission.
3. *The Womanly Art of Breastfeeding,* p. 74. Reprinted by permission.
4. Deborah Tanzer, Ph.D., and Jean L. Block, *Why Natural Childbirth?* (Garden City, NY: Doubleday, 1972), pp. 60–62. Reprinted by permission.
5. M.M.I. Liley, M.D., and Beth Day, *Modern Motherhood* (New York: Random House, 1966), p. 19. Reprinted by permission.
6. Gregory V. Smith, M.D., Lynnette J. Calvert, M.D., and William P. Kanto, M.D., *American Family Physician* (published by the American Academy of Family Physicians), vol. 17, no. 4, April 1978, p. 92.
7. *The Womanly Art of Breastfeeding,* p. 30.
8. Leviticus 12:3.
9. 1 Corinthians 7:18.
10. Thomas E. Reichelderfer, M.D., and Juan R. Fraga, M.D., *Care of a Well Baby* (New York: Lippincott, 1968); David Grimes, M.D., "Circumcision: Lack of Parental Informed Consent," *Ob. Gyn News,* vol. 13, no. 7, reported in *International Medical News Service,* says in part:

   > Parental consent is routinely given before the operation is done, but informed consent is usually lacking. Information on the benefits and risks of the surgery was not provided to about three-fourths of the parents in one study. Two-thirds of another group of parents said their physicians never said anything to them about the operation.
   >
   > Morbidity associated with the procedure is low, but complications such as hemorrhage, infection, and trauma do occur. Infection can cause scarring, deformity, and meatal stenosis. Trauma can take the form of a denuded shaft, lacerated scrotum, subglandular fistula, bivalved glans, concealed penis, and cautery burns.
   >
   > The psychological effects of circumcision should not be considered short-lived, because they may not be. Immediate behavior changes occur, such as wakefulness, fussy crying, and disturbed sleep patterns. Auditory responses of circumcised male infants have been found to be different from those of females and uncircumcised males.
11. Capt. E. Noel Preston, MC, USAF, "Whither the Foreskin? A Consideration of Routine Neonatal Circumcision," *Journal of the American Medical Association,* Sept. 14, 1970.
12. Tine Thevenin, *The Family Bed, An Age-Old Concept in Child Rearing* (Box 16004, Minneapolis, MN 55416; 1976).

23. The New Family

There was a child went forth every day,
And the first object he look'd upon, that object he became,
And that object became part of him for the day or certain
*   part of the day,*
Or for many years or stretching cycles of years. . . .
His own parents, he that had father'd him and she that had
*   conceiv'd him in her womb and birth'd him.*
They gave this child more of themselves than that,
They gave him afterward every day, they became part of him.

The mother at home quietly placing the dishes on the
*   supper-table,*
The mother with mild words, clean her cap and gown, a
*   wholesome odor falling off her person and clothes as she*
*   walks by,*
The father, strong, self-sufficient, manly, mean, anger'd,
*   unjust,*
The blow, the quick loud word, the tight bargain, the crafty
*   lure,*
The family usages, the language, the company, the furniture,
*   the yearning and swelling heart,*
Affection that will not be gainsay'd, . . .
                                        —Walt Whitman

A family is not just a group of individuals living together, but an interacting unit, modifying and shaping each others' lives. The Bible says, "None of us lives to himself, and none of us dies to himself" (Rom. 14:7, RSV), and this is especially true in the family setting.

Families are under stress these days, with husband, wife, and children struggling for their own identities, restless for "rights," "freedom," "equality," "independence." While these goals are admirable, they can be achieved only *in relation to* other human beings, for they are not the goals of an individual living in complete isolation.

Families ought not to exist to keep their members from these goals but to make their attainment possible for each member. Childbirth experiences are not the only factors in determining the extent of intimate harmony and peace within the family unit, each member being free to discover his or her own creative potential, for basic attitudes toward life precede the birth experience and are only reinforced by it in one direction or the other. It is thus likely that the couple with a healthy attitude toward childbearing and breastfeeding, who have prepared for and shared the joy of these experiences, will be a couple who have already made a good adjustment to each other as husband and wife. Their relationship will not have been only in coitus but in responding to each other in every aspect of daily living, in the very special companionship of marriage.

But when a child enters that home, his or her coming disrupts the male/female balance. It is no longer a "couple" but is now a "family," in which there are two females and one male, or two males and one female. A complex set of relationships has begun, which the new parents need to think through carefully, in relation to each other as well as in relation to the new baby.

The sex of a child is genetically determined at the moment of conception. However, there is no apparent sexual differentiation in the fetus in the early weeks. Unless the genes order the gonads to become testicles and to produce sufficient androgen, the embryo will not be a boy but a girl.[1] It is not until adolescence that the final sexual differentiation occurs.

Thus the new baby is not yet primarily male or female. He or she is primarily a *person*. But from the time of birth others may unconsciously respond to him or her in terms of his or her sexuality—disappointed that it's a boy, disappointed that it's a girl, happy that it's a boy, happy that it's a girl, placing more importance on the child's sex than on his or her essential personhood. Subtle pressures to conform to society's expectations of one sex or the other begin early. We see the tragic consequences in the high incidence of homosexuality and in the trend toward sex-change operations. Often these unhappy people have not been accepted as individuals but have been forced into an arbitrary cultural role that they were not born to fit. Their potential "personhood" has been violated.

This does not mean that there are no differences in the infant and small child, both of temperament and of interests, that may reflect his or her sex. But the child who is secure in the knowledge of being accepted as a person is better able to accept his or her own sexual identity with pride when that awareness begins to dawn.

And if the parents are to be able to accept their new baby as a person rather than as "just" a boy or girl, it would be wise for them to take another look at themselves as man and woman, both in relation to each other as well as to the baby, reaffirming the essential personhood of both husband and wife.

First a Person

The Bible makes it clear that we are male or female only secondarily. We are persons first, human beings with equal capacity for spiritual and intellectual growth and the development of creative capabilities. Genesis 1:27 says:

God said, "Let us make mankind (*adam*) in our image. . . . So God created man in his own image; male and female created he them.

If mankind (man and woman) is in God's image, what is that "image"? Jesus explains it for us when he says, "God is a Spirit, and those who worship him must worship in spirit and in truth" (John 4:24). Thus the first element of personhood is not flesh and blood but "spirit," a creative personality.

Religious leaders once tried to trap Jesus with a question about the role of men and women after death (Matt. 22:23–30), citing the hypothetical case of a woman who had been widowed seven times. To which man would she belong in heaven? Jesus' reply was that their question was foolish. "You don't know either the Scripture, or the power of God," he said, "for in the resurrection they neither marry nor are given in marriage, but are like the angels in heaven."

Paul says in Galatians 3:28 (RSV): "There is neither Jew nor Greek, there is neither slave nor free, there is *neither male nor female;* for you are all one in Christ Jesus."

Our creative personality, our real "self," our "spirit," is not bound by the limitations of sex. Only the body, which houses the spirit, comes in male or female form. The essential "personhood" of man and woman is the same.

The early church leaders were careful to explain this. In Chapter 17, "Evidence from Anthropology," some of their statements are given. Here are a few more:

Clement of Rome (A.D. 30–100):

Many women also, being strengthened by the grace of God, have performed numerous manly exploits.[2]

Clement of Alexandria (A.D. 153–217):

Let us, then, embracing more and more this good obedience, give ourselves to the Lord . . . and understand that the virtue of man and woman is the same. For if the God of both is one, that master of both is also one; one church, one temperance, one modesty; their food is common, marriage an equal yoke; respiration, sight, hearing, knowledge, obedience, love all alike.

And those whose life is common have common graces and a common salvation; common to them are love and training. "For in this world," he says, "they marry and are given in marriage," in which alone the female is distinguished from the male; "but in that world it is so no more."

There the rewards of this social and holy life, which is based on conjugal union, are laid up, not for male and female, but for mankind, the sexual desire which divides humanity being removed. . . .3

Obviously, the equal worth of a man and woman does not mean "sameness," nor do their physical differences imply superiority or inferiority as persons. There are some personality differences that reflect sex, but these are not nearly as great as we have often been led to believe.

Female hormones not only make the body softer and rounder, but they also tend to make women quieter, more receptive, more conscious of people than of things. Male hormones may make a man more restless, aggressive, explorative, more often goal-oriented than person-oriented.4 However, although male/female hormones affect temperament to a certain degree, we must not forget that every normal person is a blend of male/female qualities. The differences are a matter of *degree* rather than absolute. In God we see the perfect blend of these traits, aggressiveness without hostility, tenderness without weakness.

The temperament of a man or a woman does not just reflect the dominant bodily hormones but is also affected by his or her intellect and interests, according to the unique makeup of the individual.

Women are often referred to in one way or another as "chemical creatures" with resulting mood changes. With the consistent absence of any accompanying discussion of the same phenomenon in men, one could easily conclude that men are relatively immune from such characteristics. There is, however, no sociological, physiological or scriptural basis for this implication. To the contrary, the often ignored but richly documented fact is that men have a pronounced 30-day hormone level rhythm with mood cycles of four to six weeks in duration.5

Overall it is necessary to realize that *both* men and women respond to stresses differently at various times of the month. Fortunately these changes can be modified and even minimized by meaningful and satisfying relationships and activities.[6]

As persons, men and women are endowed with a variety of intellectual and creative potentials. The differences in creative potential among individuals are not related to their sexuality but to the gifts they have inherited from both parents, which may or may not have the opportunity to flourish, depending on the culture into which one is born and the family's position in that culture. The importance of sexual roles is primarily in relationship to others, both within the family and society at large within a given cultural setting.

Cultural Differences

In every culture there are divisions of labor, but these divisions have not always been consistent with sexual differences. In some cultures women have done all the manual labor while the men have been left free for hunting expeditions or for sudden defense against attack by neighboring tribes. In other cultures only the lower classes have worked at manual labor, while both men and women in the upper classes considered it disgraceful to use their hands at daily tasks. In such cultures, men and women servants worked in the kitchen and cared for the children, while both men and women servants toiled in the fields.

Because of such cultural variables, one cannot use biblical statements as blanket proof of certain prevalent attitudes, such as "a woman's place is in the home." Even a brief glance at the cultural settings in Bible times shows that this claim is not valid. People lived in extended families, with relatives next door or close by in the village, if not under the same roof, so that children were under the care of familiar persons all the time. In more prosperous homes both men and women performed many of the tasks, indoors and out. In poorer homes everyone worked, in the fields and in the market.

The "ideal wife" of Proverbs 31 is a beautiful example of a "working wife." She helped support the household with her income as a manufacturer, as a merchant who sold her wares in the public market, as a buyer of real estate, and as a farmer who "planted a vineyard with her own hands." Who took care of the children and housework while she was busy with all these business activities? Baby-sitters, of course. "She rose early in the morning to appoint tasks for her maidens."

Grandmothers rather than mothers often cared for the small children. When Ruth married Boaz, her baby was given to the grandmother Naomi to care for. "Naomi took the child and laid him in her bosom, and became his nurse" (Ruth 4:16). This was not unusual.

In poorer homes women worked outside along with the men. Before marrying Boaz, Ruth harvested in the fields along with the regular farm workers, who were both men and women (Ruth 2:3–9).

Frequently Paul's teaching in 1 Timothy 5:11–14 is quoted to prove that women are to be kept at home, but this could not be what Paul meant. In his time many women *had* to work out of sheer economic necessity. Priscilla worked right along with Paul and Aquila manufacturing tents.[7] Paul's teaching is that young women should not be allowed to be *"idle,* gadding about from house to house, and not only idlers but gossips and busybodies" (RSV). If he could see how many wives live today, spending idle hours on the phone or at coffee klatches or running to "sales," he would say that these idle young women would be better off finding useful employment.

Another fallacy is that women are more emotional than men and thus not suited to public life. However, emotions are a part of being human, not solely of being female. The way emotions are *expressed* is culturally determined rather than determined by sex. In current society it is considered unmanly for a man to cry or to show his feelings in public (though not unmanly for him to develop ulcers or headaches from repressed emotions). Only women are expected to let their feelings show.

. . . Cultural factors render boys and men more vulnerable to a whole spectrum of pressures. . . . His assigned sex *role*—what people expect of him—puts him at a psychological disadvantage as well. . . .

Women may be "more emotional," but more men are emotionally *disturbed*. (All over the world, more males than females have nervous breakdowns, more males than females commit suicide.) Biology again? A weaker nervous system? Perhaps. But it may be that women's very freedom to *be* emotional, to show and express their feelings, permits them to let off steam, while men are expected to sit on their emotions. No safety valve—hence *bang!*[8]

Jesus did not hide his tears and was not afraid to show tenderness in public. In Bible times it was most often the *men* who made public displays of emotion, weeping loudly, kissing and embracing other men in public, indulging openly in sorrow (Gen. 33:4; 2 Sam. 18:35; 19:4; Luke 15:20; Acts 20:36,37).

Still another mistaken concept is that women are psychologically and spiritually more gullible than men. Yet it was to the male religious leaders of his day that Jesus gave his harshest pronouncements, with statements such as "You blind guides! hypocrites! deceived and deceivers!" (Matt. 23; John 9:41).

Women were among the disciples of Jesus throughout his earthly ministry (Matt. 27:55) and followed him all the way to the cross even when the male disciples had deserted him (Luke 23:27,55,56). Women were first at the tomb and the first to see the risen Lord (Luke 24:10, 11, John 20:11–18), but when they told this to the men, "these words seemed to them an idle tale, and they did not believe them."

Women were among the hundred and twenty at the first Pentecost. When Paul later had a vision of a man calling him to Macedonia, he obeyed. And what did he find? Only a bunch of women down by the riverside. The first European convert was one of these women, Lydia, a businesswoman.

Only when we understand the essential capacity for development of the unique personhood of husband, wife, child, without false cultural impositions, are we ready to look objectively at their relationship to each other within the family. There is a biblical standard for these relationships that will not only make harmonious living together possible but when correctly carried out will in no way inhibit the unique flowering of the creative potential of any of the family members. On the contrary, it will enhance it.

The biblical standard is found in Ephesians 5:21–6:4 (RSV):

Be subject to one another out of reverence for Christ. Wives, be subject to your husbands, as to the Lord. For the husband is the head of the wife as Christ is the head of the church, his body, and is himself its Savior. As the church is subject to Christ, so let wives be subject in everything to their husbands.

Husbands, love your wives, as Christ loved the church and gave himself up for her, . . . Even so husbands should love their wives as their own bodies. He who loves his wife loves himself. For no man ever hates his own flesh, but nourishes and cherishes it, as Christ does the church, because we are members of his body. . . .

Children, obey your parents in the Lord, for this is right. "Honor your father and mother" (this is the first commandment with a promise), "that it may be well with you and that you may live long on the earth."

Fathers, do not provoke your children to anger, but bring them up in the discipline and instruction of the Lord.

The Loving Husband

God is not only a Creative Spirit but a threefold Being, who said (Gen. 1:27), "Let *us* make mankind in *our* image. . . ." The Father, Son and Holy Spirit, co-equal, co-existent, co-eternal, God in Three Persons, are in a *relationship* with one another. The Son, though equal with the Father, willingly places himself under the will of the Father (Phil. 2:3–11). The Holy Spirit, though equal with the Father and the Son, willingly places himself at the disposal of the Son (John 1:33; 16:7).

In a human family, though each member is of equal worth, there is a definite hierarchy of responsibility to be willingly carried out for the good of all. But the entire family is under the authority of God, with whom they are *not* equal.

The husband is under the authority of Christ, who shows him by his own example how a husband is to "lead" his wife. Only those are fit to lead who have first learned to obey their own leader. The Scripture says that the husband is the "head of the wife" (1 Cor. 11:3) and the "ruler of his household" (1 Tim. 3:4), but there is no command in Scripture for him to "rule" his wife. The command is: "*LOVE* your wife, *AS CHRIST LOVED* the Church. . . ."

It is a common misconception that love is only an emotion or a "feeling." Rather, love is a lasting commitment to the welfare of another, evidenced in acts of kindness and concern and carried out even to the extent of losing one's life in the other's behalf.

Christ reveals this essence of love as action when he says, "*Do* unto others as you would have them do to you" (Matt. 7:12). By this he does not mean striking a bargain: "I'll be fair to you if you'll be fair to me." Yet how many marriages are structured on this false proposition of give and take?

Christ's meaning goes far deeper. Regardless of the actions of others, we are to give of ourselves to them fully, in the way we would want them to give of themselves fully for us. He expands this further when he says, "Love your neighbor *as yourself.*" Thus he irrevocably links our loving others with *our capacity to love ourselves.* This "love" is not a self-centered interest but a deep appreciation of our own worth as a human being with a capacity for creative living. A husband who "loves himself" in this way will not be threatened by any abilities his wife may have.

The Danish philosopher Kierkegaard reminds us that our neighbor is not just some person in the abstract but the one who is *right next to us*. Thus one's husband, wife, parent, child is first of all one's neighbor, who is to be loved "as ourselves." The person who does not love any one of the family members with whom he or she lives, no matter how difficult that person may be, *does not really "love" anyone,* no matter how many others this person may seem to love. The husband who does not love his wife doesn't love anyone, for he doesn't even love himself. "He who loves his wife, loves himself."

The Old Testament gives us a beautiful picture of God as the Husband of Israel, long-suffering, generous, loving, forgiving (Isa. 54; Ezek. 16:1–14; Hos. 2:14–16). Only when the nation rebelled and deserted him did they bring trouble upon themselves, and he wooed them back and healed them again and again.

In the New Testament Christ is called the Bridegroom of believers, who loved them enough to die in their behalf. Few husbands are called upon to die for their wives, but Christ also provides the example of how to *live* for them. He says: "The kings of the Gentiles exercise lordship over them; and those in authority are called benefactors. But *not so with you;* rather let the greatest among you become as the youngest, and the leader as one who serves. For which is greater, one who sits at table, or one who serves? Is it not the one who sits at table? But *I am among you as one who serves"* (Luke 22:25,26, RSV).

Jesus not only taught this, but practiced it all through his ministry, even stooping down to wash the disciples' feet, saying to them as he did so, "You also ought to wash one another's feet. For I have given you an example . . ." (John 13:2–16).

The husband who seeks to lead his household well must even be willing to "wash the feet" of his wife and children, humbling himself to perform menial tasks for those he loves. He must not fail to love and serve not only the ideal wife, but the unlovely, unsubmissive, unthankful, complaining wife, for did not Jesus humble himself to wash the feet of Peter, who denied him, and even of Judas, who betrayed him?

A lovely example of this is the husband of a woman who was aspiring to political office in national elections. Her husband took a temporary leave of absence from his regular job in order to drive his wife to her appointments as a chauffeur, help research her speeches, and as he said, "see that she's fed, clothed, eats on time and gets to her appointments." He added, "She's the one out there making it publicly, not me. If you are a man—and a mature man—you do everything to maintain your wife's stardom."[9]

Does such a husband lose respect in the eyes of his wife and children? Not at all. Rather, he stands "ten feet tall" in their eyes. For it is a fact that the husband and father who tries to dominate invites rebellion, insubordination, and deception from his wife and children, and he often gets it. He makes a mockery of his "leadership." The humility of true greatness, on the other hand, wins their respect, devotion, and obedience.

There is another serious aspect to the leadership of the husband and father, which is that he is responsible for the spiritual welfare of each family member. The Bible warns that the man who prevents his wife or daughter from performing her duties to God "will bear *her* iniquity" (Num. 30). And in regard to little children, Jesus says that "whoever causes one of these little ones who believe in me to sin, it would be better for him to have a great millstone fastened round his neck and to be drowned in the depth of the sea. . . . See that you do not despise one of these little ones; for I tell you that in heaven their angels always behold the face of my Father who is in heaven" (Matt. 18:6,10).

Thus a husband's and father's primary responsibility is not to make a name for himself and to earn a living but to live close to God in obedience to him, giving his family an example to follow.

His secondary responsibility is to provide for their physical needs: food, shelter and clothing. This kindly protection and provision is especially needed during the months of his wife's pregnancy and during the breastfeeding years. He should not only provide for her, but stay close to her, keep involved in her interests, help with the baby, and give a lift with the chores. Washing dishes and diapering babies does not make a man "effeminate," for even God is shown as an example of a baby-sitter (Num. 11:12; Isa. 66:13).

Such loving attention on the part of the husband will set the pattern in the home. He will be the leader to whom the others look with respect. Participating in his child's life from the moment of birth will help prevent any "communication gap" from developing later. And in helping his wife to continue blossoming as a person while the children are still small, he will benefit most of all. She will not only become a better, more creative mother but will be able to develop into the kind of stimulating person he will enjoy living with after the children are grown and gone.

A Willing Wife

In Ephesians 5:21–26 (PHILLIPS) we read:

Thank God at all times for everything, in the name of our Lord Jesus Christ. And "fit in with" each other, because of your common reverence for Christ. You wives must learn to adapt yourselves to your husbands, as you submit yourself to the Lord, for the husband is the "head" of the wife in the same way that Christ is head of the Church and savior of his body. The willing subjection of the Church to Christ should be reproduced in the submission of wives to their husbands. But, remember, this means that the husband must give his wife the same sort of love that Christ gave to the Church, when he sacrificed himself for her.

The key word in this controversial passage is the word "willing." One who voluntarily yields to another is not being passive or weak. Rather, it is a positive attitude, an active, willing, voluntary granting the desires of another in order to please them. The opposite attitude is not strength, but insubordination, rebellion, and resentment. The godly wife wants to please the man she loves, doing his way rather than her own way, if this is his desire.

A wife is given to a man to be his helpmeet (Gen. 2:18–24), and not the other way around. She is to place his needs, his wishes first. It is her responsibility to encourage his leadership ability, to affirm his manliness in her children's eyes, to avoid burdening him with family demands for material things so that he becomes a slave to his job and shortens his life by overwork. She cooperates with him in permitting him to pursue the career he wants, even if it means less pay and material sacrifice for the family. She develops her own creative potentials not for her own selfish fulfillment but in order to be a better person, and thus a better wife and mother.

Such a wife is like the ideal wife of Proverbs 31, who had her priorities right. Although she was a creative, resourceful person who fully developed her own talents, she kept the interests of her husband and children first. In doing this, she found *herself* fulfilled. She encouraged her husband's endeavors and was proud of his role as a community leader. His trust in her was not misplaced, and her children were proud of her.

The ideal wife and mother is also a woman who doesn't talk too much, knowing that "actions speak louder than words." When she does speak, she has something to say worth listening to: "She opens her mouth with wisdom, and *in her tongue is the law of kindness.*" (Prov. 31:26).

Such a woman becomes qualified for larger service. Deborah, leader of the Israelites in the time of the judges (Judg. 4 and 5), earned the title "a mother in Israel," gaining the right to lead a nation. And her husband, Lapidoth, apparently did not object.

As women we tend to be defensive about the biblical commands to be submissive and to be silent at times (1 Cor. 14:34,35), because we forget that what we *are* is already speaking loudly. Our children are learning from us from the moment of birth through far more than just the words we speak. Our influence in our husbands' lives is far greater than just through the words we toss out—which they often do not seem to "hear." (Are they worth hearing?)

The greatest compliment I ever received came one evening from one of my sons when he was nine years old. I had gone to bed early, not feeling well. After a few moments he came into the room and lay down on the bed beside me. "I just love to come into your room," he said, "because there's such peace in here!"

We know our children need food, clothing, that they must brush their teeth, take baths, get to school on time, practice, do their homework. But do we ever realize that they need *peace?* It had never crossed my mind before. Perhaps there are husbands, too, who long for peace in their households, for less hustle and hurry, for fewer words.

Peter says, "Let your adorning be . . . the hidden person of the heart, even the ornament of a gentle and quiet spirit, which is in the sight of God of great price. For after this manner in the old time the holy women also, who *trusted in God* adorned themselves, being in subjection to their own husbands" (1 Pet. 3:4,5).

And then Peter adds, "so that if they [the husbands] don't obey God, your manner of life will win them over. . . ." The key to winning over even the wicked, domineering husband is not nagging, bickering, fighting, but a quiet yielding, committing the problem to God and giving him a chance to solve it in the right way. Remember that "a gentle answer turns away wrath" (Prov. 15:1).

Submission is an important biblical principle for every person to learn to follow, for it contains the secret of true victory. Jesus said, "If anyone takes away your coat, let him have your overcoat too. And whoever compels you to go a mile, go with him two." (Matt. 5:40, 41.) Christ Jesus himself is the supreme example of submission, even allowing himself to be killed because it was God's will (John 14:30):

The ruler of this world is coming. He has no power over me; but *I do as the Father commanded,* so that the world may know that I love the Father.

Christ's obedience was not out of weakness before Satan, to whom he submitted at the cross, and it led not to the end of hope but to his resurrection and the hope of salvation for all humankind.

One wife once complained, "I want to submit to my husband, but he won't take the lead. For example, he always brings the bills to me and wants me to take care of all the financial records. I don't want to do it. *He* ought to do it. *He* ought to be the man of the house!" This woman was being an unsubmissive wife, resenting her husband for his asking her to do something he knew she could do well and casting judgments on his manhood because he asked it of her. When she realized that the problem was in wanting him to lead *her* way, according to *her* notions, she changed her attitude and yielded to his desires in the matter.

This is really the key to happy relationships between husband and wife. The more the husband loves his wife, the more willingly does she yield to his every wish. The more the wife seeks to please him, the more he loves her. They may not agree in every matter, but she is willing for him to have the final say in any decision. When she respects his judgment, he is more likely to give her ideas thoughtful consideration. Through the years their tastes will become more and more in harmony until, as Longfellow says, "They were so one, none knew who ruled and who obeyed."

Obedient Children

An infant needs the love and warmth that come from suckling at the mother's breast and her continual nearness for at least the first several months of life. The father's love embraces both the breastfeeding baby and the mother, and the baby enjoys the contentment that comes from being carried in father's strong arms from the first days of life.

When baby's first steps are taken, symbolic of the move away from close attachment to the mother, reassurance is given by father's big hand enfolding the little hand, guiding the steps, until the weary toddler finds security on his daddy's shoulder. The father of small children becomes like God, the Good Shepherd, who "gathers the lambs in his arms, carries them in his bosom, and gently leads those who are with young" (Isa. 40:11).

As children grow, they need freedom to follow their individual interests. Small boys often enjoy dolls until others make fun of them. And why should they not play with dolls? It will make them better fathers. To remove dolls from boys is to intimate that fathers should not be involved with their own babies.

Some girls would rather climb trees than play dolls. Teenage sons make fine cooks if allowed the opportunity, and it is a big help for girls to know something about auto mechanics. There is no danger that these external activities will interfere with their wholesome development in their own sexual roles, in a home where mothers experience childbirth as a pleasant, natural event, babies are breastfed, and fathers are supportive of the mother and the children.

Unhappy, troublesome children are often those whose parents are in conflict. For if the parents do not really love each other, how can the child be sure that they love him or her? And the child's sexual identity becomes threatened because he or she identifies too strongly with one parent and develops hostility toward the other sex. Sexual roles become confused in the child's mind, for he or she has no adequate pattern to follow.

Because quarreling parents are disobeying God's rules for a home, a child's obedience suffers, for he or she tends to pit one parent against the other. Such children become unhappy and destructive because they are not adequately restrained and really do not know what their limits are.

A child should never be allowed to speak disrespectfully of either parent, even in a marriage that has been broken, no matter what the parent may have done. Each parent must insist that the children show respect for the other parent. Women especially tend to be at fault in this regard, causing the father to lose respect in the eyes of his children by belittling him behind his back or finding fault with him in public. But for a child to pass judgment on a parent as a person and be disrespectful is deeply harmful *to the child*. He or she will become a "difficult" child and may lose respect for all legitimate authority.

Children not only need affirmation in loving attention, cuddling when they are little, and an occasional hug and kiss when they are older. They also need discipline. A happy home is one where each person is loved and affirmed, where there are few rules and few infringements on freedom, but where *no* means *no* to the child. Safe-guards must be set for children's behavior, and these few "rules" need to provide them with the security of being consistent, for they will test these barriers to the limit. It gives them a great sense of security when they find that these barriers do not yield to their wiles or tantrums either as two-year-olds or teens.

All true authority is derived from another and not grasped for one-self. Even Christ said, "I do nothing on my own authority" (John 5:30). His authority over the church was given him by the Father. In a home, the leadership has been given by God to the husband and father, who is to yield to the authority of Christ. The wife honors her hus-band's leadership in the home, and the children are under the authority of both parents, learning both from their precept and example.

There were times when a child's whole world centered around the home. The father's work took place at or near the home; all activity, leisure, worship, education, centered around the "communal" family; and there were many playmates—brothers and sisters and cousins.

Today there are far more opportunities for individual growth and achievement but also greater stress on family relationships. The hus-band is away long hours, the children are away at school, the wife is active either in her own job or with volunteer activities, for church, P.T.A. or elsewhere when the children are no longer small. When family members lead such divergent lives, friction can more easily develop unless we follow the safe guide for happy homes, with loving husbands, willing, gentle wives, and obedient children. While this is the ideal, and life is seldom ideal, is there any happier way?

NOTES

1. "Male and Female: Differences Between Them," *Time*, March 20, 1972, p. 43.
2. *The Ante-Nicene Fathers* (Grand Rapids, MI: Eerdmans, 1951), vol. 1, p. 20.
3. Ibid., vol. 2, pp. 419 f.
4. "Male and Female: Differences Between Them."
5. *Biological Rhythms in Psychiatry and Medicine*, Public Health Service Publication No. 2088, 1970.
6. Jean R. Miller and Margaret E. Armstrong, "The Three R's of Marriage: Relation-ships, Roles, Responsibilities," *The Standard*, February 15, 1973.
7. Ruth Hoppin, *Priscilla: Author of the Epistle to the Hebrews and Other Essays* (Jericho, N.Y.: Exposition Press, 1972).
8. Albert Rosenfeld, "Why Men Die Younger," *Kansas City Star Sunday Magazine*, October 15, 1972.
9. Quoted in *Time*, March 13, 1972, p. 43.

Appendix A:
Sources of Information

Apple Tree Family Ministries. P.O. Box 9883, Fresno, CA 93795.

Apple Tree Family Ministries (ATFM) was founded by Helen Wessel in response to the requests of many readers of *Natural Childbirth and the Christian Family* for material that could be used to teach natural childbirth and other aspects of family life in churches. Among those requesting material was Kathy Nesper, at whose instigation the program was begun and who was appointed Director. The program is also based upon the book *Under the Apple Tree: Marrying, Birthing, Parenting* and several supplemental guidebooks.

Apple Tree Family Ministries offers leader certification for those who fulfill certain requirements and provides seminars for Christians who want to launch an Apple Tree program in their local community. The material is suitable for use in churches as well. For further information, write Mrs. Kathy Nesper, Director, at the address above.

American Academy of Husband-Coached Childbirth. P.O. Box 5224, Sherman Oaks, CA 91403.

The AAHCC (the Bradley Method) was founded by Jay and Marjie Hathaway to promote Dr. Robert Bradley's program of natural childbirth encouraging husband participation. The Bradley Method is based on the philosophy of Dr. Grantly Dick-Read and is in harmony with the principles in *Natural Childbirth and the Christian Family*. The AAHCC offers teacher training and affiliation.

Alternative Birth Crisis Coalition. P.O. Box 48371, Chicago, IL 60648.

The ABCC was formed to help defend parents who want alternatives in childbirth, as well as the practitioners who provide them, in the face of the medical and professional pressures against alternative birthing. Its president is Marian Tompson (a Founding Mother of La Leche League and its President for over twenty-five years).

American College of Home Obstetrics. 644 No. Michigan Ave., Suite 610, Chicago, IL 60611.

ACHO collects and publishes data on the safety and advantages of home birth, gathering data from member physicians for publication, and helping to provide encouragement and a united stand on home birth.

American College of Nurse-Midwifery. 1000 Vermont Ave. NW, Washington, DC 20005.

The ACNM is the certifying agency for nurse-midwives. It establishes curricula and standards for nurse-midwifery training programs, emphasizing excellence in preparation for its practitioners, with a focus on the childbearing family's human dignity and worth.

Birth and Life Bookstore. P.O. Box 70625, Seattle, WA 98107.

An extensive selection of books and pamphlets relating to birth and various aspects of family life is available by mail order from Birth and Life, and orders are filled very promptly. Lynn Moen, President, was formerly manager of the ICEA bookstore. A sample copy of Birth and Life's newsletter, *Imprints,* is available upon request.

Cesarean Birth Alliance. 10 Summit Drive, Manhasset, NY 11030. *Cesarean/ Support, Education and Concern (C/SEC).* 132 Adams Street, Room 6, Newton, MA 02158.

These two organizations were formed for the purpose of providing support for those desiring a vaginal birth after a cesarean and for those who must have cesarean section.

Clinical Theology Association. Lingdale, Weston Avenue, Nottingham NG7 4BA, England.

A Christian professional organization that sponsors workshops in Basic Personal Growth and Primal Integration, its growing collection of data on the relevance of the maternal-fetal distress syndrom offers new dimensions to psychotherapy and pastoral counseling.

Couple to Couple League. P.O. Box 11084, Cincinnati, OH 45211.

An interfaith organization offering married couples help with the successful practice of natural family planning, it teaches breastfeeding and the full sympto-thermal method in member groups in many localities.

The APRS Federal Monitor. P.O. Box 6358, Alexandria, VA 22306.

Published by the Alliance for Perinatal Research and Services, Inc., this publication keeps subscribers informed about state and federal activities affecting the health of women and children, with a special emphasis on childbearing.

Home Oriented Maternity Experience. 511 New York Ave., Takoma Park, MD 20012.

This national organization supporting and assisting couples who wish to give birth at home, with emphasis on safety, trains and certifies leaders who hold home birth training sessions for parents.

The Human Life Center. St. John's University, Collegeville, MN 56321.

This international center helps people of all faiths with programs for family enrichment, including natural family planning.

International Childbirth Education Association. P.O. Box 20048, Minneapolis, MN 55420.

A valuable resource agency for those who want information concerning childbirth education, the ICEA is a federation of independent childbirth education groups and instructors worldwide, sponsoring numerous regional conferences and a biennial convention.

ICEA Bookcenter. P.O. Box 20048, Minneapolis, MN 55420.

A wide range of books, pamphlets, films and teaching aids on childbirth education, for both lay and professional people, is available through the center. A sample copy of their newsletter, *Bookmarks,* is available upon request.

La Leche League International. 9616 Minneapolis Ave., Franklin Park, IL 60131.

Any woman who plans to breastfeed can benefit from contacting LLL, and it is especially helpful to those in circumstances where breastfeeding is not popular. Now more than twenty-five years old, LLL is recognized as the pioneer organization largely responsible for the resurgence of interest in breastfeeding. Local groups are active around the world and can usually be located through physicians, local newspapers, telephone listings, childbirth educators, or hospitals—or through writing or phoning the international office. Numerous publications, monthly meetings, and telephone information are available. International office telephone: (312) 455-7730.

NAPSAC International (InterNational Association of Parents and Professionals for Safe Alternatives in Childbirth). P.O. Box 267, Marble Hill, MO 63764.

NAPSAC is dedicated to implementing family-centered childbirth programs that meet the needs of families as well as provide the safe aspects of medical science. They have a number of outstanding publications available on childbirth alternatives, including a quarterly newsletter.

Pennypress. 1100 23rd Ave. East, Seattle, WA 98112.

The Pennypress has many excellent leaflets, pamphlets, and small books on childbirth and related subjects; its editor is Penny Simkin.

Read Natural Childbirth Foundation, Inc. 1300 South Eliseo Dr., Suite 102, Greenbrae, CA 94904.

A nonprofit educational organization founded to promote the philosophies and techniques of Dr. Grantly Dick-Read and to preserve his life work as it relates to childbirth.

Serena (Service for the Regulation of Natality). 55 Parkdale Ave., Ottawa, Ontario K1Y 1E5, Canada.

For over 20 years Serena has perfected and disseminated natural methods of birth regulation, especially the sympto-thermal method, as a resource for couples in controlling their fertility while deepening their relationship.

Appendix B: Bibliography of Recommended Reading

NOTE: Books under each topic are listed in the suggested reading order. Some of the books listed have portions not in harmony with *Natural Childbirth and the Christian Family*.

Marriage

Helen Wessel. *Under the Apple Tree: Marrying, Birthing, Parenting*. Bookmates International, P.O. Box 9883, Fresno, CA 93795; 1981.

Walter Trobisch. *I Married You*. New York: Harper & Row, 1971.

Ingrid Trobisch. *The Joy of Being a Woman, and What a Man Can Do*. New York: Harper & Row, 1975.

Linda Dillow. *Creative Counterpart*. Nashville, TN: Nelson, 1977.

Gordon MacDonald. *Magnificent Marriage*. Wheaton, IL: Tyndale, 1976.

Patricia Gundry. *Heirs Together*. Grand Rapids, MI: Zondervan, 1980.

Tim Timmons. *Maximum Marriage*. Old Tappan, NJ: Revell, 1976.

Ronald M. Deutsch. *The Key to Feminine Response in Marriage*. New York: Ballantine, 1968.

Ed Wheat, M.D., and Gaye Wheat. *Intended for Pleasure*. Old Tappan, NJ: Revell, 1977.

Natural Family Planning

Joseph Roetzer, M.D. *Family Planning the Natural Way*. Old Tappan, NJ: Revell, 1981.

John and Sheila Kippley. *The Art of Natural Family Planning*. 2d ed. Couple to Couple League, Box 11084, Columbus, OH 45211; 1979.

Suzanne Parenteau-Carreau, M.D. *Love and Life: Fertility and Conception Prevention*. 2d ed. Serena Canada, 55 Parkdale, Ottawa, Ontario K1Y 1E5; 1975.

Evelyn Billings, M.D., and Ann Westmore. *The Billings Method*. New York: Random House, 1980.

John Billings, M.D., and Lyn Billings. *Natural Family Planning: The Ovulation Method*. Collegeville, MN: Liturgical Press, 1973.

Ingrid Trobisch and Elizabeth Roetzer. *An Experience of Love: Understanding Natural Family Planning*. Old Tappan, NJ: Revell, 1981.

Christina Buettimer. *Natural Family Planning*. New York: Bantam, 1980.

Life Before Birth

Helen Wessel. *Under the Apple Tree: Marrying, Birthing, Parenting*. Bookmates International, P.O. Box 9883, Fresno, CA 93795; 1981.

Geraldine Lux Flanagan. *The First Nine Months of Life*. New York: Simon & Schuster, 1962.

Gail Sforza Brewer, with Thomas Brewer, M.D. *What Every Pregnant Woman Should Know: The Truth About Diets and Drugs in Pregnancy*. New York: Random House, 1977.

Gail Sforza Brewer and Janice Presser Greene. *Right from the Start*. Emmaus, PA: Rodale, 1981.

Sheila Kitzinger. *The Complete Book of Pregnancy and Childbirth*. New York and Toronto: Knopf & Random House of Canada; 1980.

Thomas Verney, M.D., with John Kelley. *The Secret Life of the Unborn Child*. New York: Summit, 1981.

Margot Edwards and Penny Simkin. *Obstetric Tests and Technology: A Consumers Guide*. Seattle, WA: Pennypress, 1980.

Elizabeth Noble. *Essential Exercises for the Childbearing Year*. Boston: Houghton Mifflin, 1976.

Madeleine Kenefick. *Positively Pregnant*. Los Angeles: Pinnacle, 1981.

Judith Miles. *Journal from an Obscure Place*. Minneapolis, MN: Dimension Books, 1978.

Susan Borg and Judith Lesker. *When Pregnancy Fails: Families Coping With Miscarriage, Stillbirth and Infant Death*. Boston: Beacon, 1981.

Penny Simkin. *Directory of Alternative Birth Services and Consumer Guide*. NAPSAC, Box 267, Marble Hill, MO 63764; 1982.

Birthing

Helen Wessel. *Under the Apple Tree: Marrying, Birthing, Parenting*. Bookmates International, P.O. Box 9883, Fresno, CA 93795; 1981.

Grantly Dick-Read, M.D. *Childbirth Without Fear*. 5th ed. Revised by Helen Wessel and Harlan Ellis, M.D. New York: Harper & Row, 1983.

Nancy Wainer Cohen and Lois J. Estner. *Silent Knife. Cesarean Prevention and Vaginal Birth After Cesarean*. South Hadley, MS: Bergin & Garvey, 1983.

Sandra VanDam Anderson and Penny Simkin. *Birth—Through Children's Eyes*. Seattle, WA: Pennypress, 1981.

Robert Bradley, M.D. *Husband-Coached Childbirth*. 3rd ed. New York: Harper & Row, 1981.

Marjie and Jay Hathaway. *Children at Birth*. New York: Academy, 1978.

David and Lee Stewart. *Compulsory Hospitalization or Freedom of Choice in Childbirth?* 3 vols. NAPSAC, Box 267, Marble Hill, MO 63764; 1979.

David and Lee Stewart. *The Five Standards for Safe Childbirth*. NAPSAC, Box 267, Marble Hill, MO 63764; 1981.

David and Lee Stewart. *Safe Alternatives in Childbirth*. 3rd ed. NAPSAC, Box 267, Marble Hill, MO 63764; 1978.

David and Lee Stewart. *21st Century Obstetrics Now!* 2d ed. 2 vols. NAPSAC, Box 267, Marble Hill, MO 63764; 1978.

Deborah Tanzer. *Why Natural Childbirth?* Garden City, NY: Doubleday, 1972.

Joy Young. *Christian Home Birth*. P.O. Box 33512, Detroit, MI 48232.

Lester Hazell. *Birth Goes Home*. Seattle, WA: Catalyst Publishing, 1974.

Gregory White. *Emergency Childbirth*. Police Training Foundation, Franklin Park, IL; 1969.

Family-Centered Maternity/Newborn Care in Hospitals. Interprofessional Task Force Secretariat, American College of Obstetrics and Gynecologists, One East Wacker Dr., Suite 2700, Chicago, IL 60601; 1978.

Diony Young and Charles Mahan. *Unnecessary Cesareans—Ways to Avoid Them*. ICEA Publications, Box 20048, Minneapolis, MN 55420.

Doris Haire. *The Pregnant Patient's Bill of Rights—The Pregnant Patient's Responsibilities*. ICEA Publications, Box 20048, Minneapolis, MN 55420.

Marilyn Moran. *Birth and the Dialogue of Love*. New Nativity Press, Box 6223, Leawood, KS 66206; 1980.

Sheila Kitzinger, ed. *Episiotomy: Physical and Emotional Aspects*. London: National Childbirth Trust, 1978.

Hermon Fitzgerald, Long, Schildroth & Ventra. *Home Oriented Maternity Experience*. H.O.M.E., 511 New York Ave., Takoma Park, MD 20012.

Breastfeeding

The Womanly Art of Breastfeeding. 3rd rev. ed. Franklin Park, IL: La Leche League, 1981.

Dana Raphael. *The Tender Gift: Breastfeeding*. New York: Schocken, 1976.

Karen Pryor. *Nursing Your Baby*. 3rd rev. ed. New York: Pocket Books, 1981.

Richard Applebaum, M.D. *Abreast of the Times*. New York: Harper & Row, 1973.

Dorothy Patricia Brewster. *You Can Breastfeed Your Baby—Even in Special Situations*. Emmaus, PA: Rodale, 1979.

Elizabeth Hormann. *Relactation: A Guide to Breastfeeding the Adopted Baby.* 1 Merrill Ave., Belmont, MA; 1971.

Norma Jane Bumgamer. *Mothering Your Nursing Toddler.* P.O. Box 5064, Norman, OK 73070.

D.B. and E.F.P. Jelliffe. *Human Milk in the Modern World: Psychological, Nutritional and Economic Significance.* Fair Lawn, NJ: Oxford University Press, 1978.

Sheila Kippley. *Breastfeeding and Natural Child Spacing: The Ecology of Natural Mothering.* Baltimore: Penguin, 1975.

Family Life

Helen Wessel. *Under the Apple Tree: Marrying, Birthing, Parenting.* Bookmates International, P.O. Box 9883, Fresno, CA 93795; 1981.

Marshall H. Klaus and John H. Kennell. *Parent-Infant Bonding.* 2d ed. New York: Mosby, 1982.

Tine Thevenin. *The Family Bed: An Age-Old Concept in Child Rearing.* Box 16004, Minneapolis, MN 55416.

Ross Campbell, M.D. *How to Really Love Your Child.* Wheaton, IL: Victor Books, 1977.

David Stewart. *Fathering and a Career.* NAPSAC, Box 267, Marble Hill, MO 63764.

Elizabeth Crary. *Without Spanking or Spoiling: A Practical Approach to Toddler and Preschool Guidance.* Parenting Press, 7750 31st Avenue NE, Seattle, WA 98115; 1981.

Selma Fraiberg. *Every Child's Birthright: In Defense of Mothering.* New York: Bantam, 1977.

James Dobson. *Hide or Seek.* Old Tappan, NJ: Revell, 1978.

James L. Hymes, Jr. *The Child Under Six.* Englewood Cliffs, NJ: Prentice-Hall, 1963.

Raymond Moore. *Better Late Than Early.* New York: Reader's Digest Press, 1975.

Raymond and Dorothy Moore. *Home-Grown Kids.* Waco, TX: Word, 1981.

Monica O'Kane. *Living With Adult Children.* Diction Books, 1981. Box 17271, St. Paul, MN 55117.

Miscellaneous

Edmund Jacobson. *You Must Relax.* New York: McGraw-Hill, 1937, 1962.

Frank Lake, M.D. *Clinical Theology.* London: Dartman, Longman & Todd, 1966.

Frank Lake, M.D. *Tight Corners in Pastoral Counselling.* London: Dartman, Longman & Todd, 1982.

Victor Frankl. *Man's Search for Meaning*. New York: Washington Square Press, 1963.

Ashley Montagu. *Touching: The Human Significance of the Skin*. New York: Columbia University Press, 1971.

Eric Fromm. *The Art of Loving*. New York: Harper & Row, 1956.

Robert Mendelsohn. *Confessions of a Medical Heretic*. Chicago: Contemporary Books, 1979.

Dorothy Gauchat. *All God's Children*. New York: Hawthorn, 1972.

Harriet Sarnoff-Schiff. *The Bereaved Parent*. New York: Penguin, 1977.

Nikki and David Goldbeck. *Supermarket Handbook: Access to Whole Foods*. New York: Signet, 1973.

La Leche League. *Whole Foods for the Whole Family*. Franklin Park, IL: La Leche League, 1981.

Index